Storied Health and Illness

Storied Health and Illness

Communicating Personal, Cultural, & Political Complexities

Jill Yamasaki
University of Houston

Patricia Geist-Martin
San Diego State University

Barbara F. Sharf
Independent Scholar/Texas A&M University

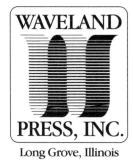

WAVELAND
PRESS, INC.
Long Grove, Illinois

For information about this book, contact:
Waveland Press, Inc.
4180 IL Route 83, Suite 101
Long Grove, IL 60047-9580
(847) 634-0081
info@waveland.com
www.waveland.com

Cover: Untitled painting by Hilda Gorenstein

Contents

Contributors

Kristian G. E. Borofka (BS, Santa Clara University) graduated from Santa Clara University in 2014 with a BS in Biochemistry. She is now pursing her dream of becoming a physician in the College of Osteopathic Medicine at Tauro University in Vallejo, CA.

Michael Broderick (PhD, Ohio University) is an Assistant Professor at James Madison University. His scholarship explores how individuals and families make health-related decisions within the strictures of corporate colonization. He explores communicative resistance to hegemony through everyday acts of resistance.

Rebekah Crawford (MA, Ohio University) is a doctoral student in the School of Communication Studies at Ohio University. Her work explores the therapeutic potential of storytelling in diverse contexts including mental illness and disability activism.

Christine Salkin Davis (PhD, University of South Florida) is Professor in the Communication Studies Department at the University of North Carolina at Charlotte. Her research interests are in the intersection of family, culture, and health communication. She publishes regularly on topics such as children's health, end-of-life communication, disability, and qualitative research methods. She specifically studies people with illnesses and conditions that are incurable as they face revisions in their personal identity and narrative and negotiate the liminal spaces between "well" and "unwell," alive and dead, and power and marginalization.

Marleah Dean (PhD, Texas A&M University) is an Assistant Professor in the Department of Communication at the University of South Florida. She studies patient–provider health communication and is currently examining genetics and risk communication in hereditary cancer. Her research has been published in *Health Communication, Academic Medicine, Patient Education & Counseling, Journal of Health and Mass Communication,* and *Qualitative Research in Organizations and Management.*

Nicole Defenbaugh (PhD, Southern Illinois University) is Director of Education at Lehigh Valley Health Network (LVHN). Prior to LVHN, she was an Associate Professor of Health Communication at Bloomsburg University. Nicole is a state and national speaker on chronic illness identity and was the national spokesperson for Celebrating UC (Ulcerative Colitis) in 2010. She is the recipient of the Norman K. Denzin Qualitative Research Award (2011), Ellis-Bochner Autoethnography and Personal Narrative Research Award (2009), and BU Teacher-Scholar Award (2009). She has a single-authored book entitled, *Dirty Tale: A Narrative Journey of the IBD Body,* in addition to articles in the *Journal of Graduate Medical Education, Journal of Health Com-*

munication, Qualitative Inquiry, International Review of Qualitative Research, Health Communication, and *Nursing Education in Practice.*

Mohan J. Dutta (PhD, University of Minnesota) is Provost's Chair Professor and Head of the Department of Communications and New Media at the National University of Singapore (NUS), Adjunct Professor at the Interactive Digital Media Institute (IDMI) at NUS, and Courtesy Professor of Communication at Purdue University. At NUS, he is the Founding Director of the Center for Culture-Centered Approach to Research and Evaluation (CARE), directing research on culturally centered, community-based projects of social change. He teaches and conducts research in international health communication, critical cultural theory, poverty in healthcare, health activism in globalization politics, indigenous cosmologies of health, subaltern studies and dialogue, and public policy and participatory social change. Currently, he serves as Editor of the "Critical Cultural Studies in Global Health Communication Book Series" with Left Coast Press and sits on the editorial board of seven journals.

Laura L. Ellingson (PhD, University of South Florida) is Professor of Communication and Women's & Gender Studies at Santa Clara University. Her research focuses on qualitative and feminist methodologies, gender within extended family networks, and communication in healthcare organizations, including: long-term cancer survivorship, interdisciplinary communication, teamwork, patient–healthcare provider communication, and intersections of gender, age, and race in healthcare. She is author of *Communicating in the Clinic: Negotiating Frontstage and Backstage Teamwork* (2005, Hampton) and *Engaging Crystallization in Qualitative Research* (2009, Sage), and coauthor with Dr. Patty Sotirin of *Aunting: Cultural Practices that Sustain Family and Community Life* (2010, Baylor University Press) and *Where the Aunts Are: Family, Feminism, and Kinship in Popular Culture* (2013, Baylor University Press). She is currently writing a book on embodiment in qualitative research.

Katherine Foss (PhD, University of Minnesota) is an Associate Professor at Middle Tennessee State University. Her 2014 book, *Television and Health Responsibility in an Age of Individualism,* connects discourse in fictional medical dramas to public perceptions of healthcare. She has also published in *Health Communication, Women & Health, Critical Studies in Media Communication, Disability Studies Quarterly,* and other peer-reviewed journals.

Elissa Foster (PhD, University of South Florida) is an Associate Professor and Director of the master's degree program in Health Communication at DePaul University. She has held academic appointments at several universities and in the Department of Family Medicine at Lehigh Valley Health Network (PA). Her principal areas of research are health communication and interpersonal relationships with special interests in communication at the end of life and at the beginning of life. She has published numerous academic articles, book chapters, and one book, *Communicating at the End of Life* (Lawrence Erlbaum, 2007). Elissa is passionate about helping to build relationships between the academy and healthcare professionals.

Patricia Geist-Martin (PhD, Purdue University) is a Professor at San Diego State University. Her research examines narratives and the process of negotiating identity, voice, ideology, and control in organizations, particularly in health and illness. She has published three books, *Communicating Health: Personal, Cultural, and Political Complexities* (2003; with Eileen Berlin Ray and Barbara F. Sharf), *Courage of Conviction: Women's Words, Women's Wisdom* (1997; with Linda A. M. Perry), *and Negotiating the Crisis: DRGs and the Transformation of Hospitals* (1992; with Monica Hardesty). She has published more than 70 articles and book chapters covering a wide range of topics related to gender, health, and negotiating identities.

Lynn M. Harter (PhD, University of Nebraska) is Professor of Health Communication in the School of Communication Studies at Ohio University. She also serves as codirector of the Barbara Geralds Institute for Storytelling and Social Impact. Guided by narrative and feminist sensibilities, her scholarly agenda focuses on the communicative construction of possibility as individuals and groups organize for survival and social change amidst embodied differences.

Satveer Kaur (MS, University College London) is a doctoral student in the Department of Communications and New Media at the National University of Singapore and a Research Assistant at the Center for Culture-Centered Approach to Research and Evaluation (CARE). Satveer conducts research on health communication in marginalized settings, with an emphasis on narrative constructions among underserved populations.

Jeanine M. Mingé (PhD, University of South Florida) is an Associate Professor in the Department of Communication Studies at California State University, Northridge. Her areas of research interest include performance studies, health communication, cultural studies, and qualitative methods. All of her work is arts-based, dedicated to cultivating social justice through use of narrative, visual imagery, poetry, installation art, and performance. Her book, coauthored with Amber Lynn Zimmerman and published by Routledge, is entitled *Concrete and Dust: Mapping the Sexual Terrains of Los Angeles.* She is currently working on her next book entitled *Tsunamis and Tidal Waves: The Transitory Radical Space of Cancer and Caregiving.*

Kristen Okamoto (MA, University of North Carolina at Charlotte) is a doctoral student in the School of Communication Studies at Ohio University. Her research reflects a commitment to understanding the ways in which we organize diverse selves, bodies, and resources for social change.

Sarah Parsloe (MA, San Diego State University) is a doctoral student in the School of Communication Studies at Ohio University. Her interests focus on the intersections of health communication, disability, identity, and uncertainty. In particular, she explores the identity politics of the autism community.

Margaret M. Quinlan (PhD, Ohio University) is an Associate Professor of Communication and a Core Faculty Member of the Health Psychology PhD Program at the University of North Carolina at Charlotte. Her scholarly work explores the organizing of healthcare resources and work opportunities for people with lived differences (such as disability and gender equality). She has published in *Health Communication, Text & Performance Quarterly,* and *Disability Studies Quarterly.*

Shaunak Sastry (PhD, Purdue University) is an Assistant Professor in the Department of Communication at the University of Cincinnati and an affiliate faculty member at the Center for Culture-Centered Research and Evaluation (CARE) at the National University of Singapore. His areas of interest are global health communication, critical theory, postcolonial studies, and culture-centered approaches to social change with a particular emphasis on HIV/AIDS interventions in the Global South. His work has been published in leading international peer-reviewed journals like *Health Communication, Culture, Health & Sexuality, Journal of International and Intercultural Communication,* and *Studies in Symbolic Interaction.* He is currently working on the manuscript for his first book, based on his ethnographic fieldwork in India, studying the health practices of long-distance truck drivers. Additionally, he has been a project manager on the Heart Health Indiana campaign under the aegis of CUAHD (Communities and Universities Addressing Health Disparities), a community-based heart-health initiative located in two Indiana counties. He is an Associate Editor for the journal *Health Communication.*

Jennifer Scarduzio (PhD, Arizona State University) is an Assistant Professor at the University of Kentucky. Her research examines the intersections of bureaucracy, emotion, violence, and wellness in a variety of organizational and health settings. Her most current research projects look at topics such as intersectionality and wellness in bureaucratic organizations and online violent victimization, such as cybersexual harassment. She is the coauthor of the textbook *Surviving Work: Toxic Organizational Communication* published by Kendall Hunt in 2014. Also, she has published in various outlets including *Communication Monographs, Management Communication Quarterly, Handbook of Health Communication,* and *Journal of Interpersonal Violence,* among others.

Barbara F. Sharf (PhD, University of Minnesota) is an independent scholar and Professor Emerita in Communication at Texas A&M University. Using qualitative forms of investigation and analysis, particularly narrative inquiry, her research interests have encompassed communication in clinical settings; patients' experiences of illness; cultural influences on healthcare; health disparities related to race/ethnicity, class, and geographic location; the portrayal of health and illness in popular media; and most recently integrative approaches to healthcare. She is currently a Research Fulbright Scholar, investigating integrative healthcare in Singapore.

Jill Yamasaki (PhD, Texas A&M University) is an Associate Professor in the Jack J. Valenti School of Communication at the University of Houston. Her research focuses on narrative inquiry and practice in health communication and aging, particularly in the contexts of creative engagement, community, and long-term care. Her work appears in journals such as *Health Communication, Journal of Aging Studies, Journal of Health Communication, Patient Education & Counseling,* and *Text & Performance Quarterly.*

Heather M. Zoller (PhD, Purdue University) is Professor and Director of Graduate Studies at the University of Cincinnati Department of Communication. She is a Senior Editor at *Health Communication* and coeditor with Mohan Dutta of the book *Emerging Perspectives in Health Communication.* Her research addressing organizing and the politics of public health appears in outlets such as *Communication Monographs, Journal of Applied Communication Research, Communication Theory,* and *Health Communication.*

Health Communication in Action (HCIA) Contributors

Peter A. Andersen, San Diego State University
Julie Apker, Western Michigan University
Lourdes Baezconde-Garbanati, University of Southern California
Wayne A. Beach, San Diego State University
David B. Buller, Klein-Buendel Inc.
Jennifer J. Bute, Indiana University-Purdue University Indianapolis
Joyee S. Chatterjee, University of Southern California
Angela Cooke-Jackson, Emerson College
Bonnie Creel, Independent Scholar
Gary R. Cutter, University of Alabama Hospital, Birmingham, AL
Mark B. Dignan, University of Kentucky
Patrick J. Dillon, University of Memphis
Marissa J. Doshi, Hope College
Tasha Dubriwny, Texas A&M University
Lauren B. Frank, Portland State University
Patricia Geist-Martin, San Diego State University
Aline Gubrium, University of Massachusetts Amherst
Evelyn Y. Ho, University of San Francisco
Shelly R. Hovick, The Ohio State University
Elaine Hsieh, University of Oklahoma
Gary L. Kreps, George Mason University
Suzanne Kurtz, Washington State University / University of Calgary
Kurt Lindemann, San Diego State University
Pamela Lutgen-Sandvik, North Dakota State University
Jennifer A. Malkowski, California State University, Chico
Summer Carnett Martin, California State University, Fullerton
Steve May, University of North Carolina at Chapel Hill
Katherine Miller, Arizona State University
Laura E. Miller, University of Tennessee
Lucy J. Miller, Texas A&M University
Michelle Miller-Day, Chapman University
Meghan B. Moran, Johns Hopkins Bloomberg School of Public Health
Sheila Murphy, University of Southern California

Jon F. Nussbaum, Penn State University
Jeffery Chaichana Peterson, Washington State University
Sandra Petronio, Indiana University-Purdue University Indianapolis
Vandhana Ramadurai, Independent Scholar
Eileen Berlin Ray, Cleveland State University
Stephanie M. Ruhl, Clemson University
Michael D. Scott, California State University, Chico
Barbara F. Sharf, Independent Scholar/Texas A&M University
Lisa M. Tillmann, Rollins College
Alexia Torke, Indiana University School of Medicine
Jillian A. Tullis, University of San Diego
Barbara J. Walkosz, Klein-Buendel Inc.
Joan B. Wolf, Texas A&M University
Kevin B. Wright, George Mason University
Jill Yamasaki, University of Houston
Amanda J. Young, University of Memphis

Foreword

Stories are powerful. Journalists get it. They always include in their articles a story that personalizes the issue. It's more difficult for scientists to "get it." They have been trained to eschew the unique for the generalizable, to present only evidence-based information, and to be completely rational and objective, never emotional and subjective.

When I was Director of Communication at the CDC, and before Dr. Andrew Wakefield's publications declaring links between childhood vaccines and autism had been debunked, our scientists were called to testify before numerous congressional hearings. Their factual, statistical testimony didn't stand a chance compared with the grieving parents and grandparents telling stories of how autism had tragically transformed their happy, responsive toddlers. Eventually my staff and I convinced the scientists to also tell stories about the decisions they made about vaccinating their own children and the positive outcomes. Experiences like these made me a believer in the importance of the narrative approach to health communication and made me excited to learn about this new book.

Not only is the focus of this book so important, but the coauthors/editors are the best ones to present it. Even though most of my own research has been quantitative, several years ago, Barbara Sharf and I collaborated on a study of an ovarian cancer narrative portrayed on the then popular TV show, *thirtysomething*. We did a thematic analysis of the content and in-depth interviews with dedicated viewers. I witnessed firsthand the rigorous methodology and thoughtful insights Barbara brings to her qualitative work, which gave me a new appreciation for that approach to research. First author/editor Jill Yamasaki is emerging as a leader in the next generation of narrative health communication researchers, especially with her creative studies of aging in the context of community. Both Barbara and Patricia Geist-Martin are senior scholars in the health communication field and well-known practitioners of the narrative approach. Even though I have not had the privilege of collaborating with Patricia, my thinking about health communication has been influenced by her work about narrative and identity in our personal and professional lives.

In addition to the chapters written by the three editors, the remaining chapters have been contributed by an array of qualitative scholars who have incorporated a variety of storied approaches to their particular topics, including ethnographic field research and critical analysis, while also guiding readers to key concepts and relevant literature. The content of this volume is comprehensive with chapters covering health communication from patient–provider interactions to entertainment-education to policy making. Topics often not explored in survey texts such as workplace health, globalized health disparities, and art as a way of communicating health are included here. Each chapter includes discussion questions and thought-provoking "Theorizing Practice" exercises that encourage readers to make sense of chapter content in circumstances that are personally relevant to them. Another aspect of this book that I find intriguing is the "Health Communication in Action" sidebars, short translational research summaries contributed by a virtual who's who in the health communication field, both senior and emerging scholars. Students who read this book will be introduced not only to a broad examination of health communication as a field of study but also to how such scholarship has significant impact in a wide variety of contexts.

The presence of this book is an innovative milestone for the study of health communication, arguing persuasively for stories as the basis for understanding and application.

Vicki S. Freimuth, PhD
Professor Emeritus, University of Georgia

Acknowledgments

We are especially grateful to Neil Rowe of Waveland Press for his enthusiasm to publish this book—and for his generosity, guidance, and patience over the two-plus years it took us to complete it. Once the book was finished, Jeni Ogilvie proved equally gracious, attentive, and patient through editing and production. We were quite fortunate to work with her.

We are indebted to our exceptional contributing authors for enriching this volume, for expending the time and effort required in working with our vision for this book, and for enabling us to showcase the quality, diversity, and relevance of health communication scholarship from a storied perspective. Thank you, also, to the many scholars who cheerfully contributed conversational translations of their published work for our Health Communication in Action sidebars.

Finally, we wanted this book to feature stories of health and illness from ordinary individuals living in the midst of extraordinary circumstances. We are honored to include their voices in the narratives featured throughout every chapter, and we are both humbled and inspired by their experiences.

About the Cover

The beautiful watercolor gracing the cover of this book is a reproduction of an untitled painting by Hilda Gorenstein (or Hilgos as she was known professionally). Hilgos completed it—and hundreds of others—in the last three years of her life while in the later stages of Alzheimer's disease. After worsening dementia seemingly ended her accomplished 75-year artistic career, Hilgos was able to resume painting with the help of students from her alma mater, the School of the Art Institute of Chicago, claiming, "I remember better when I paint." Her abstract watercolors allude to the nautical themes she specialized in throughout her career, and they represent opportunities for Hilgos—in the depths of a progressively isolating disease—to connect with others and for us, her audience, to continue to embrace and appreciate her artistic spirit and innate creative impulse. In this spirit, we are thrilled to feature Hilgos' art, courtesy of her daughter, Berna Huebner, and to support the Hilgos Foundation that Ms. Huebner created in memory of her mother. The foundation supports and encourages the ongoing process of artistic creation with people who have memory problems and/or Alzheimer's and require assistance in creating art that is meaningful and enriching.

Communicating the Complexities of Health and Illness

Jill Yamasaki

Elizabeth, a junior in college, last used cocaine on a night that started no differently than most of her evenings in 1985. She and her boyfriend, Rich, went to a local bar to listen to live music and get high, counting on the combination of alcohol and cocaine to fuel their fun into the early morning. When they ran low on cash and needed more drugs, Rich approached two dealers at the bar with a promise of smuggling cocaine into their college dorm for distribution to other students. Before long, they were in the backseat of a modified Cadillac with the two men they'd just met, cruising North Philadelphia, and snorting seemingly bottomless cocaine out of a Ziploc bag through a McDonald's straw.

Even in her altered state, Elizabeth knew the situation wasn't safe. She knew it wasn't safe to get in a car with strangers in a notoriously dangerous part of town. She knew it wasn't safe to hatch a plan to sell drugs in her college dorm. She knew it wasn't safe to do that much cocaine with abandon. And, after they finally returned to the dorm, she knew it wasn't safe when Rich started doing pushups on the ledge of the open 9th floor window. Suddenly, Elizabeth panicked. "How am I going to explain how high I am when Rich falls out of this window to his death?" Elizabeth backed away from her boyfriend. Then and there, she was done.

While seemingly outlandish, Elizabeth's story isn't all that unusual, and, as you will read throughout this chapter, it doesn't end here. Thirty years later, Elizabeth has been sober for nine years, but drug overdoses now exceed motor vehicle accidents as the leading injury-related cause of death (Levi, Segal, & Martin, 2015). Many of these deaths could be prevented with medical assistance; however, witnesses—who, like Elizabeth, are usually intoxicated themselves and scared of repercussions—often flee the scene without summoning help for the unconscious or inebriated friend they've left behind. To combat these statistics, more than 32 states, starting with New Mexico in 2007, have enacted Good Samaritan policies that provide limited immunity from arrest or prosecution for minor drug and alcohol law violations (Drug Policy Alliance, 2015). Nearly 400 college campuses, including the university Elizabeth attended, have also implemented Good Samaritan policies (Students for Sensible Drug Policy, 2015). These policies, which fall under medical amnesty laws, protect both the person who overdoses and the friend who calls 911 and stays with that person until medical help arrives.

We find it particularly fitting to begin a book about storied health and illness with Elizabeth's experiences—not only because she survived and is now a thriving adult in long-term recovery but also because her lived accounts of substance use and mental health disorders highlight the personal, cultural, and political complexities that exist when people communicate about health.[1] Good Samaritan laws and increased calls for widespread public availability of naloxone (or brand name Narcan)—an FDA-approved opioid antagonist that temporarily counters the effects of overdose—represent a growing new national response to drug use, addiction, and overdose that prioritizes medical necessities over legal consequences. This shift demonstrates one of many ways that individual physical and psychological states of being are perceived and imbued with collective social and cultural meaning (Sharf & Vanderford, 2003). As you will read throughout this book, communicating about health and illness entails a continuous negotiation of the complexities comprising this delicate balance between scientific evidence of biological disease and the subjective, nonverifiable experiences of being ill or in discomfort—in other words, in dis-ease (Morris, 1998; Sharf & Vanderford, 2003).

In this chapter, we introduce and orient you to the foundational concepts at the center of this book. As coeditors and cowriters of this collection, we are delighted to feature the detailed knowledge and specific expertise of our various chapter contributors. At the same time, we made a number of purposeful decisions to ensure overall cohesion and quality across the chapters. Specifically, we asked these authors to: (1) incorporate an engaging story from their own research or personal experience that introduces and grounds the chapter topic; (2) integrate a discussion of the personal, cultural, and political complexities in their treatment of the topic; and (3) discuss current and seminal literature related to the topic. You will see this format modeled in this chapter, with mental illness and addiction as the illustrative focus. You will also become acquainted with a number of special features included in this and every chapter throughout the book. Once you have read this chapter, we expect you to have a working understanding of the complexities, responsibilities, and consequences of communicating matters of health and illness, and we hope you will be eager to engage with what's to come.

▪ Defining Health Communication

We communicate about health on a daily basis, whether we're interacting with others, negotiating choices, making decisions, coping with uncertainty, watching TV, or surfing online. As patients, practitioners, public citizens, or private individuals, we respond to what we see and hear, engage in conversations, and create discourse that shapes our own and others' experiences of health-related situations. Refer back to the story at the beginning of this chapter. How did Elizabeth's thoughts, actions, and communication influence that evening's events? What circumstances shaped her behaviors?

Like its predecessor, this book defines *health communication* as **the symbolic processes by which people, individually and collectively, understand, shape, and accommodate to health and illness** (Geist-Martin, Ray, & Sharf, 2011, p. 3). *Healthy*

People 2010 (2000), an influential governmental report documenting the national plan for improving public health, offered a similar definition, characterizing health communication as "the art and technique of informing, influencing, and motivating individual, institutional, and public audiences about important health issues." A decade later, *Healthy People 2020* (2010) expanded objectives in this topic area to capture the many ways health communication can have a potentially positive impact on health, healthcare, and health equity:

- Supporting shared decision making between patients and providers.
- Providing personalized self-management tools and resources.
- Building social support networks.
- Delivering accurate, accessible, and actionable health information that is targeted or tailored.
- Facilitating the meaningful exchange of health information among healthcare and public health professionals.
- Enabling quick and informed action to health risks and public health emergencies.
- Increasing health literacy skills.
- Providing new opportunities to connect with culturally diverse and hard-to-reach populations.
- Providing sound principles in the designs of programs and interventions that result in healthier behaviors.
- Increasing Internet and mobile access. (*Healthy People 2020*, 2010)

As you can see, health is more than the absence of disease, and health communication is an integral component of healthcare within but also well beyond the medical milieu. Beyond the emphasis on biological vocabularies of disease (e.g., lab results, diagnoses, and medical jargon), we need to elicit and learn from individuals' personal experiences (e.g., pain, quality of life, and emotional concerns) and the words they use to speak of wellness, illness, and healing. Likewise, we must consider the overlapping, contradictory, and multiple forms of knowledge and experience that contribute to wellness and illness. Accounting for these personal, cultural, and political complexities is necessary for reaching shared understandings when we communicate about health and navigate the changing, complex landscape of healthcare.

◼ The Study and Practice of Health Communication

The field of health communication is dynamic, complex, and interesting. Researchers continue to enlarge notions of the physical, psychological, social, and spiritual dimensions of health, and scholarship has expanded to address pressing social and healthcare issues. Our own research reflects these directions, including integrative health, narrative care, humanizing practices, and innovative ways of improving well-being and quality of life in personal relationships, medical care, caregiving, the workplace, and community settings. Perhaps more so than several other areas of communication studies, health communication is an inherently applied and often interdisciplinary field of inquiry with the potential to inform healthcare delivery and health promotion practices. Importantly, health communication scholars often collaborate with health professionals, community partners, and researchers from other fields (e.g., from public health, gerontology, sociology, and medicine) with the goal of translating important insights into beneficial practices (Parrott & Kreuter, 2011).

To illustrate some of this exciting research, we have invited 36 health communication scholars to highlight their work in *Health Communication in Action (HCIA)* sidebars. These sidebars appear throughout the book, are loosely coupled with the content of each chapter, and include *Questions to Ponder* for you to engage with the featured project by considering your perspectives and examining your experiences. The first HCIA sidebar, written by Dr. Summer Carnett Martin, describes the medical, personal, and social sources of uncertainty that arise in experiences of illness and recovery—in this case, organ transplantation. We hope you will find these sidebars both engaging and enlightening as you immerse yourself in the study and practice of health communication.

HCIA 1.1

Uncertainty Related to Health and Illness

Summer Carnett Martin

The experience of illness is often accompanied by uncertainty. For example, if you wake up with a bright red sore throat, you might wonder what is causing the irritation, how long it will last and if it will get worse, whether you will be able to function normally that day or that week, whether the condition is contagious, and if you should visit a doctor. If you do consult with a healthcare professional, additional uncertainty might arise before, during, and after the appointment—including questions related to understanding the meaning of medical jargon used by the healthcare provider, managing side effects of medications, and communicating your diagnosis to others. Even acute conditions as common as a cold, the flu, or strep throat can induce short-term uncertainty. When a person is dealing with a chronic health concern, however, experiencing significant uncertainty often becomes a way of life.

In a research project that spanned the course of several years, we explored the uncertainty of individuals facing a particular type of chronic health issue: organ transplantation. Going on the waiting list for an organ is often necessitated by a chronic health condition (such as heart or liver disease). Moreover, even after a person undergoes a transplant, health concerns persist. Rather than being seen as a one-time "cure," transplantation is typically viewed by healthcare professionals and patients as a treatment that entails long-term maintenance, including years of medications and medical appointments. We suspected this journey from pre- to post-transplantation to be fraught with many forms of uncertainty but found, in our review of relevant literature, that sources of uncertainty across the entire transplant experience were not well documented. Therefore, in our project, we aimed to identify sources of uncertainty experienced by individuals across the trajectory of transplantation and to examine how transplant patients manage their uncertainty. Understanding more about the causes and management of uncertainty in transplantation can provide insight about what to expect throughout this process and how to manage uncertainty in ways that minimize negative outcomes.

To investigate these issues, we conducted in-depth interviews with individuals who have had, or who are waiting for, an organ transplant. We invited participants who had received, or who were waiting for, any type of organ (e.g., kidney, heart, liver, pancreas). Some participants were new to the waiting list, while others had undergone an organ transplant years ago. This considerable range allowed us to explore transplantation across the trajectory. In one of the articles published from these data, we identified significant sources of uncertainty experienced prior to and after the transplant. After thematically analyzing interview transcripts, we determined that the uncertainty discussed by our participants could be broadly categorized as stemming from *medical*, *personal*, and *social* sources. Based on our data, we developed an extensive categorical system to identify subcategories within each main type of uncertainty in transplantation.

We found that pre-transplant medical forms of uncertainty are a result of *insufficient information about the diagnosis, complex decisions about transplantation, unknown organ availability,* and *unclear expectations about medical procedures and outcomes*. Participant Audrey described the uncertainty she had before the surgery about her future health: "What's it going to be like... when the operation is done; is it going to work?" She explained, "You hear about people getting the transplant, then the organ being bad, or rejecting right away, so to go through all that and then have it not work is uncertain." Medical forms of uncertainty continue after the transplant and include uncertainty related to *complex medication regimens* and *unpredictable future health*.

In addition to stemming from medical sources, uncertainty in transplantation has personal causes. Personal forms of uncertainty experienced pre-transplant stem from *ambiguity in the meaning of life, complex role and identity challenges,* and *unclear financial consequences*. Regarding ambiguity in the meaning of life, participant Autumn said, "What does it mean if all I end up doing is going back and forth to dialysis, recovering that day and the next day feeling better? Then I go back to dialysis." She continued, "I think, like most people, certainly, I want to feel like I'm doing something more." Participants also reported personal forms of uncertainty after the transplant, due to *unclear financial consequences* and *complex role and identity challenges*.

Uncertainty in transplantation is also social in form. Prior to the transplant, individuals experience social forms of uncertainty, including *unclear relational implications* and *questioning from others*. The post-transplant experience continues to be marked by social uncertainty, including *possible stigmatizing interpersonal reactions, unclear relational implications,* and *complex interactions with the deceased donor's family*. For example, regarding this latter category, some participants agonized over the decision of whether to write to the deceased donor's family. Participant Charlotte explained, "I thought, 'They're grieving, maybe they don't want to hear about this person who's living and doing well,' and it turned out that they were like, 'We were waiting. We were hoping you would write to us.'" In sum, these results demonstrate that uncertainty stems from a variety of sources across the transplant experience and underscore the importance of medical care that attends to issues extending beyond physical health.

QUESTIONS TO PONDER

1. Consider your own experiences with uncertainty related to health and illness. What forms of uncertainty have you experienced related to a specific health challenge?

2. In what ways do you imagine that uncertainty might be *detrimental* to people's health?

3. Although uncertainty is typically viewed as negative, some scholars suggest that this is not *always* the case. Under what circumstances might uncertainty be *beneficial* to people's health?

Source: Martin, S. C., Stone, A. M., Scott, A. M., & Brashers, D. E. (2010). Medical, personal, and social forms of uncertainty across the transplantation trajectory. *Qualitative Health Research, 20,* 182–196.

■ Thinking with Stories

Importantly, we learn from stories of health and illness—the stories we tell, the stories others tell, and the stories we construct in conversation. These stories offer coherence to "wounded storytellers" (Frank, 1995), whose lives have been disrupted by illness and possibility to those who bear witness. When we think *with* stories—rather than thinking *about* stories—we imaginatively attend to the lived experiences of others. In so doing, we can examine and better understand our own lives, as well as give voice to and offer empathy for the suffering of others (Frank, 1995; Morris, 1998).

Critical to learning from these stories is encouraging people to tell their own stories of being silenced, discredited, stigmatized, and excluded, as well as those of being heard, encouraged, comforted, and included. For example, consider the beautiful watercolor gracing the cover of this book. The artist, Hilda Gorenstein (or Hilgos as she was known professionally), painted this image in her early 90s while in the later stages of Alzheimer's disease. After worsening dementia seemingly ended her accomplished, decades-long, artistic career, Hilgos was placed in a Chicago-area nursing home. There, she resumed painting with the help of students from her alma mater, the School of the Art Institute of Chicago, claiming, "I remember better when I paint." To be sure, the hundreds of abstract watercolors she painted in the final three years of her life allude to the nautical themes she specialized in throughout her career. But they also represent opportunities for Hilgos—in the depths of a progressively isolating disease—to connect with others and for us, her audience, to continue to embrace and appreciate her innate creative impulse and artistic spirit (see Huebner, 2011).

Chapter 2 highlights the storied nature of health and illness, the importance of narrative to the study of health communication, and the narrative sensibilities comprising the heart of this book. We ask that you embrace this core premise as a way of thinking about, analyzing, and reconsidering your own and others' health beliefs, behaviors, and communication.

First, as this chapter progresses, you will read more about Elizabeth's experiences with substance use disorder and mental illness. Then, in the chapters that follow, we invite you to think with the stories of individuals living with the inherent challenges and unexpected opportunities of other health-related situations, including aging, cancer, dialysis, sexual harassment, miscarriage, obesity, alopecia, breastfeeding, health threats to immigrant workers, developmental disabilities, and youth violence. Once you've read and absorbed these stories, we suspect you'll find yourself thinking, feeling, and acting in previously unimagined ways.

■ Theorizing from Everyday Health Practices

The sincere desire to learn about, theorize from, and understand the complexities of our own and others' experiences is vital to communicating matters of health. Thus, this book is premised on the notion that we are constantly *theorizing* (i.e., guessing, predicting, or explaining) from the stories we tell, hear, and see about everyday health practices. See Theorizing Practice 1.1 for the first in a series of *Theorizing Practice* boxes that appear throughout the book. These exercises in each chapter will encourage you to examine significant stories or experiences in your own and others' lives in

---

Theorizing Practice 1.1
Health Communication Assessment

To gain firsthand knowledge of health communication, keep a journal about your own health-care beliefs and behaviors. Write an entry each day that describes the following:

- Describe one behavior you engaged in today that you believe contributes to or detracts from your health (e.g., taking or not taking vitamins, exercise or sedentary activities, smoking, meditating, or eating particular foods).

- Explain why you do this behavior and how you believe it contributes to or detracts from your health.

- Describe how communication was part of engaging in this behavior today (e.g., retelling the behavior to a friend or healthcare provider, talking with someone while engaging in the behavior, sharing your experiences with someone who also engages in the behavior).

- Describe how you might ensure continuing this healthy behavior or reducing/eliminating this unhealthy behavior.

Once you have faithfully journaled for a month, examine the frequency and nature of your healthy and unhealthy behaviors. Write a short analysis of these patterns. Try to provide an understanding of the multiple influences, such as culture, family, work, and politics, on your behaviors (Geist-Martin et al., 2011, p. 17).

---

order to respond to questions, test assertions, and, hopefully, enlarge your viewpoints in ways you haven't considered.

At this point, we return to Elizabeth's story as an illustration for exploring the personal, cultural, and political complexities integral to—and integrated within—all health-related communication. The discussion that follows will assist you in recognizing, appreciating, and understanding these complexities at work in both your daily life and in the chapters to come.

■ Personal Complexities

Elizabeth tasted her first sip of wine at age 5, was sneaking alcohol daily by age 8, and was a polydrug user by age 12. "It changed how I felt. It was the only thing that helped me sleep. It was the only thing that calmed me and quieted the constant chatter in my head," she recalls. The "chatter" in Elizabeth's head—that she didn't measure up, that she didn't fit in, that she didn't feel right, that she didn't belong—stemmed from her family's frequent criticisms and lofty expectations, and was exacerbated by the sexual abuse she never reported. "Alcohol—and later marijuana, pills, cocaine, and anything else I could get my hands on—felt like my solution," continues Elizabeth. "And it felt like my solution for 33 years. I started drinking before I learned my multiplication tables, before I learned long division. It was before I developed any coping systems, before I finished developing as a person, and that made it extraordinarily difficult to stop."

Despite her addictions, Elizabeth graduated college, moved to England, and began working with hard-core heroin addicts at a needle exchange program. She was no longer using cocaine or stealing pills, but she was drinking alcohol and smoking large amounts of cannabis resin every day. Elizabeth smoked resin through her first two pregnancies and in her eventual position as a drug educator. "That's when I really started to get in a position of being trapped," says Eliza-beth. "My job was to provide drug education to the community as a whole, and it was marvel-ous, and I loved it. But I was high the entire time, and I had to be high at work because no one had ever seen me straight. I remember interviewing people to work on the team, and this girl came in totally high and, after she left, Paul, my manager, turned to me and said, 'Why would anyone come high to do this?' And I was sitting there thinking, 'I'm so messed up right now.' I was trapped."

Elizabeth's husband's career eventually brought them back to the United States. Now a stay-at-home mom of three, Elizabeth could no longer score other drugs, so her alcohol use increased substantially. "That's when I really started to hide how much I was drinking because I operated under the delusion that I would be happy if only I managed well," remembers Elizabeth. "Everything had to be about the outside. Martin had a great job. My house looked like Martha Stewart's. I had to have certain cars. We had to live this certain lifestyle. Just like my father's mother, who was an alcoholic, I figured if I look so good on the outside, you're never going to look at the inside."

Until, finally, Elizabeth's outside cracked. She was drinking around the clock, constantly starting fights with Martin, and lashing out violently at her teenage children. She broke her arm falling out of bed drunk, woke up on the kitchen floor covered in her own waste, and passed out in the driveway. After five or six stints in detox, none of which she remembers, Elizabeth checked into a residential treatment center, where Martin and her counselor confronted her. "I was get-ting sober, but I was angry, and Martin had enough. He screamed in my face, 'You don't bring anything to the table!' Well, in my world, I was the table. I had always been the table. I had been the center of the universe, and no one had ever challenged me. And they were challenging me. I said, 'You have no right to say this.' My counselor screamed, 'He has every right to say this. He's done.' And I cried, 'How can you say this? Martin, you're not done.' And he said, 'I'm done.' So I got my angry little self into group, and then I too was done." At age 42, Eliza-beth came clean. She's been in long-term recovery ever since. "I had used for 33 years, and that was enough," says Elizabeth. "Now at almost 51, it feels a lot better to not feel like the walking dead. I never had to be that person again—and that was a choice as long as I never used. I had the power to build skills and be a stronger, better person. But I had to be clean."

Elizabeth's story highlights some of the many personal complexities of substance abuse and addiction. Her family roles, relationships, and dynamics as a child and adult; her strategies for coping with stress and managing habits; her feelings of being trapped and entitled; and her decades-long journey to sobriety all reflect and influence her subjective experiences of illness. Although multiple people may share the same diagnosed disease (in this case, substance use disorder), an inside understanding of another's suffering helps to personalize and contextualize each person's unique illness experience (Pierret, 2003; Vanderford, Jenks, & Sharf, 1997).

We live and communicate about health-related issues in social relationships across a myriad of contexts, including home, the workplace, and the public arena. *Home* is the site in which health practices are negotiated and maintained, relationships are enacted, and the effects of cultural and community contexts are most strongly felt. Despite the primary influence of home, family, and friends, *the workplace* is where many people spend much, if not most, of their waking hours. It is the site of organiza-tional resources, occupational hazards, and influential interactions. More of a socially formulated environment than actual physical site, the *public arena* serves as a major informational channel for health promotion and educational campaigns, as well as a conduit for marginalization and discrimination. Given the complex nature of our participation in personal relationships spanning these discrete, but overlapping, social contexts, the same illness will be experienced differently by others who, "from their separate perspectives, observe different aspects of its truth" (Morris, 1998, p. 5). Thus, what might be true for one person will not be true for another. Martin would have a different story of his subjective experiences with Elizabeth's addiction, as would her children, colleagues, and counselor.

■ Cultural Complexities

It wasn't long before Elizabeth's counselor suspected that she might have bipolar disorder. Elizabeth resisted. "No! That can't be. My father was bipolar, and I didn't want to believe that this was who I was and what my problem was, but she just kept after me and after me and after me until I finally had no alternative but to acknowledge that this was an issue." A psychiatrist officially diagnosed her. The dual diagnosis (i.e., co-occurring mental health and substance use disorders) wasn't that surprising, given Elizabeth's family history and the propensity for people to self-medicate with alcohol or drugs when they experience troubling mental health symptoms or to develop mental health disorders when they regularly abuse alcohol or drugs. Still, while Elizabeth had no qualms acknowledging her substance abuse, she found it very difficult to admit publicly that she was mentally ill. "No one really thinks of addiction or mental illness as a disease, but there's this idea—this stigma—that you're going to go nuts and harm somebody if you're mentally ill," says Elizabeth. "It was very tough at first. People's reactions were 'Oh. You, you have a mental health problem?' But today I'm quite happy to be an advocate and a face: This is what bipolar looks like. I live with it on a daily basis."

According to the Substance Abuse and Mental Health Services Administration (2014), one in four U.S. adults experiences mental illness in a given year, and one in 17 lives with a serious mental health condition such as schizophrenia, bipolar disorder, or major depression. All told, an estimated 54 million Americans of all ages contend with some form of mental illness in any given year (Substance Abuse and Mental Health Services Administration, 2014). Further, the National Institute on Drug Abuse (2010) reports that people with mental disorders are twice as likely to also have substance use disorder, just as people with substance use disorders are twice as likely to have a mental disorder—a phenomenon characterized as *dual diagnosis, comorbidity,* or *co-occurring disorders.* People with dual diagnosis, like Elizabeth, require a comprehensive approach to treatment that identifies and evaluates each disorder concurrently (National Institute on Drug Abuse, 2010). However, as with other health-related issues, cultural assumptions influence whether people seek help, the types of treatment they seek, their coping styles, available support systems, and the *stigma* (i.e., deeply discrediting attribute) they attach to mental illness.

Despite anti-stigma campaigns and advances in public knowledge, misconceptions about mental illness continue to perpetuate harmful stereotypes that depict people with mental health disorders as unpredictable and dangerous (Pescosolido et al., 2010). Violence is a major cause of this stigma. Graphic media coverage of mass shootings by people with a history of serious mental illness (e.g., the horrific massacres at the Newtown elementary school and the Aurora movie theater), followed by heated debates of national gun control policies, fuel many of these negative perceptions (McGinty, Webster, & Barry, 2013). Widespread discrimination also contributes to strong feelings of *internalized stigma* (i.e., self-belief in negative stereotypes) among people with serious mental illness (Livingston & Boyd, 2010; Quinn, Williams, & Weisz, 2015). Thus, it is not uncommon for people to avoid or delay seeking professional help due to shame, fear of disclosure, concerns about confidentiality, and beliefs that they can (or should be able to) handle their problems on their own (Clement et al., 2015).

By defining ourselves—or being defined by others—as healthy or unhealthy, we may affiliate with particular cultural communities. At the most general level, *culture* can be defined as a group or community of people who share a set of beliefs, values, and attitudes that guide their behavior (Geertz, 1973; Kreps & Kunimoto, 1994). We each develop our own idiosyncratic, multicultural identities through the combination of different cultural orientations and influences of the many cultural communities to which we belong (Kreps & Kunimoto, 1994). Take a moment to consider your own membership in multicultural communities based on your age, language, friendships, year in school, birthplace, region of upbringing, hobbies, intellectual interests, religion, gender, political affiliation, and the many other factors that lead you to talk and to act in certain ways. Then, check out Theorizing Practice 1.2 for an examination of mental illness and "the culture of anxiety" on college campuses.

Theorizing Practice 1.2
Students in Crisis on College Campuses

The following excerpt is from Yahoo Global News Anchor Katie Couric's 2015 report entitled *Students in Crisis: Mental Health & Suicide on College Campuses* (http://news.yahoo.com/mental-health-suicide-on-college-campuses-katie-couric-141742009.html). As you read it, consider your responses to the following questions:

1. Can you relate to the ways students are characterized in this report? Why or why not? How is the culture on your campus similar to or different from what is described here?

2. Are you aware of the different resources available for psychological and emotional help on your campus? What about informal ones? How would you assist a friend in distress?

3. In what ways does social media connect you to others? How might it prevent you from connecting to others?

Campus Culture of Anxiety

College students are reporting that they're more depressed and anxious than ever before and are pouring into overwhelmed college counseling centers for help, often waiting weeks for appointments. Universities are attempting to respond but haven't kept up with the crisis.

"We know that colleges have actually increased their staffing and increased their budgets in many, many cases," said Dr. Victor Schwartz, the medical director for the JED Foundation and the former medical director of counseling services at New York University. "It hasn't kept up with the demand. As much as they seem to increase, students are coming in. There does seem to be a very, very large need."

It's unclear what's driving the dramatic decrease in emotional health on campus. It's possible more students now feel comfortable seeking help in the first place, instead of bottling up their problems. Dr. Allison Baker, a child psychiatrist with the Child Mind Institute, also pointed out that more young people are receiving mental health treatment as children, which allows them to go to college in the first place. But many college counseling centers are ill equipped to deal with these students' more complicated mental health issues. "Colleges are slammed, and services are lacking," she said.

Stopping the Stigma

But there's also clearly a societal and cultural element at play. *New York Times* columnist Frank Bruni, author of "Where You Go Is Not Who You'll Be: An Antidote to the College Admissions Mania," said that college administrators overwhelmingly describe today's students as "fragile." They're seeing less resilience and adaptability in students today than even those from a decade earlier. Some blame over-involved parenting styles that put intense pressure on kids to succeed.

"There's an intense economic anxiety . . . that filters from parents to kids and has a whole generation of kids worried about what their future is going to hold," Bruni said. "And then you have this kind of parenting and this kind of atmosphere that often exists in certain communities right now where kids are following this very exacting script through high school that their parents have written for them. And then they get to college and they're on their own in a very real way for the first time. And the script isn't there for them."

Some college counseling centers have started mandating that students take "resilience workshops" before they access the overburdened counselors in the first place, Yahoo News National Affairs Reporter Liz Goodwin said. The workshops teach them basic coping skills and how to "self soothe" after an ordinary setback such as a bad grade.

Schwartz highlighted the role of social media, which has been a part of campus life for a decade now but continues to grow. The technology is meant to connect people, but it might not actually increase feelings of closeness and intimacy that can help a young person survive a crisis. "There's data that, in fact, students feel less connected to their friends than they did 10 and 20 years ago," Schwartz said.

Margaret Kramer, a graduating senior at the University of South Carolina who has been a mental health advocate on her campus, said that social media creates tremendous pressure to present oneself as perfect. "We're constantly online, constantly having to create several personas for ourselves within our classroom, within our professional life, if we have that as a student," she told Couric via Skype. "There's a perfection expected. I've definitely been affected by that."

Couric also spoke to two grieving parents of bright and promising college students who took their own lives after battling mental illness. Sue Cimbricz, the mother of Sam Freeling, who died by suicide as a senior at the University of Rochester less than two years ago, told Couric that something changed in her son, suddenly, and that she still doesn't know what happened. "He said he didn't have the same feelings of joy and happiness that he had before," she said.

Though Freeling was in treatment, Cimbricz thinks the social stigma around mental illness may have made the emerging disease even harder for her son to deal with. He tried to hide his pain. "I think to a large degree a lot has to do with the social stigma attached with this and that feeling of isolation," Cimbricz said.

Donna Satow, who founded the JED Foundation to educate people about suicide after her son took his own life in 1998, agreed that stigma is still an issue but that it's slowly getting better. She hopes to spread the message that suicide is preventable and that mental illness is treatable, just like other diseases. "We just felt that with the people we knew and the knowledge we had, we should try with all of our might to combat this," Satow said. "It is preventable if young people can get the right help. The help is there."

■ Political Complexities

It took a team of professionals to help Elizabeth get well. "I started AA, and I went every day at 7 A.M. for 3 1/2 years. Got a sponsor, did what I was supposed to do, and started working the steps, for which I'm forever grateful," recalls Elizabeth. "They were the rule book that I never thought I had. I never knew how to say I was sorry. I never knew how to take responsibility for things. And I needed 12 ways to live life as a responsible adult." Elizabeth welcomed the community provided by AA, but also needed intensive emotional, mental, and physical treatment to regain her health. "I went from just having AA to having a team comprised of my therapist, a psychiatrist, nutritional guidance, exercise support, my regular physician, and, eventually, family and marriage therapists," she explains. "I built this team around me, all of whom worked together, which was ideal. That's why when I think today about what is important about treatment—when you look at effective outcomes, at what should be offered to everyone—it's so much more than just a 12-step model. That's all very well and good, but the people you see in AA are just as broken as you are. They're not therapists, and AA has never claimed to be that. AA provides the community and teaches people to be accountable, but I also needed the skills, the coping mechanisms. I got that from a variety of different options."

However, Elizabeth is quick to acknowledge that people with dual diagnosis don't often have knowledge of or access to the variety of professional resources available to her. "I was really lucky. I went to a lot of therapy. I dealt with the underlying issues. I have really good coping skills. Not everyone gets that, and they end up just going back out," she says. "And that's just alcohol use. If you look at someone who's using opiates, their options are even fewer. It's so unfortunate." Elizabeth's prior work in methadone clinics and the needle exchange program reflects her training in harm reduction risk management, a concept she continues to champion today. "These people were coming into the needle exchange who were really, really ill. They were stealing to fund their habit or they were sharing dirty needles. You want them doing something that is safer. Because what is the alternative? Dying? As long as someone's alive, there is an option, there is hope, that they will be able to be well someday. That's what you want—to keep people alive," explains Elizabeth. "The line between a high and death is really close. So having paramedics carry Narcan or naloxone is really important because they can reverse the overdose. Or implementing Good Samaritan laws because it's so much better than dumping them in front of the ER where they may not get noticed or leaving them on the couch to die. You know, they're not in a room full of sober people, and they're going to be making decisions that aren't safe. That's not a nice way to die. That's not how you want to die."

Elizabeth's comments harken back to the beginning of this chapter and the story she told about her college dorm room in 1985. President Nixon declared war on drugs in 1971, but the 1980s and 1990s marked the height of the political hysteria associated with it. Zero-tolerance policies and mandatory minimum sentences criminalized addiction and dramatically increased rates of incarceration for nonviolent drug law offenses. Even as I write this chapter, nonviolent drug abuse violations remain the highest arrest category nationwide. According to the most recent FBI report, more than 1.5 million drug-related arrests occurred in 2013; of those, possession accounted for 82.3%, and sale or manufacturing comprised 17.7% (United States Department of Justice, Federal Bureau of Investigation, 2014). Now, by many accounts, the war on drugs has been a trillion-dollar failure that has deepened racial and socioeconomic divides, overpopulated prisons, and shattered young lives, while ultimately doing little to prevent or treat drug abuse and addiction (e.g., Dana, 2015; Porter, 2012).

What would happen if we treated addiction as a public health crisis rather than a criminal justice issue? What if we provided more funding for drug treatment instead of drug law enforcement? Eric March, an online blogger, echoed the calls of many citizens, including law enforcement officers, healthcare professionals, and policy makers, when he wrote, "We need to rethink the way we handle drug addiction nationwide. It's easy to lock someone up, throw away the key, and forget about them forever. It's harder to try and understand the complicated forces that underlie their addiction and try to get them the help they need" (March, 2015, para 10).

This brief foray into the controversies surrounding substance use disorder reveals some of the political complexities involved when we communicate about health or illness. When we share our views on health issues, we often discover that others see the topic from a different perspective. As we read and talk more about any one particular health issue, we find that negotiating these politics can be difficult because of the very different perspectives people may have based on their gender, race, ethnicity, age, and other factors.

Politics can be defined as the structure of diverse interests about a particular issue, or it can be defined as the process of communicating those interests. Politics as structure operates in the position or authority people have regarding an issue (e.g., the authority of a physician, lawyer, or activist), or in the way people view an issue (i.e., their philosophy or ideology), as well as their interests or stakes in that issue. Politics as process includes the ways people communicate their interests, speak about an issue, try to persuade others to see their point of view, and make possible or impossible certain actions aligned with that issue. Politics are never as simple as being for or against something—communication becomes instrumental in every aspect of almost any health issue as people take positions and communicate in ways that attempt to change others' points of view or to resist how their own positions are being characterized by others. To negotiate politics and transcend imbalances, we must consider diverse voices, perspectives, and opinions. Moreover, as patients, family members, and healthcare professionals, we must speak to the inequality we encounter when communicating matters of health and illness.

■ Negotiating Politics and Transcending Imbalances

Communication is central to negotiating identities, interests, and issues in ways that transcend stigma, contradictions, and marginalization. The politics of medicine and healing can be the arts of making possible what seemed impossible *and* of making impossible what seemed possible. To ensure the former and prevent the latter, we need to consider the directions in which we are moving and continue to answer questions such as:

- What are we trying to make possible through our communication?
- Whose interests are at stake?
- What authorities must be challenged?
- What or who makes impossible what we thought was possible?

Answering these questions requires that we continually seek and incorporate diverse forms of knowledge into our understandings of health and illness. Learning more about the differing needs and interests of people based on their race, culture, gender, religion, sexual orientation, and age is one way to do so. Another way is to identify the interests of structures or stakeholders that may marginalize, discriminate against, restrict access, and/or fail to reach various populations. This knowledge moves us to see more clearly the politics of emotional and physical isolation, the magnitude of negative personal and societal messages, and the perpetuation of disenfranchisement and marginalization through communication. In addition, we gain an understanding of the power of communication to include, to empower, and to advocate for those persons and groups whose healthcare needs have not been considered or addressed.

Consider Chief Leonard Campanello of the Gloucester, Massachusetts, police department, who, in June 2015, made the bold decision to no longer arrest drug users who seek help. He posted an official statement of the new policy on Facebook, part of which follows:

> Any addict who walks into the police station with the remainder of their drug equipment (needles, etc.) or drugs and asks for help will NOT be charged. Instead, we will walk them through the system toward detox and recovery. We will assign them an "angel" who will be their guide through the process. Not in hours or days, but on the spot . . . Lives are literally at stake. I have been on both sides of this issue, having spent 7 years as a plainclothes narcotics detective. I have arrested or charged many addicts and dealers. I've never arrested a tobacco addict, nor have I ever seen one turned down for help when they develop lung cancer, whether or not they have insurance. The reasons for the difference in care between a tobacco addict and an opiate addict are stigma and money. Petty reasons to lose a life. (Gloucester Police Department, 2015, May 4)

The Facebook post drew 2.1 million supporters in less than two weeks and was met with positive acclaim from local, state, and national organizations. Less than three months later, the aptly named Gloucester Police Angel Initiative had partnered with more than 40 recovery and treatment centers and had successfully placed in treatment programs all 109 people who voluntarily presented for help at the police department (Gloucester Police Department, 2015, August 14). During that brief time, Chief Campanello and businessman John Rosenthal also launched The Police Assisted Addiction and Recovery Initiative (PAARI), which supports other local police departments as they replicate aspects of The Gloucester Police Angel Initiative. According to Chief Campanello, "We are thrilled by this momentum and are committed to assisting more people struggling with the disease of addiction" (Gloucester Police Department, 2015, August 14).

As Chief Campanello demonstrates, the knowledge we gain from analyzing and understanding the political complexities of communicating matters of health should move us to change policy. Personal stories can raise social awareness, destigmatize disease, celebrate survivors, commemorate the dead, *and* inspire or affect policy decisions (Sharf, 2001). Sharf's research on breast cancer demonstrates how survivors' biographies and narratives can work as a catalyst for reform and political motivation when the *pathos* (emotional proofs) and *ethos* (character-related proofs) giving force to these stories are effectively combined with the third form of rhetorical proof, *logos* (logic, the rational). Theorizing Practice 1.3 invites you to consider the power of shared personal stories for breaking the silence and eliminating the stigma surrounding mental illness and addiction.

Theorizing Practice 1.3
Breaking the Silence through Shared Stories

A number of social movements recognize the power of personal stories to break the silence and eliminate the stigma surrounding mental illness and addiction. Here are a few:

- *Heroes in Recovery* (http://heroesinrecovery.com/share) "aims to eliminate the social stigma that keeps individuals with addiction and mental health issues from seeking help, to share stories of recovery for the purpose of encouragement and inspiration, and to create an engaged sober community that empowers people to get involved, give back, and live healthy, active lives."

- *Project Semicolon* (http://projectsemicolon.org) "is a global faith-based non-profit movement dedicated to presenting hope and love to those who are struggling with depression, suicide, addiction, and self-injury." Originally, people were encouraged to draw a semicolon on their bodies as a symbol of continued life (just as a semicolon continues a sentence that could have ended); however, it quickly grew into something greater and more permanent. Today, people all over the world are tattooing the mark as a reminder of their struggle, victory, and survival.

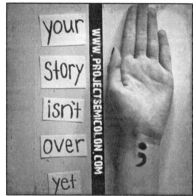

- *New Recovery Advocacy Movement* (http://manyfaces1voice.org) "shines a light on the personal and societal value of recovery through the moving stories of people who are public about what their lives are like now that they're no longer using alcohol or other drugs" in both *The Anonymous People*, a feature-length documentary, and its companion book, *Many Faces, One Voice*.

- *Addiction Obituaries* (http://nyti.ms/1Mnwdbc) are "part of a trend toward a greater degree of acceptance and de-stigmatization about issues pertaining to mental illness, including addiction." While not the result of an organized effort, a growing number of families are writing obituaries that drop euphemisms (e.g., "died unexpectedly") and instead "speak unflinchingly, with surprising candor and urgency, about the realities of addiction" by disclosing overdose as the cause of death and describing the pain, outrage, and devastation felt by survivors. These obituaries circulate widely on social media, spurring public dialogue and prompting an outpouring of messages in which strangers share similar experiences.

Peruse some of the stories on these websites and choose a few favorites. What makes them compelling? How do they appeal to credibility (ethos) and emotional response (pathos)? What rational evidence (logos) do they incorporate? Are you aware of other social movements locally, nationally, and/or internationally?

■ Linking Complexities and Shared Understandings

Hopefully, at this point in the chapter, it is apparent that personal, cultural, and political complexities operate simultaneously to shape our health beliefs and practices. Cultural conceptions of mental illness and substance use disorder perpetuate secrecy, shame, and the criminalization of addiction; however, more voices are calling for change in the way we think about, treat, and manage these disorders. These differing vantage points comprise a range of assumptions and understandings that then inform our interactions with others.

The Culturally Sensitive Model of Communicating Health (Sharf & Kahler, 1996) offers a helpful method for making sense of these perspectives. The model consists of five complex layers of meaning that participants bring to their relationships and conversations about health and illness (see Figure 1.1). Importantly, while all five layers operate simultaneously, one or more layers may predominate in conversation, and the layer that is salient at one point for one person may not be for another. A brief examination of these layers of meaning demonstrates how the model can work to explain the subtleties and complexities that underlie communication about mental illness and addiction.

The *ideological layer of meaning* comprises the core values, philosophical "truths," and ethical underpinnings of society. As you've read in this chapter, pervasive myths contribute to social and internalized stigma that frame the experiences of individuals living with mental illness and addiction at all levels of the model. When dual diagnosis is viewed as a matter of poor self-control or moral failing rather than as a chronic

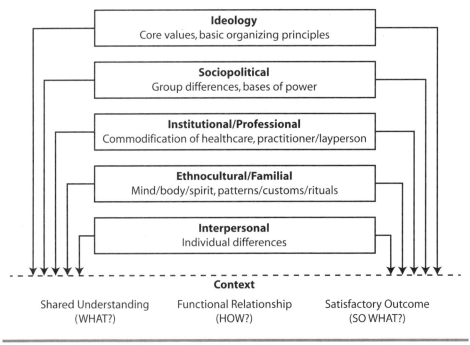

Figure 1.1   The Culturally Sensitive Model of Communicating Health

disease requiring long-term care, people are often more reluctant to seek help or to support those needing help.

The *sociopolitical layer of meaning* encompasses the politics surrounding primary social bases of power, such as race, class, age, and gender. Within these social categories, certain groups of Americans have traditionally enjoyed privileged status. Addiction conjures stereotypes of deviant individuals engaged in high-risk behaviors. In reality, however, substance use disorder affects a wide spectrum of demographic groups—young to old, poor to affluent. Heroin abuse is soaring, due primarily to its inexpensive price and widespread availability for people already addicted to prescription opiates. Indeed, four in five people today who start using heroin began their opioid addiction on prescription painkillers (Pollack, 2014), largely due to problematic prescribing practices for the treatment of chronic, non-cancer pain, such as osteoarthritis. Still, research demonstrates that racial, ethnic, and socioeconomic disparities persist in the successful treatment of substance use disorders and mental health issues (Saloner & Cook, 2013). Minorities living in poverty generally have access to fewer or lower-quality treatment options than those in predominately white communities. They also have higher dropout rates from treatment due to external environmental factors such as high social distress, weak social support, and few economic opportunities (Saloner & Cook, 2013).

The *institutional/professional layer of meaning* involves the organization of healthcare and related services, as well as professional understandings of health problems and issues. Between 2009 and 2012, states cut $5 billion in mental health services, ultimately paring away both the community services designed to keep people healthy and the hospital care needed to help them heal after a crisis (Szabo, 2014). As a result, 60% of adults with any mental illness go untreated in a given year, leading some to believe we have replaced hospital beds with jail cells, homeless shelters, and coffins (Szabo, 2014).

The *ethnocultural/familial layer of meaning* incorporates the cultural traditions, customs, rituals, and values that (1) form patterns of everyday living, expression, and social interaction, and (2) are often learned through the family. Research demonstrates that the stigma of mental illness disproportionately deters ethnic minorities, youth, men, military personnel, and perhaps surprisingly, health professionals from disclosing concerns or seeking help (Clement et al., 2015). For many families, including Elizabeth's, the stigma of mental illness compels family secrecy, silence, and shame, resulting in maladaptive coping behaviors.

The *interpersonal layer of meaning* focuses on the dynamics of style, intimacy, emotion, and roles played out in human interactions. Although we are socialized in terms of expected role behaviors (e.g., patient, doctor, addict, or officer), the styles and sensibilities of specific people filling these roles may differ (Sharf & Kahler, 1996). Chief Campanello, who you've learned views addiction as a public health crisis rather than a crime, will likely communicate very differently with an addict seeking help than other officers might.

Differences in race, ethnicity, socioeconomic status, education, age, and life experiences can create distance, lack of understanding or shared meaning, and problematic communication when we consider matters of health and illness. Chapter 2 explicitly examines the personal, cultural, and political complexities of aging in our society, and we purposefully return to these complexities again in Chapter 14. In the intervening chapters, you will see some complexities at play more than others; however, we recommend that you refer to this model and its five layers when you consider how people communicate matters of health and illness in different contexts with different results.

HCIA 1.2

Connecting Substance Use and Health with Personal Stories

Michelle Miller-Day

After the curtain came down.
The actors, the director, and I—the writer—
stand with lights shining in our faces,
talking with the audience
about HEALTH.
"Health is about more than just not being sick,"
says the middle-aged white woman, speaking with lips pink
as sorbet.
She sits clutching a program in her hand.
"It's more about being and feeling well,
energized,
with a reason to live."
"I have a healthy body," she says.
"My mind is healthy too
(most of the time)" [audience laughter]
"But this hasn't always been my life."
Grabbing chairs and crouching to sit on the edge of the stage, we collectively
Look
Listen
Ask her what her story is and has been.
Oh the power of stories!
We wrap narratives around ourselves to make sense of the world.
Laying personal accounts over others to spread our experiences,
our meanings.
Layered thickly with culture.
She looks to her left, her right,
clears her throat.
"My story is my story, I won't bother," she says.
A voice from behind interrupts.
"No," he says, voice cutting through her hesitation.
"Include us in your story."
Eyes turn to her, asking to see, and ears open to hear.
We long to see ourselves in what she has to say. Stick it in our pockets
to pull out for another day.
She looks down at her lap.
Then bravely
tells a story of her younger self who needed a shot of tequila to get to sleep one night . . .
and the next.
A larger glass with ice.
No ice.

Half a bottle.
Switch to vodka.
Soon a bottle was needed to get relief.
Other than trouble with sleep, she was "healthy" but
Not happy
Not rested
Unless drunk
In recovery for 20 years.
Only after her doctor promised
(threatened)
That if she didn't stop she would need a liver
transplant
At the age of 31.
"Now," she says, "I know what it is to feel well."
Wellness in body, mind, and spirit.
Wellness in relation to others.
Wellness not merely absence of infirmity.
"That is my story," she says, and sits.

This story is based on an event I experienced several years ago. This one woman's story touched the hearts of many in attendance that evening. I believe that by touching their hearts, her story also activated their brains, encouraging them to think about their own alcohol use, their own mind-body-spirit connection, and their own sense of wellness. People left the theatre that evening considering that health is more than "just not being sick."

My research has convinced me that when we make health decisions we tend to base our decisions on the narrative story lines available to us. Story lines we learn through listening to specific others (e.g., my Aunt Mary and her struggle with weight loss) and generalized others in ongoing cultural dialogues around issues of health and well-being (e.g., in the U.S. you can't be overweight, nor can you be too thin, you cannot eat fat, but oh! except for those good fats, did you hear about what happened to Cathy when she went on the all grapefruit diet?). Stories surround us and influence us, help us to understand the often-contradictory information we receive from a variety of sources. Narratives are particularly useful when developing health messages because they can increase engagement of less involved audiences and provide concrete examples of experience, providing audience members with possibilities.

In one recent project, my colleague and I discuss a narrative approach to designing programs to prevent adolescent alcohol, tobacco, and other drug use and abuse. This "from kids, through kids, to kids" approach to designing health messages has been very successful and relies on collecting stories of youth and then creating health promotion messages based on these stories ("from kids"). In doing so, recipients see themselves as engaged and connected in a personally relevant and meaningful way with the messages. Adolescents will then create media from those collected stories (e.g., videos, posters, radio ads, songs) to be included in the program ("through kids") and then delivered to other youth ("to kids"). To date, this prevention program titled *"keepin' it REAL"* has urban, rural, suburban, and multicultural U.S. versions, a British version, and a Nicaraguan version. This health communication program has been taken to scale and reaches nearly two million youth annually.

In the end, adolescent substance use is a tricky health issue to address. There are competing cultural stories about the use of alcohol and tobacco (by whom and at what age?), marijuana (it's harmless/harmful, medically necessary), and other substances such as those storied as "healthy alternatives" such as vaping pens (e.g., e-cigs). As the debates on these issues continue on the national stage, the power of stories can—at a minimum—reveal how the use of illicit substances affects individual lives.

(continued)

QUESTIONS TO PONDER

1. The woman in the story above used alcohol to help her sleep, but there is a current trend to mix energy drinks with alcohol to help individuals (often students) stay awake. Can you think of any stories of other students, friends, or family whose alcohol use has impacted their sleep cycles or other aspects of their health? When do you believe that alcohol use crosses over from use to abuse?

2. Watch the following video (The Journey of Quitting from Jefferson County Public Health: https://www.youtube.com/watch?v=BwLJsthrvu0). What is your emotional reaction to these stories? Which, if any, of these stories do you identify with? Why or why not? Do these stories encourage you to consider quitting tobacco if you currently use? Or to try to convince a loved one to quit? Why or why not?

3. The *keepin' it REAL* prevention program reaches nearly two million adolescents annually. Find other examples of health communication campaigns or programs being implemented to the public (outside of academia).

Source: Miller-Day, M., & Hecht, M. L. (2013). Narrative means to preventative ends: A narrative engagement framework for designing prevention interventions. *Health Communication, 28,* 657–670.

■ Health Citizenry

During her 9th year of recovery, Elizabeth took the Shatterproof Challenge and rappelled down a 26-story building in the heart of Houston. According to the Shatterproof website (http://shatterproofchallenge.org), "Addiction is a disease that shatters lives. It's time to say enough. The Shatterproof Challenge is a collection of fundraisers benefiting Shatterproof, a national organization committed to protecting children from addiction to alcohol or other drugs and ending the stigma and suffering of those affected by the disease." Before the event, Elizabeth raised funds and posted on Facebook: "It really does feel so similar to when I was faced with getting sober—having to trust that it was going to be OK, that these people know what they are doing. That I'm not going to die doing this."

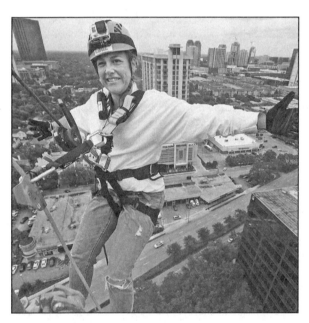

The Shatterproof Challenge illustrates Elizabeth's ongoing commitment to health activism, which we define as the wide range of behaviors

Elizabeth ready to begin the Shatterproof Challenge. (Photo courtesy of Elizabeth Lockyer.)

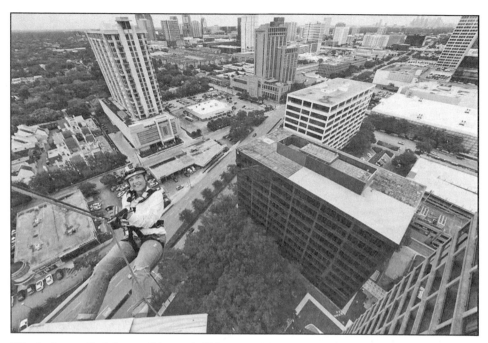

Elizabeth rappelled down a 26-story building to celebrate her sobriety and advocate for others. (Photo courtesy of Elizabeth Lockyer.)

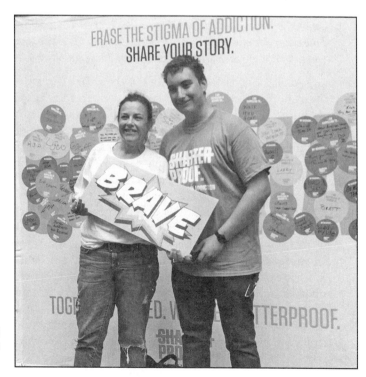

Elizabeth with her son, Boone, after completing the Shatterproof Challenge. (Photo courtesy of Elizabeth A. Lockyer and Rhys Boone Dylan Lockyer.)

people choose for becoming consciously engaged in health-related issues. As mentioned previously in this chapter, Elizabeth's early professional career included innovative, multidisciplinary drug work as a counselor, program planner, outreach director, educator—and addict. Her ever-increasing use of cannabis resin fueled constant paranoia, self-doubt, and anxiety, even while she exceeded expectations and effected community change. First, she worked directly with clients (i.e., heroin addicts) in an agency that delivered a range of open-access, treatment, and recovery services, including a telephone helpline, crisis drop-in center, street outreach, and needle exchange program. "So much of what we did was about keeping people alive and moving them toward recovery, shaping behavior, rewarding positive change, and looking for underlying causes," recalls Elizabeth. "It informs what I believe today and certainly what I created for myself in my own recovery." Then, she worked with community and governmental groups to develop and establish a drug education project that targeted youth through participatory photography, art, screenplays, and puppet shows.

Once Elizabeth was sober and no longer capable of handling her former levels of stress, her psychiatrist suggested she apply for disability. Instead, Elizabeth retrained as a peer support specialist. "So many people said, 'That's such a step down. How can you do that?' But I didn't see it that way," says Elizabeth. "It's going out in the community as someone who has mental health issues and substance abuse issues and saying, 'This is how I operate. This is how I stay stable. This is how I handle my status. And here are some suggestions for how you can function, as well. Let's work on getting to a point where you can function in the community.'"

As someone with mental health and substance use disorders, Elizabeth also learned to advocate for herself. "I had to learn how to cope with my life. I had to regain skill sets. I had to learn how to function in the world. And I had to learn how to speak to doctors," says Elizabeth. "I had to learn how to say I'm an addict. I'm an addict, and I have mental health issues. I have to out myself. I have to learn sometimes to educate physicians about what is an appropriate medication. For example, after shoulder surgery, I had to say 2 pain pills were not going to be enough. I advocated for myself and said, 'Here is what I will do to manage my medication, and here is what I've done in the past without issue, and here's a physician you can call to prove that.'"

Addict. Counselor. Educator. Director. Peer. Advocate. Elizabeth's story highlights the many identities and roles that characterize her lived experiences as a *health citizen* (Arntson, 1989; Rimal, Ratzen, Arntson, & Freimuth, 1997). When it comes to the identities that individuals assume as health communicators, the descriptive vocabulary can be quite limiting. We can be experts or professionals (i.e., providers, policy makers, researchers) who provide medical care, formulate standards of practice and rules for the receipt of care, or study the medical science and social delivery of care. Alternatively, we can be patients or health consumers—that is, the recipients of healthcare, as well as those who pay for it.

However, these identities do not speak to the much broader contexts of health communication. Elizabeth, like all of us, interacts with others in a full range of health-related activities—sometimes as a practitioner, sometimes as a patient, but always as an engaged participant (Rimal et al., 1997). We use the term *health citizen* to convey this sense of universality among all members of a society, as well as the rights, responsibilities, and privileges that accompany such participation. Our book highlights several specific kinds of *communication competencies*—combinations of knowledge and skills—aimed at helping you to become a dynamic health citizen in a number of different contexts. As you read, we encourage you to consider and strengthen the various ways in which you enact your own health citizenry.

HCIA 1.3

Seeking and Sharing Family Health Histories

Shelly R. Hovick

In 2004, the U.S. Surgeon General designated Thanksgiving Day to be National Family Health History Day. Every year on this day, families are encouraged to talk about and record their family health histories. While most people understand that family history is an important disease risk factor, research shows that many people have *not* sought family health information. Although 96% of people consider family health histories to be important to their health, fewer than 30% have actively collected this information. These findings, as well as increased evidence of the importance of family history on health, have inspired health communication research and interventions to help individuals collect and record family health history.

Despite increased health communication efforts, researchers still know little about what drives family members to seek and share health information, and whether individuals have *adequate* knowledge of their family health history. Many of us, particularly those whose disease risk is average, assume we have a good understanding of diseases that run in our family. Only in rare situations, such as a doctor visit, are we asked to provide a complete family history. As a result, we may not have a true understanding of our family history and, thus, our potential disease risk.

The idea that individuals may not have a complete understanding of their family health history motivated my own research into the factors that facilitate and deter families from seeking and sharing valuable family health information. In particular, my colleagues and I wanted to gain the perspectives of older adults, who often act as gatekeepers of family health information. Through our discussions with individuals, four unique patterns emerged in regard to the ways families may manage communication of health information. Some reported that their families communicated *openly*, freely sharing information about their family's health. As one participant shared with us, "When one is going through something, we try and support each other. We openly share information with one another." In contrast, several participants reported their family members were *noncommunicative* in regard to family health information. Noncommunication was due to concerns about privacy and gossip ("people talking") within the family, fears of burdening others, or generational norms for communication of health information. One participant said, "Older people at the time didn't really tell you—well, mine certainly didn't tell me the different things they had."

While the majority of participants told us their families openly communicated health information, some said that they communicated more *selectively*, whereby they restrict the sharing of family information to certain topics or people. Not wanting to worry others often drove participants' decisions to communicate selectively, and they communicated most often with family members with whom they were physically or emotionally close. The final pattern that emerged was *one-way* communication. Many older adults felt their communication regarding family health was often unacknowledged or unreciprocated by other family members. Participants told stories about attempts to communicate family health history to their children, who weren't interested in the information. As one participant told us, "I don't think it even gets in their ear."

While we still have much to learn concerning where these patterns of communication originate, we did find that the secrecy of prior generations in regard to health had a lasting impact on families' present-day communication, and even drove some individuals to enact different health communication behaviors with their children. Thus, a topic as seemingly simple as family history communication is complex and can be impacted by a wide variety of individual and social factors.

These studies, as well as calls from several public health agencies, suggest that health communication efforts must continue to encourage individuals to seek and share family health information. Asking individuals to record a family health history may be an effective strategy for revealing gaps in knowledge and increasing information seeking. Because family conversations about health history are not necessarily common, individuals may not realize they lack information about family health until they are asked to provide it. Several online tools have been developed by federal agencies, health departments, hospitals, and universities to help individuals collect family health information, share it with others, and even assess disease risk (including the Surgeon General's *My Family Health Portrait*). However, research is still needed to evaluate these tools and their impact on family communication, knowledge, and even disease risk perceptions. Furthermore, these tools do not necessarily address potential family communication barriers or attempt to influence patterns of communication regarding family health. Future health communication efforts must take the unique patterns of health communication within families into account, as well as individual willingness to disclose private health information. Given the increased focus on genetics and personalized medicine in healthcare, family health history continues to be vital information.

QUESTIONS TO PONDER

1. How often do you talk to your own family members about health conditions within the family? What are some of the reasons you or members of your family might be hesitant to talk about health issues?

2. What style of communication (open, closed, selective, or one-way) is most similar to the communication patterns within your own family regarding health? Why?

3. What are some potential communication strategies to encourage families like yours to maintain or increase family health history communication?

Sources: Hovick, S. R., Yamasaki, J. S., Burton-Chase, A. M., & Peterson, S. K. (2014). Patterns of family health history communication among older African American adults. *Journal of Health Communication, 20*, 80–87. Yamasaki, J., & Hovick, S. R. (2014). "That was grown folks' business": Narrative reflection and response in older adults' family health history communication. *Health Communication, 30*, 221–230.

■ Conclusion

This book features the work of uniquely qualified, highly recognized scholars who attend in various ways to the complexities, difficulties, and joys of communicating about health and illness. In the chapters that follow, we invite you to complicate your thinking as individuals who live and embody the many issues addressed in health communication scholarship. You will read about foundational health communication topics from a variety of perspectives and within a variety of contexts. As you do, you will immerse yourself in the applied work of health communication scholars, think with the stories of others, and theorize from everyday health practices. Throughout, we challenge you to think and act as informed practitioners, patients, and health citizens.

Discussion Questions

1. Have you or has someone close to you struggled with mental illness and/or substance use disorder? How does Elizabeth's story fit with your lived experiences and understandings? What, if anything, surprised you?

2. What does health mean to you? Could someone with a diagnosed disease have good health? Could someone practice unhealthy behaviors and still be healthy? Could someone seem in good health and yet be unhealthy? Explain your reasoning, including the personal, cultural, and/or political influences informing your opinions.

3. Which layer(s) of meaning in the Culturally Sensitive Model of Communicating Health do you find yourself considering most in times of health or in times of illness?

4. What other health issues signify "moral failing" rather than illness in our society? How does stigma influence behaviors and policies at personal, organizational, and societal levels? What could be done instead to make the impossible seem possible for these health issues?

5. What are some of the identities, roles, and behaviors that comprise your personal experiences as a health citizen?

NOTE

[1] Although this book is a stand-alone edition with distinct title and content, it began as a second edition to *Communicating Health: Personal, Cultural, and Political Complexities* by Patricia Geist-Martin, Eileen Berlin Ray, and Barbara F. Sharf (2003, 2011), and it emphasizes some of the same complexities and competencies. Foundational concepts from that title are included in this chapter with permission.

REFERENCES

Arntson, P. (1989). Improving citizens' health competencies. *Health Communication, 1,* 29–34.

Clement, S., Schauman, O., Graham, T., Maggioni, F., Evans-Lacko, S., Bezborodovs, N., . . . Thonicroft, G. (2015). What is the impact of mental health-related stigma on help-seeking? A systematic review of quantitative and qualitative studies. *Psychological Medicine, 45,* 11–27.

Dana, W. (2015, June 25). The war on drugs: 'A trillion-dollar failure.' Retrieved December 1, 2015, from http://www.rollingstone.com/culture/features/the-war-on-drugs-a-trillion-dollar-failure-20150625

Drug Policy Alliance (2015, August). State legislation: Overdose prevention. Retrieved September 1, 2015, from http://www.drugpolicy.org/sites/default/files/Fact_Sheet_State_based_Overdose_Prevention_Legislation_August2015.pdf

Frank, A. W. (1995). *The wounded storyteller: Body, illness, and ethics.* Chicago, IL: The University of Chicago Press.

Geertz, C. (1973). *The interpretation of culture.* New York, NY: Basic Books.

Geist-Martin, P., Ray, E. B., & Sharf, B. F. (2003). *Communicating health: Personal, cultural, and political complexities.* Belmont, CA: Wadsworth. Reprinted: (2011). Long Grove, IL: Waveland Press.

Gloucester Police Department (2015, May 4). *Gloucester police chief announces major drug policy changes* [Facebook status update]. Retrieved August 22, 2015, from https://www.facebook.com/GloucesterPoliceDepartment/posts/697808590329673

Gloucester Police Department (2015, August 14). *The Gloucester Initiative surpasses 100 participants* [Press release]. Retrieved August 22, 2015, from http://gloucesterpd.com/2015/08/14/the-gloucester-initiative-surpasses-100-participants/

Healthy People 2010 (2000). 2nd ed. Washington, DC: U.S. Department of Health and Human Services, Office of Disease Prevention and Health Promotion.

Healthy People 2020 (2010). Washington, DC: U.S. Department of Health and Human Services, Office of Disease Prevention and Health Promotion. Retrieved from www.healthypeople.gov

Huebner, B. G. (Ed.). (2011). *I remember better when I paint: Art and Alzheimer's: Opening doors, making connections.* Glen Echo, MD: Bethesda Communications Group.

Kreps, G. L., & Kunimoto, E. N. (1994). *Effective communication in multicultural healthcare settings.* Thousand Oaks, CA: Sage.

Levi, J., Segal, L. M., & Martin, A. (2015, June). *The facts hurt: A state-by-state injury prevention policy report.* Washington, DC: Trust for America's Health.

Livingston, J. D., & Boyd, J. E. (2010). Correlates and consequences of internalized stigma for people living with mental illness: A systematic review and meta-analysis. *Social Science & Medicine, 71,* 2150–2161.

March, E. (2015). *One town came up with a genius plan for dealing with drug users: Stop arresting them.* Retrieved June 18, 2015, from http://www.upworthy.com/one-town-came-up-with-a-genius-plan-for-dealing-with-drug-users-stop-arresting-them

McGinty, M. S., Webster, D. W., & Barry, C. L. (2013). Effects of news media messages about mass shootings on attitudes toward persons with serious mental illness and public support for gun control policies. *American Journal of Psychiatry, 170,* 494–501.

Morris, D. B. (1998). *Illness and culture in the postmodern age.* Berkeley: University of California Press.

National Institute on Drug Abuse. (2010, September). *Comorbidity: Addiction and other mental illnesses.* Retrieved September 20, 2015, from http://www.drugabuse.gov/publications/research-reports/comorbidity-addiction-other-mental-illnesses/letter-director

Parrott, R., & Kreuter, M. W. (2011). Multidisciplinary, interdisciplinary, and transdisciplinary approaches to health communication: Where do we draw the line? In T. L. Thompson, R. Parrott, & J. F. Nussbaum (Eds.), *The Routledge handbook of health communication* (2nd ed., pp. 3–17). New York, NY: Routledge.

Pescosolido, B. A., Martin, J. K., Long, J. S., Medina, T. R., Phelan, J. C., & Link, B. G. (2010). "A disease like any other"? A decade of change in public reactions to schizophrenia, depression, and alcohol dependence. *American Journal of Psychiatry, 167,* 1321–1330.

Pierret, J. (2003). The illness experience: State of knowledge and perspectives for research. *Sociology of Health & Illness, 25,* 4–22.

Pollack, H. (2014, February 7). *100 Americans die of drug overdoses each day. How do we stop that?* Retrieved June 18, 2015, from http://www.washingtonpost.com/news/wonkblog/wp/2014/02/07/100-americans-die-of-drug-overdoses-each-day-how-do-we-stop-that/

Porter, E. (2012, July 3). *Numbers tell of failure in drug war.* Retrieved December 1, 2015, from http://www.nytimes.com/2012/07/04/business/in-rethinking-the-war-on-drugs-start-with-the-numbers.html?_r=0

Quinn, D. M., Williams, M. K., & Weisz, B. M. (2015). From discrimination to internalized mental illness stigma: The mediating roles of anticipated discrimination and anticipated stigma. *Journal of Psychiatric Rehabilitation, 38,* 103–108.

Rimal, R. N., Ratzan, S. C., Arntson, P., & Freimuth, V. S. (1997). Reconceptualizing the "patient": Health care promotion as increasing citizens' decision-making competencies. *Health Communication, 9,* 61–74.

Saloner, B., & Cook, B. L. (2013). Blacks and Hispanics are less likely than Whites to complete addiction treatment, largely due to socioeconomic factors. *Health Affairs, 32,* 135–145.

Sharf, B. F. (2001). Out of the closet and into the legislature: The impact of communicating breast cancer narratives on health policy. *Health Affairs, 20,* 213–218.

Sharf, B. F., & Kahler, J. (1996). Victims of the franchise: A culturally sensitive model of teaching patient-doctor communication in the inner city. In E. B. Ray (Ed.), *Communication and disenfranchisement: Social health issues and implications* (pp. 95–115). Mahwah, NJ: Erlbaum.

Sharf, B. F., & Vanderford, M. L. (2003). Illness narratives and the social construction of health. In T. L. Thompson, A. Dorsey, K. I. Miller, & R. Parrott (Eds.), *The handbook of health communication* (pp. 9–34). Mahwah, NJ: Erlbaum.

Students for Sensible Drug Policy (2015, August). Good Samaritan policy reference document. Retrieved September 19, 2015, from http://ssdp.org/campaigns/call-911-good-samaritan-policies/

Substance Abuse and Mental Health Services Administration (2014). *Results from the 2013 National Survey on Drug Use and Health: Mental health findings.* NSHUH Series H-49, HHS Publication No. (SMA) 14-4887. Rockville, MD: Substance Abuse and Mental Health Services Administration.

Szabo, L. (2014, May 12). Cost of not caring: Nowhere to go. *USA Today.* Retrieved September 1, 2015, from http://www.usatoday.com/story/news/nation/2014/05/12/mental-health-system-crisis/7746535/

United States Department of Justice, Federal Bureau of Investigation (2014, November). *Crime in the United States, 2013.* Retrieved June 18, 2015, from https://www.fbi.gov/about-us/cjis/ucr/crime-in-the-u.s/2013/crime-in-the-u.s.-2013/cius-home

Vanderford, M. L., Jenks, E. B., & Sharf, B. F. (1997). Exploring patients' experiences as a primary source of meaning. *Health Communication 9,* 13–26.

2

Communicating Health through Narratives

Barbara F. Sharf

*Hilda is a 5'1", petite, well-dressed, silver-haired 91-year-old. Six years ago she went through knee replacement surgery, and endured a long, difficult recovery. She certainly wasn't planning on repeating the experience, but over the past year she had been having increasing periods of intractable pain in the opposite knee. After finally making an appointment with the orthopedic surgeon who performed the first operation, she encountered great reluctance on his part to repeat the procedure because of her age. Having considered her alternatives, which she concluded meant constant pain, little sleep, and needing to walk with a cane or even being confined to a wheelchair, she confronted the surgeon's resistance. "Doctor, it was a beautiful day on Sunday, and my husband suggested we go for a walk, but I was unable to move. I understand the risks involved, but I want to enjoy the life I have left to me, and I **don't** want to be relegated to a wheelchair. Yes, I'm 91, but I am not just a number. I've been through this before, I have a positive attitude going into this, and I believe it will turn out well." Following this conversation and an in-depth examination of Hilda's MRI, confirming severe bone-on-bone arthritis, the surgeon relented and agreed to do the surgery.*

Increased risks of surgical complications, hospital-generated infection, and more difficulties with rehabilitation for a person in their ninth decade is a statistical reality that physicians must consider. That such risks are worth taking in order to maintain one's quality of life is a matter of individual assessment and personal choice. The recounting of this incident brings to mind several issues related to how people age in the U.S. These may include social theories about the preference for aging in place with personal independence and dignity; ethical guidelines about the importance of autonomy in medical decision making; and political considerations about the cost of healthcare and the ways in which cost is measured. For instance, would the charges for this surgery and rehabilitation amount to less than the financial and psychological expenditures for disability and pain control?

Hilda's vignette is a brief story about health and aging that highlights a specific patient–physician interaction while simultaneously invoking social, cultural, and political conceptions, meanings, and attitudes about aging in the U.S. Using well-being in the context of aging as an illustrative focus, my intent with this chapter is to explain what the importance of narratives is to the study of health communication and why we decided to take a narrative approach. This examination entails a continuation of the personal story begun in this introduction, while simultaneously including broader narratives from the American context that exemplify cultural and political complexities and, in turn, have bearing on both social policy and individual lives.

■ The Meaning(s) of Aging

"Age is just a number." "You're only as old as you feel." "50 is the new 35." All these common aphorisms are ways of saying that age is a personal state of mind, that mere chronology is not a determinant. As the Baby Boomer generation who embraced the rebellious prescriptive to "never trust anyone over 30" in the 1960s now advances into their 50s, 60s, and 70s, this cohort leads a demographic trend toward the "graying" of America, equating to 10,000 people a day reaching the age of 65. The cultural impact of the Boomers can be seen in the plethora of movie action heroes, like Liam Neeson, Bruce Willis, Sylvester Stallone, Pierce Brosnan, and Denzel Washington, all in their 60s. Similarly, cosmetic and apparel companies, and magazines, have acquired senior models and spokeswomen such as actresses Helen Mirren, Jessica Lange, Anjelica Huston, and Jane Fonda (Simon & Jaffe, 2015). By 2029, more than 20% of the U.S. population will be over 65, and even as the "Boomer" demographic starts to diminish through mortality, the growing aging trend will continue into the next generation. Thus, by 2056, the population age 65 and older will outnumber the segment under 18 (so, dear readers, eventually this evolution will include you and those close to you, as well!) (Colby & Ortman, 2014).

Given these numbers, questions of how to "do" aging well are increasingly discussed (Poo & Conrad, 2015). But aging is not only a matter of personal will and self-perception. It would be sheer denial to fail to recognize the material reality of physiological and mental changes, including decline of some bodily organs and functions, as people get older. As a former student was able to joke when both her parents were diagnosed with cancer soon after their 60th birthdays, "their warranties expired."[1] In addition to somatic changes, self-perceptions interact with cultural characterizations, social labeling, and institutional regulations (Yamasaki, 2014). Thus, a 65-year-old person may not regard herself as elderly, but rather as a vibrant, active individual. Even so, she may still be required to use Medicare for health insurance or choose to purchase a senior bus pass to save money. Alternatively, as Yamasaki (2014) describes in an analysis of a contestant on the popular reality show *The Biggest Loser*, a 49-year-old woman, ironically named Liz Young, chose to portray herself repeatedly as a "Southern grandmother of nine." Though she had the distinction of being the oldest female to make it to the "final four" competition, other contestants several years her senior had competed on the show. To get to this point in the competition, Young persevered through several challenges with a considerable amount of weight loss. Yet rather than embodying a revitalized, affirming persona, she chose to continue a lackluster self-characterization, stating the show was her "last chance" since she likely had only "a good twenty years left."

The television audience strongly responded very negatively to what was perceived as her unseemly, premature embracing of age as defeatism. Furthermore, viewers argued strenuously with Young's portrayal of aging through self-description and appearance, providing many counterexamples of people with more chronological years but much younger, forward-thinking spirits. At the same time, she was also perceived as behaving immaturely in certain, annoying ways. The bottom line is that this public performance of advancing age, equated with a primary self-identification of "grandma,"[2] was perceived as inconsistent with people's contemporary understanding and personal experiences of what it means to be 49 and to experience *healthy* aging. Though these are not necessarily typical, consider the contrast of Liz Young's depiction of aging at 49 with such public images as the fit vivaciousness of Michelle Obama at age 50, the vitality and wisdom of Pope Francis at 78, and even—or especially—the beauty and activity of comedienne Betty White at 93! How one looks, feels, and personifies age is certainly individual and subjective, but the biology of increased longevity and cultural role modeling shape popular expectations of what it now means to get older. How those meanings of age are communicated results in stories that help instill and promulgate ideas about well-being and decline, autonomy and protectionism.

Now, take a moment to assess some of your own responses to perceptions of aging.

Theorizing Practice 2.1
Adapting Communication to Age

Communication scholars have long recognized that people rely on age-related stereotypes when meeting and interacting with people of different generations. Visual cues, interpersonal context, and prior (or lack of prior) experiences call forth expectations of age that influence the resulting communication. Initial messages based on these perceptions may be (1) *affirming* (i.e., normal adult-to-adult talk), (2) *overly nurturing* (i.e., patronizing in infantilizing ways, such as baby talk), or (3) *directive* (i.e., patronizing in cold and controlling ways). Ideally, people of all ages will strive for intergenerational communication through a person-centered rather than category-based approach in which both partners consider one another's individual characteristics, engage in appropriate adaptations, and reassess the interaction as it progresses (Hummert, Garstka, Ryan, & Bonnesen, 2004).

- Who are the two or three oldest people you know? What ages are they? How do you know or estimate age? Now choose which of these individuals you are closest with in order to answer the following questions: How frequently do you talk with this person? Under what circumstances? Which of the following modes of communication do you use for these conversations: face-to-face on site, telephone, written letters, emails, text messages, face-to-face via Skype or other digital programs, or social media sites like Facebook, Instagram, or Twitter?

- In what ways are you mindful of adapting your communication with this person? For example, are there certain topics that you stay away from? Are you mindful of what language you use and what kind of humor you think is appropriate?

- Are there other ways in which your interactions with this person are distinctive? How so? To what degree, if any, do you think these choices are related to age, specifically the age of the other person, and/or differences in age between the two of you? Conversely, in what ways is age not an important factor?

■ The Essential Nature of Health and Illness Narratives

While the concept of "narrative" was at one time the province of literary scholars and other academics, it now is frequently included in ordinary discourse and has become embedded in everyday situations. We noted a pivotal example during the period of time in which this chapter was being written, as political pundits discussed the distressing phenomenon of disaffected youth throughout Westernized countries being recruited to ISIS (Islamic State), the violent extremist militant organization. Described by one commentator as "the most critical communication problem of our time," an army general on another news program portrayed the situation as a battle in which the U.S. and its allies need to create a better narrative using social media to counter the apparently wildly successful narrative being put forth by ISIS. To hear a military expert discussing international warfare in terms of dueling narratives demonstrates the pervasiveness—and importance—of this word and the ideas it represents.

The Narrative Turn

Though narrative has always existed as an essential literary form in the humanities, it can be argued that the more recent popularization of the term had its roots in the "narrative turn" that occurred throughout the social sciences in the 1960s and '70s (Polkinghorne, 1988) when scholars from diverse disciplines argued for recognizing story creation as the basis for human understanding. In communication studies, it was asserted that to conceptualize and articulate experience in story form is an innate human capacity such that narrative constitutes a paradigm or significant mode of thought that encompasses most human communication (technical discourse being an exception) (Fisher, 1987). Concurrently, narrative also became a focus for humanistic medicine as a novel and insightful way of understanding clinically-related communication including "stories of sickness" (Brody, 2003), "illness narratives" (Kleinman, 1988), "doctors' stories" (Hunter, 1991), medical records (Poirier et al., 1992), physician-patient communication (Sharf, 1990), and family response to serious illness (Anderson & Geist-Martin, 2003). In both communication and medicine, as well as in education and many of the social sciences, narrative inquiry, "the systematic study of narrative data," (Riessman, 2008, p. 6) became a viable form of interpretive scholarship alternative to the standard positivistic, measurement-driven approach to investigating and conceptualizing issues related to interpersonal and organizational discourse (Bochner, 2014; Charon, 2008; Harter & Bochner, 2009).

Story Elements

In simplest terms, a narrative is a story. Stories are one of the earliest and most favored forms of communication, enriching the development of individual lives from childhood through adulthood and old age. Stories are also ubiquitous in every faith tradition, culture, and nation-state, providing familiar touch points for its adherents/citizens that can be unifying or divisive. They are the means through which we record history and memories, and derive shared values. Thus, understanding communication as narrative entails focusing on such familiar story elements as

- *characters*, the people or beings that enact the events of the story;
- *motives*, the thoughts, emotions, and circumstances that impel characters to make certain choices and take particular actions;

- *plots or dramas*, how key events and characters' actions are configured in relation to one another, typically resulting in tensions or conflicts that need to be resolved in some way;
- *scenes*, the locale and surroundings in which events transpire;
- *time or chronology*, the sequence in which the plot is revealed, as well as the temporal (past, present, or future) orientation of the characters;
- *perspective*, the voice and viewpoint of the narrator and other characters;
- *morals and life lessons*, the value-laden implications and consequences of how the plot is resolved.

It's also important to realize that these internal story elements are inevitably colored by the style, context, and circumstances in which the story is told or re-told.

Narrative Functions

In fact, whenever we tell a story that explains what has occurred or what we hope will happen, that illustrates a point of view or exemplifies the kind of person we are or want to be, we are putting narrative to use. While narrative is an integral aspect of communication in all contexts, it has a special salience for communication in health-related situations. Stories are often generated in response to a rupture or turning point in the course of a person's life (Bruner, 1990). Because threats to people's health can be life changing and even life threatening, illness narratives that contribute to understanding and articulating the meanings of illness both for the teller and listeners may serve several important functions.

Personal stories provide a way of *sensemaking* in uncertain or chaotic circumstances, such as a serious diagnosis or health risk. Narratives *provide implicit explanations* to account for causation, remedy, and outcomes of health problems; *infer warrants or reasons for decisions* made; and *enable a sense of control* in the face of threat and disorder. They can help a great deal in the face of life-changing circumstances to enact transformations in *personal identity* in terms of how individuals view themselves and are perceived by others. Furthermore, narratives can help create identification among people experiencing similar problems, thus building a *sense of community* in place of social isolation (Sharf & Vanderford, 2003). Several narrative theorists have underscored the importance of stories as a form of *witnessing individual and community suffering and trauma* (Frank, 1995; Kleinman, 1988). To the extent that health professionals have been trained to listen to and acknowledge illness narratives as testimonials to suffering, such storytelling and story listening helps to *humanize the practice of medicine* (Charon, 2008; Sharf, Harter, Yamasaki, & Haidet, 2011). Finally, creating and sharing narratives may *result in beneficial physical and psychological health outcomes* (Pennebaker, 2000).

Illness Narrative Types

In the course of a person's experience of living with illness, interactions with health professionals often comprise only an infrequent, at times minor, part. The degree to which illness pervades a life or recedes into the background is often not a matter of choice, and thus illness, disability, changes in body image, and efforts to heal all may become an integral feature of that individual's personal narratives (Frank,

2002). Sociologist Arthur Frank (1995) presented a narrative typology based on his study of writings of people with life-threatening conditions, whom he called "wounded storytellers." His categories of *restitution* (stories of striving to return to pre-illness "normality"), *chaos* (stories of disorder and lack of control brought on by diagnosis, onset, and recurrence of illness), and *quest* (stories of searching for the deeper existential significance of undergoing illness and suffering) have proven a useful framework for the work of many fellow scholars. Such personal stories often include plotlines focused on family and partner relationships, struggles with an individual's own body, internal and social identity transformations, and confronting mortality. Still, these particular story types may not be applicable for all illness situations, such as living with chronic but less serious ailments, nor do they readily account for types of stories that may commemorate or celebrate recovery or continuation of good health and well-being.

Narrative Scholarship

Communication scholars have broad interests in health-related narrative phenomena in a wide variety of contexts and formats. Health, of course, entails components of recovery and healing, prevention, and well-being at many levels. Health narrative studies span an incredible range. Ways in which individuals and communities heal from violence and trauma; health and disability in the workplace; coping with the reactions of others to health impairments; dealing with impending death and grief; popular media depictions of illness; cross-cultural understandings of health risks and remedies; healthcare team interactions; formulating community health problems and resources are all examples of the many issues that have been examined (see, for example, Ellingson, 2004; Geist-Martin, Ray, & Sharf, 2011; Harter & Assoc., 2013; Harter, Japp, & Beck, 2005). At this juncture, Theorizing Practice 2.2 asks you to start applying some of this information about illness narratives to a specific example. Let's see what you've learned so far!

Theorizing Practice 2.2
Narrative Analysis

Professor Eileen Berlin Ray from Cleveland State University has been a productive health communication scholar for the past 30 years. Recently, she has had to contend with a serious personal health problem that has affected all aspects of her professional and family life. In the brief excerpt that follows, Dr. Ray narrates some pertinent recollections of changes she's experienced as a professor. After reading her story, formulate your response to the following questions:

- What are the main story elements that characterize her recollections?
- Which functions do you think this brief narrative may serve (and for whom)?
- Using Frank's typology of illness narratives, how would you classify this story, and why?

Transitioning to a New Normal

I've been a college professor for over 30 years. I have always been someone who walks fast, talks fast, thinks quickly on my feet, and is known for my humor. This carries over into my classes. I facilitate discussion, sit, stand, move around, write on the board. My classes were known for high energy, high movement, and high interaction.

In the fall of 2009, I noticed a couple of changes. One was with my walking. Sometimes it was hard to control my movement and my gait appeared spastic. The other was with my hands and fine motor movement. Sometimes things would slip from my fingers, like chalk when I was writing on the board or a bottle of water. Once or twice I fell for no apparent reason. I mentioned it to my husband, who suggested I see my doctor. I didn't. Denial is powerful.

Then, at a professional conference that November, things got worse. While walking to a restaurant with friends, I couldn't control my walking. I kept banging into my friends and lamp posts. I couldn't deny it any longer.

The diagnosis was cervical myelopathy. Essentially bone spurs were strangling my spinal cord. It was progressive. Surgery was imperative. Without it, I would end up flat on my back. The goal was to stop the progression of symptoms. That was the definition of success. There was no way to know what or how much, if any, functioning I would get back. The surgery involved making a wedge between my spinal cord and 7 cervical vertebrae. Every day I was losing more functioning. Surgery was scheduled for January.

After taking spring semester and the summer off to recover, it was time to return to my full schedule in the fall. The good news was my symptoms were not progressing. The not-so-good news was I hadn't gotten much functioning back. I was teaching the same classes I always taught. But now I walked into the classroom slowly behind my new companion, a red walker. I felt like it was the most conspicuous thing in the room. I felt very old. I was sure students were wondering what was up with this disabled, old prof. They may have been wondering if I was recovering from something and if my walker was temporary. I had no way to know. What I did know was that in the months off since the surgery, I had lost my professional sea legs. I felt vulnerable, uncertain, nervous, and tired. It was very hard to focus and took me four times longer to do everything from getting ready in the morning to prepping my classes. My energy level was low, and I was angry at my forced dependence on my husband and friends. For the semester, my goal was modest, to just get through my classes.

I did make it through. I wasn't happy about my classes. I knew what I could have been giving my students and what they were missing. But much to my surprise, my teaching evals were good and no one mentioned the walker or my disability. Were they just being polite? Politically correct?

In the four years since I returned to the classroom, some things have changed. While I still use the walker, I park it at the front of the room and ignore it. Early in the semester, I tell my students what happened (especially relevant in my health communication class) and answer questions. I cannot walk steadily, so I ask students to hand out and collect papers for me. I have to alternate between sitting on a table and standing, and I tell my students about my condition the first day and ask them to signal me when I've sat or stood for more than 15 minutes. I tease them if they forget (which isn't often), and they seem protective of me.

Some days my walking is better than others, but my walker or a cane is always nearby just in case. Some days I can write legibly and type; other days not so much. It's unpredictable. So far the surgery has been a success. The best news is that I haven't gotten worse. I can't say I've fully accepted my new normal. I keep trying to do what I used to do and get very frustrated when my body won't let me. What I have found is that 99% of the time people are more than happy to help. Addressing my disability up front makes me feel more comfortable, and teaching has been a lifesaver.

(continued)

What means the most to me, however, is that when I hear students asking others who I am, I hear words like "curly hair" and "short." When I hear students asking others about my classes, I hear words like "really interesting," "relevant," and "she's very funny." I don't hear, "She's the one with the walker." Maybe they do say it, but if so, it's not the first thing out of their mouths. And that makes me very happy.

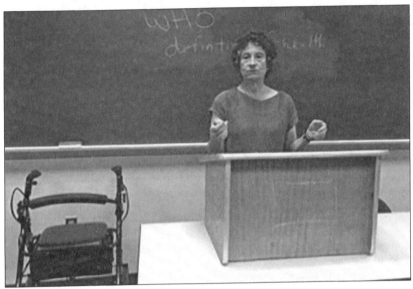

Parking the walker, while teaching. (Courtesy of Eileen Berlin Ray, personal collection.)

■ From Illness to Well-Being

Because good health is frequently taken for granted and less dramatic than serious illness, stories that depict well-being are less common and tend to be not as recognized or memorable as those about serious illness and disability. Furthermore, what constitutes well-being is an expansive, changeable, and relative concept, especially in the context of aging. Can a person with symptoms of reduced vision, hearing and/or mobility, heart disease, or advanced diabetes or arthritis be in a state of well-being? Sociologist Kathy Charmaz (1991) describes in detail how everyone who suffers from a chronic illness has "good days, bad days" that inevitably include struggles and life losses, as well as physical and existential kinds of suffering. In large part, it is in how individuals construct their life stories that it becomes apparent whether they are maintaining a state of comparative well-being, some people more than others, some times better than others. Related to this point, in her ethnographic studies of everyday life, nursing care, and relationships in assisted living communities, Yamasaki (2013) points out the power of communicating, encouraging, and honoring narratives that "celebrate the unique personhood and biographical continuity of each [resident]" (p. 122), even when those people have compromised physical and mental capacities. In other words, eliciting and listening to individuals' stories about the details of their lives, accomplishments, and cherished memories is essential to preserving who they are as valued human beings versus lumping seniors together in homogenous, depersonalized, and frequently negative categorizations, such as references to senility and diminished capacities or derogatory allusions to "old geezers" and "blue hairs." In fact, the preservation of personal identity through storied portrayals may be an essential coping strategy for surviving and even thriving in a long-term care situation (Yamasaki & Sharf, 2011). But what is the impact when "the truths" of personal narratives bump up against prevalent meanings conveyed in dominant cultural narratives repeated through public media, private conversations, and other means? As we continue the personal narrative of Hilda, the woman introduced at the start of this chapter, and her husband, Gene, we examine broader social meanings of well-being in the context of advancing age.

◼ Cultural Narratives about Aging

From their spacious, seventh-floor condominium, Hilda and Gene can look out over leafy Philadelphia Main Line suburban streets from the balcony. They often take the #44 bus that stops a block from their condo building to travel to center-city, or Gene drives his Hyundai Sonata to shop at the local supermarket and take Hilda to the hair salon. The couple sometimes enjoys musical concerts, frequently attends local films and theatre performances, and even occasionally will travel to New York City to see a Broadway play. Typically once a week, they have dinner out at their favorite Chinese restaurant or one of the other neighborhood eateries. Other nights, they have simply prepared, healthy meals at home, or get together with friends. They take walks in the nearby city park or use the equipment in the condo exercise room. In short, they are living the fortunate, seemingly unremarkable life of urban, middle-class American retirees.

Beneath these surface images, the couple represents a more interesting phenomenon. As mentioned earlier, Hilda had her 91st birthday this year, and Gene will be celebrating his 95th. Hilda, a former legal secretary, and Gene, a pharmacist by profession, remained employed until well into their seventies. The couple does their own housekeeping, are quite capable of getting around, and are mentally sharp with excellent memories. They do have regular visits to various doctors and occasional serious health problems that arise. In the past two years, Hilda suffered a compression fracture in her spine as a result of a fall, and, more recently, underwent a second knee replacement, and had a growth removed from inside her mouth. Other than occasional dental problems, Gene has been remarkably healthy. His one major medical crisis occurred at age 79. This was a sudden, serious bout of diverticulitis, a very painful intestinal inflammation that required major surgery, which was followed by a life-threatening postsurgical infection that he fortunately survived. This period of illness forced his retirement from more than 50 years of working long hours as a pharmacist in a variety of professional settings that included owning his own neighborhood pharmacy as a younger man to his last position managing a methadone clinic for addicted veterans at the local VA hospital.

To his family's surprise and pleasure, Gene has displayed unknown talents and interests in his post-retirement activities. He taught himself the craft of making stained glass windows, creating beautiful, original designs.

Though he first used a computer at work, at home he emails and has a Facebook page, as well as accounts on both LinkedIn and Twitter. He's written several brief essays that recall his experiences growing up in Philadelphia and as a Bronze Star-awarded medic and infantry sol-

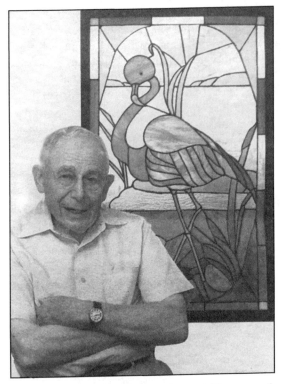

Gene featured with his stained glass art. (Courtesy of Philadelphia Corporation for Aging; Originally published in *Milestones* newsletter, January 2008.)

dier in *World War II. Along with his 92-year-old brother, Irv, he was interviewed on the local public radio station to discuss their impressions of how their home city of Philadelphia has changed over the course of many decades. Most recently, he wrote the "saga" of his extended family, declining a gift subscription to Ancestry.com, and instead working entirely from his own memory and knowledge dating back two generations prior to his own and encompassing subsequent generations into the present. This work was honored with an extended family celebration by the relatives who live in the area.*

A weekly highlight for Gene, Hilda, and Irv is attendance at a community center about a 30-minute drive away from their neighborhood for a meeting of a group called REAP (Retired Executives and Professionals). Comprised of some 90 members, aged 60 through mid-90s, with backgrounds in healthcare, business, engineering, education, the arts, and other professions, this group combines friendly social interaction with a regular schedule of presentations. Members commit to being presenters on an annual basis (in reality, some may not be a speaker every year, while others may give more than one talk) with the caveat that the topics of their presentations must be something different than what they'd done or studied in their professional careers. These talks require quite a bit of individual research and effort to create interest across an eclectic audience, including the use of sophisticated electronic media.

"I look forward to hearing about different topics each week," states Gene. "While not every talk is of A-1 quality, many are." As an example, he recalls one woman's history of rival worldwide manufacturers of musical cymbals, a competition between two brothers separated by a family dispute. Gene continues, "Just this week, the presenter 'impersonated' the artist, Frida Kahlo, talking about her 'husband,' the Mexican painter Diego Rivera. This speaker is so good, she's been invited to give this presentation to several other audiences."

Hilda has spoken about famed Washington Post *publisher Katherine Graham. Gene, a lover of history and the arts, has given biographical presentations that have included industrialist/adventurer Howard Hughes, artists Norman Rockwell and Marc Chagall, and several early and mid-20th-century popular composers such as Oscar Hammerstein. In the process of preparing his talks, Gene taught himself how to create PowerPoint slides, as well as to incorporate music in conjunction with the visuals. He muses, "I think one of my most successful talks was one I gave on Jerome Kern, the composer of the musical* Show Boat. *I incorporated 20 of his best-known songs, like 'Old Man River.' Several people came to tell me later how much they enjoyed hearing about that music."*

REAP members also organize annual group outings to visit neighboring regional destinations with interesting museums, historical sites, and other cultural events. In addition, there are separate meetings of subgroups with specific shared interests, such as the Songbirds, a choral group in which Gene participates. "You get to know people very well. This summer [while regular REAP meetings are on hiatus], a woman who has a music room at her house has invited the Songbirds to get together to rehearse."

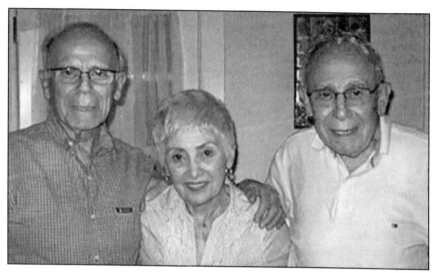

Irv, Hilda, and Gene. (Courtesy of Barbara Sharf, personal collection.)

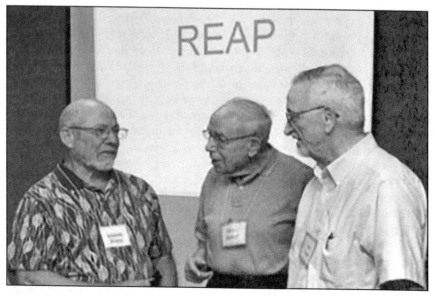

Lively discussion at a REAP meeting. (Courtesy of Irving Sharf, personal collection.)

This narrative offers a partial portrayal of Gene, depicting a plotline of relatively good health and well-being for a man in his ninth decade. He continues to live a fulfilling life that incorporates literary and artistic accomplishments beyond the expertise developed through a lengthy professional career, a happy marriage, and active social interaction, as well as a willingness to learn new technical skills and engage with contemporary social media. Perhaps most notably in this rendition, Gene is a main character or protagonist whose perspective blends long, detailed memories—of family, hometown, history, music, and art—with modern modes of living and communication. It is a depiction of longevity, well-being, and self-fulfillment. There is no inherent rupture or tension that is evident. However, an alert observer might point out that a rupture occurs for the reader because this personal story contrasts strongly with the predominant cultural narrative of advanced old age as synonymous with disease, decline, and disability.

Literary scholar and cultural commentator David Morris (1998) asserts that aging bodies are continuously inscribed and reinscribed—that is to say, symbolically marked and molded—with cultural meanings, including "cruel stereotypes of old age" (p. 235) in part based on the alarming acceleration of seniors suffering from Alzheimer's disease. Perhaps the epitome of this negative portrait of growing old was recently characterized in a controversial essay published in *The Atlantic* by well-known physician, bioethicist, and health policy contributor Ezekiel J. Emanuel (2014). Emanuel, aged 57, proclaimed "why I hope to die at 75," based on his belief that by that age, he will already have lived a full life. He argues that by age 75, creativity and productivity have been biologically curtailed for most people, and that his personal wish is to be remembered by his loved ones as a vital, independent individual, rather than as a disabled or poorly functioning person who necessarily becomes a family burden. Though Americans have extended life expectancy, he contends they are more likely to be incapacitated through aging; in other words, better *quality* of life doesn't extend. He makes clear that he is not advocating active euthanasia or assisted suicide. Rather, he has a clear plan in mind for himself that he will no longer submit to vaccinations and tests for early detection of health problems, undergo treatment for major diseases like cancer, or even take antibiotics for more routine infections. He asks "whether our consumption is worth our contribution." Emanuel's bleak but precisely clear depiction of his own wishes portrays old age, or at least years beyond age 75, as life on a downhill slope that impedes the available resources and quality of existence for younger generations.

Though perhaps blunter and more adamant in his description, Emanuel's general perspective about old age is widely held; that is, old age is to be avoided as much as possible. Morris (1998) observes that aging in the U.S. has acquired an attitude of "postmodern timelessness" (p. 236), referring to considerable efforts to mask the appearance of age (prime examples include cosmetic surgeries, as well as skin and hair treatments), as well as the desire to appear "healthy, sexually active, engaged, productive, and self reliant" (Cole, 1992, p. 229) for as long as possible. To the degree that these ideas dominate social thinking about the meaning of aging, they constitute a *master narrative*, an account that underlies, reflects, and perpetuates mainstream cultural values and assumptions about the way the world functions (Sharf et al., 2011). *Counter narratives* are stories that engender ways of thinking and worldviews that vary from or directly disagree with the dominant ideas embodied within the master narrative.

HCIA 2.1

A Wicked Spin on Aging

Stephanie M. Ruhl

"Getting out of an old story requires telling a new one," writes sociologist Arthur Frank. The old story I had been living within was focused on the frustrations that often accompany the process of aging (i.e., physical limitations, diminishing social circles, illness). My weekends had been spent fully immersed within the physical and cognitive decline that filled the spaces of a full-time geriatric healthcare facility. My grandfather was a resident, living with an advanced Alzheimer's diagnosis. My world was narrowly fixated on aging and illness as deterioration and decline. Medical narratives and deficit perspectives continually threatened to overwhelm the good that was still a part of my grandfather's story. The energies I had so desperately devoted to pursuing creative, innovative approaches of caring now were attempting to run on the fumes of an empty tank once full of hope.

My grandfather died, as to be expected by his diagnosis, leaving a tremendous void in my life. As truly painful as the experience was—still is—I stumbled upon another story that begged to be told. This story spoke truth of the realities of growing older, but it did so in a manner that refused to be defined or confined by the inherent changes that comprise the life course. Only four and a half months before Grandpa's body ultimately failed him and my family had to begin preparing for his funeral, I was introduced to a unique community of senior citizens who actively challenged my perceptions of aging. Chair volleyball, a hot and competitive sport popular among senior citizens in Southeast Ohio, became my favorite new pastime.

In May 2011, I entered a gymnasium where 12 senior citizen chair volleyball teams, comprised of individuals ages 60 to more than 100 years old, eagerly gathered to see their placement in the state tournament bracket. Edward, the tournament director, who was dressed as the ultimate referee with a whistle around his neck and stopwatch in hand, read the rules to team captains and volunteers, sternly emphasizing the "one-cheek rule," indicating that one cheek must remain on the chair at all times, the yellow and red card rulings for coaches/spectators/players, and no spiking from the front row. I found these quite excessive at first, and then absolutely necessary once the first game was underway.

Virgil, known for his wicked spin of the ball that opposing teams could not return, played front-center position and stubbornly refused to let the no-spiking rule compromise his competitive game. Players passionately raised their voices when I made mistakes in scorekeeping duties—one sarcastically yelled, "What game are you watching?" They mocked my protective instincts, gasps, and rescue attempts to save senior citizens from falling off of their chairs, assuring me, "It's all a part of the game." I was thrust into the lively, energetic world of chair volleyball. It was an unexpected whirlwind of laughter, fun, exercise, and competition in the midst of white and graying hair, tight perms and balding heads, wheelchairs and walkers, wrinkled skin, wide smiles, and oversized brightly colored team T-shirts accessorized with matching jewelry, bright lipstick, and suspenders.

I quickly realized that chair volleyball puts its own wicked spin on the experience of aging. Even as bodies and minds age, experience illnesses, recover from surgeries, and confront declining physical abilities, players participate on the court to their fullest ability. They laugh, tease, remain unbelievably competitive, and poke fun at their old age by attributing mistakes to "senior moments" and slowing reflexes. This sport, or perhaps more specifically the inclusive spaces characterized by a wide spectrum of ranging abilities, invites those living with the corporeal aspects of growing old—chronic illness, weakened physical capaci-

(continued)

ties, loneliness—to collectively perform a story that challenges the dominant narrative of aging as decline. These individuals enjoy active lifestyles, edifying relationships, and social engagement in an environment they describe as "fun, fun, fun." Although embedded within a society that too often excludes and marginalizes senior citizens, these players empowered themselves to reconstruct the experience of aging in fulfilling ways. Each time they take their seats on the court, with every volley of the multicolored beach ball, they make powerful statements to themselves and all who witness—they are still living, still contributing, still a meaningful and important part of something good.

QUESTIONS TO PONDER

1. How have you witnessed society excluding or marginalizing senior citizens?
2. What creative activities can you envision that might promote positive social experiences for aging individuals?
3. In what ways might society at large benefit from constructing more inclusive spaces in which multi- and inter-generational interactions are encouraged? What would it take to make this a reality?

Source: Ruhl, S. M. (2013). Dialogic moments and a wicked spin on aging. *Health Communication, 28,* 853–855.

All cultural stories related to aging agree on the importance of quality of life. The plotline of the cultural counter narrative doesn't escape, avoid, or disguise the aging process but attempts to improve upon it. A lengthy essay in the same issue of *The Atlantic* as Emanuel's opinion piece asks, "What happens when we all live to 100?" (Easterbrook, 2014), referring to a trend stretched over nearly two centuries of human life expectancy steadily increasing three months a year, the so-called "escalator effect." From a number of vantage points, the focus of science and medicine is now on increasing the *"health span,"* in lieu of only increasing the life span (Easterbrook, 2014). This change includes taking the emphasis away from trying to cure or eliminate particular diseases toward redirecting scientific efforts to slow the aging process at the cellular or genetic levels, which indirectly will ward off the development of certain diseases (Easterbrook, 2014; Gifford, 2015). From a public health perspective, "muscle wasting with age is the second leading cause of nursing home admissions after Alzheimer's disease" so that "sitting is [now] the new smoking" (Davies, 2015), meaning that inactivity is currently regarded as a major life-shortening health risk. There has also been great interest in identifying the global "blue zones," those places throughout the world where significant numbers of people live extraordinarily long lives with a high quality of functioning. These zones then are being examined to understand how the local diets and lifestyles, particularly the notion of "living with purpose," contribute to the well-being of their citizens (Buettner, 2015).

Another important aspect of the master cultural narrative of aging has to do with care and housing for the very frail or ill elderly who can no longer live on their own. Continuing care communities that include independent apartments, assisted living units, full-time nursing care, and specialized care for dementia, and allow for mobility of residents among these units, as needed, is an excellent concept. However, in practice well-understood, agreed-upon, and enforceable standards of caregiving, safety and facility requirements, and sufficient, appropriately trained staffing provided for residents often falls alarmingly short (Hawes, 2013; Hawes, Phillips, & Rose, 2000). While skilled nursing care and better regulated assisted living facilities will continue to be needed and necessarily improved, the counter narrative emphasizes ways of *aging in place*, meaning individuals growing older in their own homes and not having to move elsewhere. This vision includes housing designed for easier interior access and mobility; an emphasis on communities that may incorporate collective financing for mobile home healthcare, shared recreational amenities, availability of continuing education; and municipal integration of citizens of all ages through public transportation (both walkable and mass transit options) and thoughtfully designed activities and facilities (*Partners for Livable Communities*, 2009). To counter the considerable problem of malnourished seniors who can no longer shop for and prepare their own meals, there is even a fledgling business of "drop in" chefs who will bring ingredients to an individual's home and prepare a week's meals for a moderate cost (Jaffe, 2015).

The personal story of Gene and Hilda is a positive contrast to the master narrative of decline, dependence, and disability, but not exactly a fit with the counter narrative of new emphases and directions. They, like many of their fellow members of REAP, have developed their own pathway to comparatively good health and well-being, likely aided by fortunate genetics, as well as education and socioeconomic status. Now take a few minutes to reflect about how your own personal life story coexists in relation to master cultural narratives.

Theorizing Practice 2.3
Accounting for the Personal in Relation to the Cultural

Consider what the concept of well-being means for your own life. What are the important issues that help to define what that means for you right now: Good health? Ways of earning money? Supportive relationships? Career options? Lifestyle choices?

- What have been the major ruptures, tensions, or turning points that are essential to how your personal plotline has developed so far? Has there been a particular story told by someone else that had a significant impact on your own life story?

- What is the mainstream master narrative for people in your demographic? How does your personal story fit or differ from this cultural narrative? What happens if and when your personal story differs from or conflicts with the dominant perspective?

- How does your personal story fit or differ from existing cultural counter narratives?

Political Complexities of Aging

Political complexities in the health arena range from national policy deliberations to the micro-politics of how power is exerted in healthcare interactions to unpacking the assumed meanings in how health is discussed and understood. Political narratives use story formats to transform abstract or difficult-to-understand issues into concrete, specific terms that most people are able to grasp, and even become emotionally invested in.

Probably one of the first entities that comes to mind when thinking about politics and aging is AARP,[3] one of the largest advocacy groups in the U.S. As soon as most Americans turn 50, they receive a recruitment package from AARP. This group is known for its strong efforts to defend and maintain post-retirement benefits like Social Security and Medicare health insurance, both of which are forms of financial payments to qualified individuals who contributed a portion of earnings through a required tax during their working years. The economic solvency of these benefits are continuously in dispute and danger of running short due to the much increased life span of the population. Other threats to the integrity of the Medicare system include rising costs for hospitalization and pharmaceuticals, fraudulent charges, and refusal of healthcare professionals to accept set Medicare payments deemed as insufficient reimbursement. The AARP narrative concedes that cost containment is necessary but that this form of health insurance must be kept intact for the hard-working citizens who paid into the system for decades, and particularly for the elderly indigent who do not have other resources on which to depend. Simultaneously, there is a counter narrative that raises the concern that maintaining current levels of expenditures for today's elders is being subsidized by current younger, healthier workers who may be left inadequately covered for their own future medical needs.

■ From Well-Being to Quality of Life

The story of AARP's advocacy is a clearly recognizable illustration of a political master narrative. However, when it comes to some of the more sensitive issues related to aging, politics are frequently enacted in family settings, centered on possible limitations to individual voice, autonomy, and decision making due to age-related factors. Such a change in narrative plot and scene becomes apparent as we return to Gene and Hilda.

Mobility, having the means to transport individuals to desired locations, especially outside one's home, is an essential aspect of modern living, an integral part of well-being, and one of the most important aspects to be addressed at a policy level to encourage healthy aging. In an urban environment, walkable destinations and mass transit such as buses and taxis enable mobility for the elderly. There are also limitations on these forms of transportation, depending on availability in particular locations, weather, time of day, and threat of crime. In suburban and rural locations, possibilities for mass transit are limited or nonexistent. Bottom line, being able to drive a car is an important, if not essential, element of American life; many aspects of living may need to be radically altered or limited without the use of a car.

As mentioned earlier, Gene still drives, mainly for local errands and social activities. Even at age 95, driving remains his right and privilege as long as the Commonwealth of Pennsylvania grants him a license. Because he is aware that his night vision is not as good as his daytime eyesight, he voluntarily curtails driving much after dark. Both of Gene and Hilda's daughters reside in other states. The closest family, including grandchildren and, most recently, a great-grandchild, live in North Carolina, approximately an eight-hour drive. Airplane flights are reasonably priced and take only 90 minutes. However, Hilda has a severe fear of flying and refuses to go by plane. There is an available train route, but Gene and Hilda prefer to travel in their own car, at their own pace, typically dividing the trip into two days of easy driving with an overnight stay. The last few visits, Gene's "younger" brother Irv, also in his 90s, accompanied the couple and shared the driving (Hilda does not drive). However, their daughters and grandchildren are very uneasy with these long road trips and have tried to convince them to consider the alternatives, to no avail. Neither daughter feels that she has the authority to stop her dad from long-distance driving, so this conflict can be understood as an ongoing family disagreement. But from another vantage point it is also an example of a social policy dilemma. At what point might an advanced senior driving on an interstate present a danger to self, passengers, and other drivers? (Arguably, the same questions can be asked of young teenage drivers.)

Since age alone seems a prejudicial and insufficient basis upon which to tackle such a question, what other factors should be taken into consideration, if any? Upon what criteria does individual judgment and autonomy trump public health concerns, and vice versa?

Probably the greatest threat that accompanies the continued expansion of an aging population, specifically the increase of life span without concomitant increase in health span, is Alzheimer's disease (AD) and related forms of dementia. Once this dreaded ailment is the focus, we are no longer in the realm of healthy aging. What becomes most at stake is quality of life, in these circumstances, primarily for the unfortunate individuals with this illness and also for the people who become their caretakers. The tag line of the Alzheimer's Association is "everyone with a brain is at risk for Alzheimer's" (www.alz.org). People as young as late 40s to early 50s have been diagnosed with early onset AD, but mostly this is a disease associated with advancing age, and it is the sixth leading cause of death in the U.S. One in three seniors dies of AD, and in 2015 more than five million people over 65 were diagnosed, but in 10 years, that statistic will change to more than seven million, a 40% increase. Statistics are sobering if we stop to let their rational impact take hold and sink in. The power of narrative, of course, is that if stories are told or presented well, recipients of the story are engaged, involved, and swept along, intellectually and emotionally, at times achieving vicarious or empathic understanding of a situation that is otherwise unknowable.

The film *Still Alice* (Glatzer & Westmoreland, 2014) is an effectively moving portrayal of a 50-year-old, brilliant, Columbia linguistics professor (played by Julianne Moore, for which she won the Academy Award for Best Actress in 2015) who is overcome with inherited AD. As audience, we are able to see the onset and impact of the disease as it overtakes Alice's life and family. She uses her computer for reminders, to quickly obtain forgotten information, to test her grasp of life as she has known it, and failing her own self-created reality-testing, to leave herself explicit instructions about when and how she should end her life (a plan foiled by unforeseen circumstances). We look on as her classes become disorganized and she loses her job, tries valiantly to maintain relationships with her husband and adult children, gives a heart-rending, frank talk at an Alzheimer's Association conference, and is unable to find the bathroom in her own home. By the end of the film, this person, who had been defined by her intellect and her understanding of language, has lost most of her ability to use words and, in the process, to exercise her judgment and choices about her predicament. In effect, the title *Still Alice* is a double entendre, referring to the disappearance of language and the remainders of a person's essence.

Though the film is a fictional portrayal, in many ways it is strikingly similar to another first-person account of experiencing AD from the inside out. Journalist Greg O'Brien, also diagnosed with early onset AD, has written an autobiographical account of his struggle (O'Brien, 2014), along with participating in a series of interviews broadcast on National Public Radio (Hersher, 2015a, b, c, d). Describing in compelling detail the most difficult and routine moments of living with AD, Greg tells of breaking the news of his diagnosis to his children, having to sign over his house ownership and all other business affairs to his wife, and his compulsion to continue running on a daily basis, despite physical degeneration, as a way of trying to clear his mind. Though what he discusses is very serious, flashes of humor engendered by his situation come through:

> I know I shouldn't be driving, but I just hate to give it up. At least my wife knows where I am. After I had an accident a couple months ago, she found this computer thing—an app on your iPhone that can tell people where you are at all times. So I gave it to my wife, I gave it to my kids. It's like piece by piece, stripping yourself away of your identity. I know I'm not supposed to be driving, but it's a country road, and I'm going to the gym, because that's just what I'm going to do. There's [going to be] a day when I can't do it. . . . But . . . what I do just to piss [my family] off sometimes, is, I turn the phone off, and then they don't know where I am. (Hersher, 2015b)

The ironic tone of Greg's storytelling reveals his frustration with the relentless surrender of life and freedom, all the things he has worked for and are dear to him. Perhaps contrary to stereotype, with much effort, he is still able to articulate his experiences and perspectives but is powerless to stop the onslaught of indignities that result from the ever-encroaching dementia that diminishes his ability to think and act for himself.

While it is an essential first step that these depictions help many more people to understand what AD is, how it progresses, and what happens to those who are afflicted, this is not enough. Narratives that challenge, expand, or modify widely ascribed accounts of reality are necessary aspects of social advocacy and activism that can be used in the service of changing health policy. The Alzheimer's Association (2016) emphasizes that AD is the only one of the top 10 causes of death in the U.S. that "cannot be prevented, cured, or slowed." The implication that there is no progress in addressing this affliction, in comparison to other life-endangering conditions, and in light of expanding prevalence and skyrocketing costs to the nation is certainly motivation to change the status quo. Why so little progress? Has the federal government given enough resources and attention to this health threat? When the sufferers are cognitively impaired and the time and energies of their loved ones are devoted to caregiving, who can step forward to press for changes in priorities and policies?

At one point in the film, Alice tells her husband that she wishes she had cancer instead of AD, because having cancer is not perceived as something shameful. Her point is well taken when understood in light of another statistic—that 45%, less than half, of people with AD and their caregivers have been specifically given the diagnosis, as compared to 90% of people with cancer diagnoses. If AD carries this kind of stigma with health professionals, what is its impact within the general population? Commenting on his tremendous effort to publish his memoir, Greg said, "There are millions more [people] out there who are suffering. . . . If I could give them that voice so maybe things get a little better for them, then that's good" (Hersher, 2015a). But in a difficult, tearful moment during a subsequent interview, he admits:

> This fight? I don't know how much longer I can do it. You got the Alzheimer's thing, that the progression goes, and then there's the toll that it takes on you. I don't know how much longer I can keep this fight up. It's 24-7. It sucks. And there's days when I just want to go home [to heaven].

Alice tried to carefully plan her death when she had lost her capabilities to act meaningfully, but her more impaired self could not manage with unexpected contingencies. Greg is not giving up but hints that there may come a time when he will—but will that point be a matter of his autonomous, informed choice? Such questions raise significant issues about how hopeless suffering is dealt with in our society and, implicitly, the possibility of planned, humane suicide.

This brief analysis of two stories that depict the circumstances of having AD points to the intricate, compelling difficulties of restricted voice, autonomy, and public policy; how these problems can best be communicated to the larger population, which itself may be implicated, directly or indirectly; and the potential effectiveness of using narrative for advocacy.

HCIA 2.2

Privacy Management Conundrum: Making Healthcare Decisions for Someone Else

Sandra Petronio ■ Jennifer J. Bute ■ Alexia Torke

Suppose you received a call from a relative asking if you would help your aunt. You are the closest to the hospital where she is receiving care. All of the other relatives live too far away to help. You have not seen your aunt for some time, probably since your mother, her younger sister, passed away. You were never that close but out of respect for your mother, you go to the hospital. As you enter the hospital it takes you some time to locate where your aunt is and find her physician so you can determine how you can help her. The physician tells you that she is unable to make healthcare decisions for herself because she is cognitively impaired due to having Alzheimer's disease and the physician needs a surrogate to make those decisions. You stand there reeling. You know little about your aunt's condition or her wishes about medical care. Yet, you want to help.

Acting as a Surrogate

Situations in which hospitalized patients are incapable of disclosing their choices about medical care options due to dementia, Alzheimer's disease, or injury are more common than people might think. Such circumstances have included, for example, whether to consent to a particular treatment, such as chemotherapy, to address the patient's cancer, whether the individual would want extraordinary end-of-life care or opt for "do not resuscitate," and overall, whether the patient has the ability to have a say in choices about the kind of care provided in the course of their illness. Research shows that approximately 47% of patients in the hospital are partially or completely unable to communicate, compromising their medical decision making.

(continued)

When a patient is unable to effectively communicate with the medical team, family or individuals close to the patient often serve as surrogates. As surrogates, they provide health and personal information to clinicians and engage in medical decision making on behalf of the patient, performing two important communicative roles. An important aspect of the surrogate–clinician interactions leading to ethical treatment is how the patient's private medical information is managed.

Communicating the Patient's Private Information

Surrogates often experience difficulty communicating with clinicians, leading to problems with successful medical decision making for the patient. The question is how best to understand interactions about privacy management and disclosure within this type of stressful circumstance. Studies utilize Communication Privacy Management (CPM) theory (Petronio, 2002) to get a better grasp on the way surrogates navigate interactions with clinicians in the best interest of a loved one.

CPM theory highlights certain issues that influence best practices for managing private information within the surrogate–clinician context. In general, people believe they own and have the right to control their private information. The notion of "privacy boundaries" is used to mark degree of ownership of information. The regulation of these boundaries is accomplished through "privacy rules" that can shift and change as situations require different levels of maintaining the desired level of control over the information.

Proxy Information Co-Owners

We also know that once private information is intentionally disclosed to others, they become "authorized co-owners," meaning the individual as owner of this information wanted these designated individuals to know the information. As such, original owners entrust co-owners to take good care of their information in ways that fit with the expectations of original owners. In considering surrogates, research suggests co-ownership roles closely align with serving as a "proxy" or agent for the patient regarding disclosure of private information. This means that surrogates not only fulfill an obligation as a co-owner, they also have to make judgments about decisions patients *might* have made about their medical treatment. Examining the "medical proxy co-owners" and management of patients' private health information gives insights into the evermore complicated position surrogates face in helping family or friends. Surrogates may or may not be well informed about the wishes of the patient, which complicates decision making. Similar to the opening case in which the individual knew little about his aunt's wishes, surrogates must frequently make difficult decisions.

Surrogate Interactions

Considering how surrogates navigate interactions with clinicians related to the patient's private medical information and decision making, research offers insights into their struggles. As an overview, surrogates often expect that they will have an open line of communication with the medical team, yet in reality they tend to find that getting access is difficult and frustrating. While surrogates may not have legal "power of medical attorney" (POA), they are called upon to aid in the decision making as an advocate for the patient and often the patient's family. Part of fulfilling a proxy owner role presumes the right to know the clinicians' findings concerning tests and general assessments of the patient's health issues. Yet, surrogates are often shut out of the conversational loop. As a result, they must work diligently at gathering information to fulfill their role and help the patient. Nevertheless, the clinicians make demands on them for information that they might not know. As this overview suggests, more insight is needed to aid surrogates as they communicate to help incapacitated patients when they adopt a proxy ownership role.

■ Conclusion

This chapter has provided a brief introduction to what it means to take a narrative approach to the study of health communication. I've used issues related to health and aging as a way of demonstrating how narratives work to communicate complexities at personal, cultural, and political levels of analysis. Why have we decided to emphasize narrative? A simple answer is that we consider ourselves narrative scholars in our own respective work. This means we ask research questions in ways consistent with narrative purposes or functions; we seek qualitative data, whether from interviews, focus groups, or written or visual texts, which can be elicited in story form; and we pay particular attention to narrative elements (Yamasaki, Sharf, & Harter, 2014). Those personal interests are based on the strong belief that the resulting storied data and analyses are powerful enactments of theoretical ideas and statistical generalizations. They enable us to see in depth how communication processes and relationships play out in the context of health-related problems and contexts. Finally, and not least, we believe that incorporating typical textbook materials—theories, concepts, literature reviews, particular studies—in narrative frameworks is simply more interesting for readers.

As we invited contributors to this text, other scholars whose works we admire and feel have been influential in the study of health communication, we explained our emphasis on narrative and requested that a storied approach be somehow incorporated in the chapters or sidebars they agreed to write. The results are varied. You will find chapters written as stories, as more straightforward explanations with interesting examples and case studies, and as research reports that confirm the importance of storytelling processes and narrative forms in healthcare, health promotion, community support, organizational wellness, entertainment education, and other health-related sites of interest. We hope that you learn from, engage with, and enjoy what's to follow.

Discussion Questions

1. Imagine that you and a group of your classmates are functioning as a social marketing team with an assignment to create a media campaign to improve social perceptions of "the elderly." What aspects of the stigma might you want to address? What are some strategies this campaign would incorporate?

2. Have you personally known anyone with a diagnosis of Alzheimer's disease? How did the stories of Alice and Greg fit with your preconceptions of this illness? What, if anything, surprised you?

3. What is an example of a health or illness narrative (real or fictional) that has made a significant difference to you personally, to cultural understandings of a healthcare issue, or to the politics of how a health problem has been handled?

4. Brainstorm one or two questions related to health communication that you might want to investigate for a final paper in this class. How do you think you'd go about doing this research with a narrative approach?

NOTES

[1] Attributed to Dr. Rachel Jumper.

[2] We don't believe that the audience reaction had to do with negative attributions to being a devoted grandmother, but rather that many expect a 49-year-old woman to have additional forms of primary identification.

[3] AARP has been the popular acronym for the organizational name American Association for Retired Persons. The full name has now been dropped, probably because many members are not retired and because the organization seeks to maintain a more contemporary, less stodgy image (once again avoiding the narrative of aging as decline and disability). In addition to being one of the largest congressional lobbying entities in the U.S., it also serves as a broker for services and products for older constituents, especially Medicare health insurance supplements.

REFERENCES

Alzheimer's Association (2016). 2015 Alzheimer's Association facts and figures. Retrieved February 3, 2016, from http://www.alz.org/facts/overview.asp#quickFacts

Anderson, J. O., & Geist-Martin, P. (2003). Narratives and healing: Exploring one family's stories of cancer survivorship. *Health Communication, 15,* 133–143.

Bochner, A. P. (2014). *Coming to narrative: A personal history of paradigm change in the human sciences.* Walnut Creek, CA: Left Coast Press.

Brody, H. (2003). *Stories of sickness* (2nd ed.). New York, NY: Oxford University Press.

Bruner, J. (1990). *Acts of meaning.* Cambridge, MA: Harvard University Press.

Buettner, D. (2015). *The Blue Zones solution: Eating and living like the world's healthiest people.* Washington, DC: National Geographic.

Charmaz, K. (1991). *Good days, bad days: The self and chronic illness in time.* New Brunswick, NJ: Rutgers University Press.

Charon, R. (2008). *Narrative medicine: Honoring the stories of illness.* New York, NY: Oxford University Press.

Colby, S. L., & Ortman, J. M. (May, 2014). The baby boom cohort in the United States: 2012 to 2060. *Current Population Reports: U.S. Census Bureau.* Retrieved February 8, 2015, from http://www.census.gov/prod/2014pubs/p25-1141.pdf

Cole, T. R. (1992). *The journey of life: A cultural history of aging in America.* Cambridge, UK: Cambridge University Press.

Davies, D. (2015, Feb. 26). From naked mole rats to dog testicles: A writer explores the longevity quest (interview with Bill Gifford). *Fresh Air*, National Public Radio. http://www.npr.org/blogs/health/2015/02/26/389261354/from-naked-mole-rats-to-dog-testicles-a-writer-explores-the-longevity-quest

Easterbrook, G. (2014, Oct.). What happens when we all live to 100? *The Atlantic*. Retrieved May 6, 2015, from http://www.theatlantic.com/features/archive/2014/09/what-happens-when-we-all-live-to-100/379338/

Ellingson, L. L. (2004). *Communicating in the clinic: Negotiating frontstage and backstage teamwork.* New York, NY: Hampton Press.

Emanuel, E. Z. (Oct., 2014). Why I hope to die at 75. *The Atlantic*. Retrieved May 4, 2015, from http://www.theatlantic.com/features/archive/2014/09/why-i-hope-to-die-at-75/379329/

Fisher, W. R. (1987). *Human communication as narration: Toward a philosophy of reason, value, and action.* Columbia: University of South Carolina Press.

Frank, A. W. (1995). *The wounded storyteller: Body, illness and ethics.* Chicago, IL: University of Chicago Press.

Frank, A. W. (2002). *At the will of the body: Reflections on illness* (2nd ed.). Boston: Houghton Mifflin.

Geist-Martin, P., Ray, E. B., & Sharf, B. F. (2011). *Communicating health: Personal, cultural, and political complexities.* Long Grove, IL: Waveland Press.

Gifford, B. (2015). *Spring chicken: Stay young forever (or die trying).* New York, NY: Grand Central Publishing.

Glatzer, R., & Westmoreland, W. (Directors). (2014). *Still Alice* [Film]. Los Angeles, CA: Sony Pictures Classics.

Harter, L. M., & Associates. (2013). *Imagining new normals: A narrative framework for health communication.* Dubuque, IA: Kendall Hunt.

Harter, L. M., & Bochner, A. P. (Eds.). (2009). Healing through stories: A special issue on narrative and medicine. *Journal of Applied Communication Research, 17*.

Harter, L. M., Japp, P. M., & Beck, C. S. (Eds.). (2005). *Narratives, health, and healing: Communication theory, research, and practice.* Mahwah, NJ: Erlbaum.

Hawes, C. (2013, July 30). Assisted living is "a ticking time bomb." Life and death in assisted living. *Frontline*. Public Broadcasting System.

Hawes, C., Phillips, C. D., & Rose, M. (2000). *A national study of assisted living for the frail elderly: Final summary report.* Washington, DC: U.S. Dept. of Health & Human Services.

Hersher, R. (Jan. 24, 2015a). 'How do you tell your kids that you've got Alzheimer's?' *All Things Considered*, National Public Radio. Retrieved May 10, 2015, from http://www.npr.org/blogs/health/2015/01/24/379381706/how-do-you-tell-your-kids-that-you-got-alzheimers

Hersher, R. (Jan. 31, 2015b). After Alzheimer's diagnosis, 'the stripping away of my identity.' *All Things Considered*, National Public Radio. Retrieved May 10, 2015, from http://www.npr.org/blogs/health/2015/01/31/382240633/after-alzheimers-diagnosis-the-stripping-away-of-my-identity

Hersher, R. (Feb. 28, 2015c). One man's race to outrun Alzheimer's. *All Things Considered*, National Public Radio. Retrieved May 10, 2015, from http://www.npr.org/blogs/health/2015/02/28/389593868/one-mans-race-to-outrun-alzheimers

Hersher, R. (March 7, 2015d). Supporting a spouse with Alzheimer's: 'I don't get angry anymore.' *All Things Considered*, National Public Radio. Retrieved May 10, 2015, from http://www.npr.org/blogs/health/2015/03/07/391242734/supporting-a-spouse-with-alzheimers-i-dont-get-angry-anymore

Hummert, M. L., Garstka, T. A., Ryan, E. B., & Bonnesen, J. L. (2004). The role of age stereotypes in interpersonal communication. In J. F. Nussbaum & J. Coupland (Eds.), *Handbook of communication and aging research* (2nd ed., pp. 91–114). Mahwah, NJ: Erlbaum.

Hunter, K. M. (1991). *Doctors' stories: The narrative structure of medical knowledge.* Princeton, NJ: Princeton University Press.

Jaffe, I. (2015, April 27). Drop-in chefs help seniors stay in their own homes. *Morning Edition*, National Public Radio. Retrieved May 10, 2015, from http://www.npr.org/blogs/health/2015/04/27/401749819/drop-in-home-chefs-may-be-an-alternative-to-assisted-living

Kleinman, A. (1988). *The illness narratives: Suffering, healing, and the human condition.* New York, NY: Basic Books.

Morris, D. B. (1998). *Illness and culture in the postmodern age.* Berkeley: University of California Press.

O'Brien, G. (2014). *On Pluto: Inside the mind of Alzheimer's.* Cape Cod, MA: Codfish Press.

Partners for Livable Communities. (2009). *Redesigning communities for aging in place: Developing a livable San Antonio for all ages.* Retrieved May 10, 2015, from http://livable.org/livability-resources/reports-a-publications/159-redesigning-communities-for-aging-in-place-developing-a-livable-san-antonio-for-all-ages

Pennebaker, J. W. (2000). Telling stories: The health benefits of narrative. *Literature and Medicine, 19,* 3–18.

Poirier, S., Rosenblum, L., Ayres, L., Brauner, D. J., Sharf, B. F., & Stanford, A. F. (1992). Charting the chart—An exercise in interpretation(s). *Literature and Medicine, 11,* 1–22.

Polkinghorne, D. E. (1988). *Narrative knowing and the human sciences.* Albany: State University of New York Press.

Poo, A. J., & Conrad, A. (2015). *The age of dignity: Preparing for the elder boom in a changing America.* New York, NY: The New Press.

Riessman, C. K. (2008). *Narrative methods for the human sciences.* Los Angeles, CA: Sage.

Sharf, B. F. (1990). Physician-patient communication as interpersonal rhetoric: A narrative approach. *Health Communication, 2,* 217-231.

Sharf, B. F., Harter, L. M., Yamasaki, J., & Haidet, P. (2011). Narrative turns epic: Continuing developments in health narrative scholarship. In T. L. Thompson, R. Parrott, & J. F. Nussbaum (Eds.), *Handbook of health communication.* (2nd ed., pp. 36–51). New York, NY: Routledge.

Sharf, B. F., & Vanderford, M. L. (2003). Illness narratives and the social construction of health. In T. L. Thompson, A. Dorsey, K. I. Miller, & R. Parrott (Eds.), *Handbook of health communication* (pp. 9–34). Mahwah, NJ: Erlbaum.

Simon, S., & Jaffe, I. (2015, May 23). This summer, a "mature" season for action stars and fashion models. *Weekend Edition*, National Public Radio. Retrieved June 5, 2015, from http://www.npr.org/2015/05/23/408996510/this-summer-a-mature-season-for-action-stars-and-fashion-models

Yamasaki, J. (2013). The poetic possibilities of long-term care. In L. M. Harter & Associates, *Imagining new normals: A narrative framework for health communication* (pp. 107–124). Dubuque, IA: Kendall Hunt.

Yamasaki, J. (2014). Age accomplished, performed, and failed: Liz Young as old on *The Biggest Loser. Text & Performance Quarterly 34,* 354–371.

Yamasaki, J., & Sharf, B. F. (2011). Opting out while fitting in: How residents make sense of assisted living and cope with community life. *Journal of Aging Studies 25,* 13–21.

Yamasaki, J., Sharf, B. F., & Harter, L. M. (2014). Narrative inquiry: Attitude, acts, artifacts, and analysis. In B. B. Whaley (Ed.), *Research methods in health communication: Principles and application* (pp. 99–118). New York, NY: Routledge.

3

Communicating in Patient–Provider Relationships

Marleah Dean

Mrs. Stanley was a healthy 62-year-old patient until she was diagnosed with Stage III ovarian cancer less than a year ago. Since her diagnosis, she has undergone a bilateral salpingo oopherectomy (the removal of the fallopian tubes and ovaries) and chemotherapy. Her physicians have been monitoring her health, and so far, her recovery has been going well.

Before the cancer, neither Mrs. Stanley nor her family was very concerned about health problems; now, her family is extremely conscious about cancer. When Mrs. Stanley was diagnosed, her oncologist asked her whether there were other family cases of cancer. Mrs. Stanley explained that her mother died of ovarian cancer at age 43 and her older sister died of breast cancer at age 54. Thus, Mrs. Stanley's oncologist referred her to a genetic counselor.

After discussing her family history of cancer with the genetic counselor, Mrs. Stanley tested for the BReast CAncer gene (BRCA)—a genetic mutation that greatly increases one's risk for hereditary breast and ovarian cancer [Friedman, Sutphen, & Steligo, 2012]. Her results, unfortunately, came back positive for one of the genetic mutations called BRCA1. Because this gene is inherited, the genetic counselor recommended that Mrs. Stanley's two daughters undergo genetic testing as well. Mrs. Stanley and her family have been thrown into a struggle between health and illness.

In the story above, Mrs. Stanley and her family must interact with a variety of healthcare providers. According to Sparks and Villagran (2010), the *patient–provider interaction (PPI)* is defined as "creating shared meaning about healthcare and conditions in medical encounters" (p. xii). In other words, patients and providers must work together to understand each other's situations and perspectives. This is true for the interactions that Mrs. Stanley and her daughters have with their providers. Because of this familial gene, they will have to communicate their needs and desires as well as negotiate care based on their preferences.

This chapter examines the patient–provider relationship and the communication between healthcare providers and patients. To help illustrate the ways in which communication is so essential to the PPI, I use Mrs. Stanley's case throughout the chapter. First, I present a model of communication that describes the PPI in relation to various contexts. Then, I explain two models of medicine that frame patient care, leading to a discussion about relationship-centered and patient-centered care. Finally, I discuss how communication can lead to better health outcomes in direct and indirect ways.

HCIA: 3.1

Veterinary Medicine:
A Parallel World of Communication in Healthcare

Suzanne Kurtz

When we think of communicating with our healthcare providers, most of us think of communicating with the physicians, nurses, and other providers who work with us as patients. For many years, health communication researchers, educators, and students; healthcare professionals; and the schools and funding agencies that supported the work of all these folks, followed the same path—all focused their attention on communication between healthcare professionals and patients in *human* medicine.

But there is another world of healthcare communication out there, one that certainly impacts human health, but where the patients are not human beings and the doctors are not physicians. That world is the world of *veterinary* medicine, where patients come in a wide array of shapes, sizes, and species that may present individually or in herds or flocks or other groupings. Unquestionably, veterinarians must become competent at interacting with their patients from the animal kingdom, and the interspecies communication they engage in is a fascinating field of study and practice. However, veterinarians must also communicate well with the human clients who accompany those patients in order to gather information, plan, make decisions, and ensure follow-through and optimal care of their patients. Undeniably, in both human and veterinary medicine, a basic unit of care is interaction between people. While veterinary–client and physician–patient communication is central, communication with the patient's significant others and with other members of the professional team is also vital.

There are, of course, differences between human and veterinary medicine. Nevertheless, the goals we are trying to achieve through communication in either healthcare context are remarkably similar:

- More effective consultations for patients, clients, and clinicians, characterized especially by greater accuracy, heightened efficiency, and enhanced supportiveness and trust
- Relationships characterized by collaboration and partnership
- Better coordination of care (between healthcare professionals and with patients and clients, families, significant others)
- Improved outcomes of care

Happily, using communication to achieve these goals is more than wishful thinking. More than 40 years of research and educational development in human medicine have shown that improving communication in *specific* ways significantly impacts the very goals and outcomes delineated above. Recognizing that communication between people plays a similarly important role in veterinary medicine, researchers, educators, and practitioners in that field are building on the work accomplished in human medicine. As a result, a small but growing body of research on communication in veterinary medicine demonstrates that the communication skills, capacities, and processes shown to be effective in human medicine, as

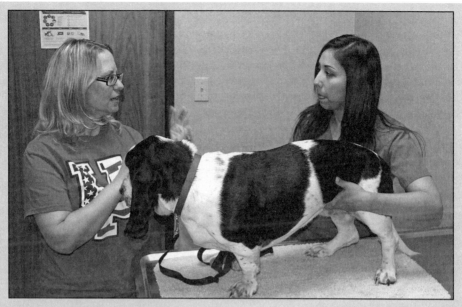

(Photograph by Torrence Washington.)

well as the developments regarding communication education, are equally applicable to veterinary medicine.

In response to these developments, veterinary schools are employing a variety of approaches to increase veterinary students' communication competence. Of course, even the best of these educational programs will be rendered less than effective if there is no consistent follow-through in the "real world" of practice. Yet, because communication research and education are relatively recent developments in veterinary medicine, both practicing veterinarians and faculty may not have had the opportunity to participate in formal communication training. Consequently, communication programs often also aim to enhance these experienced veterinarians' communication skills.

Given the common ground between human and veterinary medicine, it is not surprising that the same evidence-based communication concepts, capacities, and skills enhance communication and form the foundation for educational programs in both contexts. Whether we are professionals or students in training, patients or veterinary clients ourselves, it is useful to conceptualize communication in terms of three slightly overlapping and highly interdependent categories of skills:

- Content Skills—what you say and understand others are saying
- Process Skills—how you communicate
  - How you structure interaction
  - How you relate to others
  - How you use and interpret nonverbal skills/behaviors
- Perceptual Skills—what you are thinking and feeling
  - Clinical reasoning, problem solving, and other thought processes
  - Attitudes, biases, assumptions, intentions

(continued)

  – Emotions and what you do with them

  – Capacities such as compassion, mindfulness, integrity, respect, etc.

Left to our own devices, we tend to give the least amount of conscious attention to our process skills despite their importance. But just what are the specific, evidence-based communication process skills that make a difference? While a number of skills models attempt to answer that question, one of the most comprehensive and applicable for both veterinary and human medicine is the Calgary-Cambridge Communication Process Guide. Summarizing 45 years of research, the C-C Communication Process Guide is comprised of 72 evidence-based communication skills. These skills are organized around an intuitive framework that corresponds to tasks important in any healthcare consultation: initiating the session, gathering information, providing structure, building relationship, explaining and planning, closing the session. The skills on the guide are applicable across the specialties in human and veterinary medicine and to an array of complex and routine issues. Originally developed in Faculties of Medicine at the University of Calgary (Canada) and, with later collaboration, Cambridge University (UK), the guide is widely recognized and used worldwide in human medicine and for the last dozen years in a variety of veterinary contexts. The communication skills on the C-C Communication Process Guide are not only for enhancing communication between physicians and patients or veterinarians and clients, but also between professors and students or between colleagues or between friends—wherever accuracy, efficiency, trust, and supportiveness matter.

QUESTIONS TO PONDER

1. Skilled communication is clearly significant in both human and veterinary medical contexts. Think of a time when you were the patient in human medicine or the client in veterinary medicine, and the interaction between you and the doctor was especially effective. Jot down notes for a few minutes about the situation and what each of you was doing, particularly specific communication skills and capacities each of you demonstrated that contributed to this being such an effective interaction. Also include bits of the dialogue you recall. Pair up with a colleague and take turns telling each other in detail about your experience, highlighting what was working so well (let one person describe her/his experience completely before the other responds with comments and questions; then do the same with the other person telling his/her story). What did you learn about effective healthcare communication from this exercise?

2. Locally, nationally, and globally, the health of people, animals, and the environment requires the integrative effort of multiple disciplines, since the health of each part of this triad is inextricably linked to the others. Identify one health issue that has emerged at the intersection of human and animal health or at the intersection of all three parts of the triad. Discuss the ways in which communication might contribute to managing or resolving this health issue; include communication skills and capacities individuals might need to develop as well as knowledge about communication concepts and how communication works. Given the situation you have identified, discuss how communication specialists or you as a student might impact or otherwise work with: (a) healthcare professionals and policy makers who are responding or need to respond to this health issue or (b) students in these areas (including your own training), so that you and they might be better prepared to contribute to such integrative efforts in the future.

Source: Adams, C., & Kurtz, S. (2012). Coaching and feedback: Enhancing communication teaching and learning in veterinary practice settings. *Journal of Veterinary Medical Education, 39,* 217–228.

■ Ecological Model of Health Communication

Because of Mrs. Stanley's positive genetic test results, her daughters now worry about their cancer risk. Two months ago, after visiting the MacDonald Cancer Risk Evaluation Center at Penn Medicine in Philadelphia, both daughters decided to undergo genetic testing. The daughters decided to go to this cancer risk center not just for its genetic testing and clinical care services but also because it is associated with the Basser Research Center for BRCA—a new research center dedicated to only patients and families with BRCA gene mutations.

Mrs. Stanley and her daughters wait for the genetic counselor. It seems like all they do is wait. They wait for the support letter from Mrs. Stanley's oncologist for her daughters to undergo genetic testing. They wait for the insurance company to approve the genetic testing. And now, they wait huddled together on a bright orange couch. Despite the room's warmth and familiarity, anxiety lurks. Mrs. Stanley is holding both of her daughters' hands. Hannah, age 37, reviews the notes and questions she brought with her to the appointment. Mrs. Stanley's younger daughter, Alison, who is 28, stares out the three-story window, daydreaming.

After waiting 40 minutes, the genetic counselor enters the room. "Well, unfortunately, the results are not what we had hoped for. Both of you tested positive for the BRCA1 genetic mutation—that means you have 87 percent risk for developing breast cancer sometime during your lifetime and 50 percent risk of developing ovarian cancer during your lifetime."

Hannah, not surprised by this news, immediately begins asking questions. She stresses that she wants to see a breast surgeon and talk about preventative surgical options. Hannah explains that, while using the Internet to search for information about BRCA, she found an organization called FORCE (Facing Our Risk of Cancer Empowered http://www.facingourrisk.org/index.php) where she connected with several BRCA+ women who have undergone preventative surgeries to reduce their cancer risk.

In contrast to Hannah's active participation and direct communication with the genetic counselor, Alison continues to stare out the window. She is convinced there must be a mistake with the test results. She thinks, "I'm too young. I haven't lived. I don't have a boyfriend or even started contemplating wanting a family unlike Hannah!" Alison stands abruptly. "I have to go," she informs the genetic counselor, and without even looking at her sister or her mother, she leaves. Mrs. Stanley tries to stop her, but Alison refuses. This news is clearly affecting Hannah and Alison in different ways. As for Mrs. Stanley, she is overwhelmed with feelings of devastation and guilt for passing on this gene that significantly heightens her daughters' (and now potentially her grandchildren's) cancer risk.

We all have experiences with healthcare providers. Whether attending a checkup with our hometown primary care provider, visiting an emergency department for stomach pains, or accompanying our grandparent to an appointment, each of us knows generally what to expect in a health encounter. As patients, we understand that we must describe all relevant background history and explain our current symptoms, and we know that providers are often busy, overwhelmed, and pressed for resources. Yet what we frequently do not think about are the various contextual issues that influence the PPI. To understand this, it is essential to learn what factors influence patient–provider health communication.

Street's (2003) *ecological model of communication in medical encounters* (see Figure 3.1) provides an excellent starting point for understanding communication in healthcare interactions. Ecology is the examination of relationships between organisms and

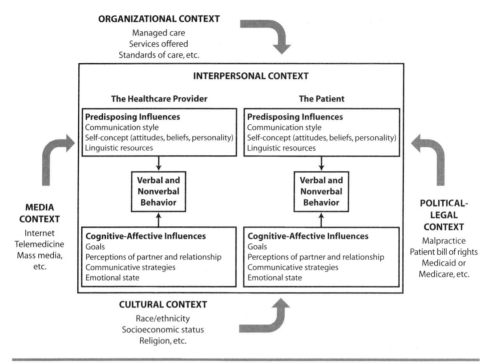

Figure 3.1   Ecological Model of Communication in Medical Encounters

their environment. Employing an ecological perspective in the health encounter means examining communication interactions between healthcare providers and patients in a variety of different social contexts—organizational, media, cultural, political/legal, and most important to this chapter, interpersonal. That is, this ecological model emphasizes "the importance of individual choices and also contextual factors as being layers of influence on the patient–provider interaction" (Dean, Oetzel, & Sklar, 2014, p. 1619). In the following section, I explain each context of the ecological model. As you read, think about what factors have influenced your own healthcare encounters over the years.

The first and most important context to patient–provider communication is the *interpersonal context* (Street, 2003). The interpersonal context encompasses the healthcare provider and the patient. Messages are key to health encounters. Messages encompass both verbal exchanges (i.e., talk) as well as nonverbal communication such as posture, body language, eye contact, and the use of space and touch. For example, a patient may tell the provider she does not have questions, but avoids eye contact and does not leave, indicating a desire to talk more. Likewise, when breaking bad news to a patient, the provider may disclose the diagnosis, while gently touching the patient's hand to display comfort.

The patient's and the provider's individual features influence messages communicated in their relationship. *Cognitive factors* include the perceptions they have of each other and of their relationship, while *affective factors* involve the emotions they experience and interpret during health encounters. Additionally, each individual comes to an encounter with particular goals. Of course, the main goal of any health encounter for the provider is to heal, cure, or manage the patient's condition or symptom. Moreover, providers want their patients to adhere to their medical advice and suggestions. However, patients also desire to be heard, respected, and validated. In addition to their individual goals, patients and providers engage in communication styles that influence how they interact with each other as well as make meaning out of the health encounter. For instance, a patient who actively participates by explaining her goals and asking questions encourages the provider to offer information and check understanding, producing an effective and satisfied encounter. On the other hand, a patient who passively listens to the provider may leave the encounter feeling confused and unsatisfied.

The second context in the ecological model of communication in health encounters is the *organizational context* (Street, 2003). Organizational factors that influence the interpersonal context include the healthcare services offered to patients and families, standards of patient care, managed care (i.e., organizations that coordinate costs and delivery of healthcare services), work environment climate, and the health facility's size and location (du Pré, 2013). For example, physical environments can influence communication. Typically, medical spaces are often sterile, cold, and uncomfortable with their white walls, cramped quarters, and florescent lights. However, recent efforts by organizations like Planetree, a nonprofit organization, reveal innovative commitments to developing aesthetically pleasing and empowering environments (http://planetree.org/reputation/). Recent research regarding the effects of space on health communication advocate for attention to healing environments (see, Barbour, Gill, & Dean, 2016, for a review). Environments that incorporate warm tones, provide access to nature, include art, and make room for families, foster nurturing and produce therapeutic effects such as reduced anxiety, increased recovery rate, and improved emotional well-being (du Pré, 2013).

The third context is the *media context* (Street, 2003). From media-based health campaigns to popular TV shows such as *Grey's Anatomy* to mobile health applications like MyFitnessPal (i.e., a free application that tracks fitness and diet), media influences the PPI. Yet presently, the Internet is perhaps the most influential medium. Forty to 80% of individuals now use the Internet as a major source to seek health information for themselves or for family and friends (Ayantunde, Welch, & Parsons, 2007). Using the Internet to seek health information can increase knowledge, enhance communication, and encourage patient involvement in health encounters, yet providers are often put off when patients present online health information due to credibility concerns and problems with self-diagnosis and treatment. Because Internet-informed patients often are viewed as a threat to providers' power in the health encounter (Caiata-Zufferey & Schulz, 2012), patients can introduce the information in a "face-saving" way by appealing to the physician as the expert, while also presenting the information assertively (Bylund et al., 2007). By engaging in these strategies, providers are more likely to validate patients' efforts, which results in less disagreement, higher satisfaction, and reduced concerns (Bylund et al., 2007).

The fourth context is the *cultural context* (Street, 2003). Communication between patients and providers is also influenced by culture (Sparks & Villagran, 2010). Culture is defined as the set of beliefs, norms, and behaviors that are shared and held by a group of individuals and passed down to each generation (du Pré, 2013). Previous research on patient–provider communication and culture has focused largely on ethnicity. At the surface level, ethnic backgrounds are often associated with different languages (e.g., Chinese vs. English), which can complicate the PPI. Yet even when individuals speak the same language, there are often unknown cultural-specific metaphors, idioms, and stories (Geist-Martin, Ray, & Sharf, 2011). Also, ethnic groups have different explanatory models. Explanatory models (EMs) explicate how individuals not only perceive but also experience health and illness (Kleinman, 1988). In other words, EMs are meaningful within particular social-cultural contexts because they highlight how individuals and their families make sense of, respond to, and cope with illness and healthcare experiences. In the PPI, a provider's EM dictates "clinical behavior" such as formulating diagnoses and enacting curing therapeutic plans. Similarly, the patient's EM guides "illness behavior," such as explaining symptoms, making decisions to seek care, and adhering to treatment plans (Ashton et al., 2003).

Many times, the provider's EM can be in conflict with the patient's EM. For example, in the book *The Spirit Catches You and You Fall Down*, Fadiman (1997) explores two explanations for the same health condition. According to the healthcare providers, Lia Lee (a Hmong child) suffers from epilepsy, but her Hmong family and culture perceive her condition as the result of "spirits catching her soul." The providers' EM reveals a preference toward scientific explanations and modern medicine, while the Hmongs' EM emphasizes the importance of spirituality in healing. So while ethnic factors are important to the PPI, culture is not simply defined by ethnicity.

In addition to ethnicity, cultural groups may form based on individuals' religion, sexual orientation, geographic location, generation, and other characteristics. That is, a cultural group is simply one that shares similar beliefs, values, attitudes, perspectives, and behaviors (Oetzel, 2009). For instance, one of the ways culture influences communication is in terms of high-context and low-context communication (Dean, Oetzel, & Sklar, 2014; Hall, 1976). Communication that is high-context centers on the ways in which messages, and thus meaning, are created in indirect or ambiguous ways; as such, high-context communication relies on nonverbal messages (e.g., touch, eye contact, and other features of nonverbal behavior). Communication that is low-context focuses on the ways in which messages are created in direct or explicit ways, which commonly manifests as verbal messages. For example, providers tend to use low-context communication because of their preference for clear, relevant, and efficient information (Dean & Oetzel, 2014), whereas patients commonly engage in high-context communication. Overall, the clashing of cultures can produce miscommunication and impact health outcomes.

The fifth and final context is the *political-legal context*, and it is the least studied of the contexts (Street, 2003). This context refers to the patient bill of rights, malpractice claims, and insurance issues such as Medicaid and Medicare coverage. The patient bill of rights was created to ensure healthcare organizations provide fair and optimum care to all patients (Lare, 1997). Such laws are needed because medical errors are often a result of miscommunication, which leads to malpractice claims (Rider & Keefer, 2006). Yet perhaps the most current, and widely debated, issue in the political-legal context is the Patient Protection and Affordable Care Act. The Affordable Care Act seeks to insure the millions of Americans who do not have healthcare coverage;

however, there are concerns about the quality of and access to such care, staff short-ages, technology issues, and costs (see Zoller & Sastry, this volume). This law dramat-ically changed the U.S. healthcare system, as it enacted national universal coverage. Universal coverage means that all U.S. citizens are guaranteed healthcare coverage in some form or fashion (du Pré, 2013). But it has yet to be seen how this law will affect the PPI, and only time will tell. In sum, with an understanding of the various contexts that impact patient–provider communication in health encounters, I now turn to models of medicine that frame patient–provider communication and overall care.

Biomedical vs. Biopsychosocial Models of Medicine

Referred by the genetic counselor, Hannah scheduled an appointment with a breast surgeon. Dr. Thompson is based out of a group in New York City. After waiting for more than an hour, the surgeon finally enters the room. Avoiding eye contact, Dr. Thompson briefly introduces herself and explains that she has examined Hannah's medical records and doesn't understand why she is here. Hannah states that she recently tested positive for BRCA, but before she can finish, Dr. Thompson interrupts, "I know you have the gene, but you do NOT have cancer; therefore, you do NOT need surgery."

Hannah starts to provide her family's history of cancer and her mother's current condition, but again, Dr. Thompson objects. The debate continues back and forth. Finally, Dr. Thompson throws her hand down on the exam table saying, "You are just another Angelina Jolie!" Silence. "I have other patients to see now. My nurse will discuss your options with you."

Shocked and hurt, Hannah leaves Dr. Thompson's office feeling like a child who has been reprimanded for taking too many cookies. As she drives home to Philly, Hannah realizes that even though she tried to argue that she wanted this preventative surgery for a variety of rea-sons—her Ashkenazi Jewish ethnic heritage, her family's history of cancer, the emotional distress she has experienced since hearing her test results, and the psychological trauma she experienced watching her mother's cancer treatment and side effects—ultimately Dr. Thompson could not see past her physical body, which at the present, did not have cancer.

This section explains the two prevailing models of medicine for healthcare prac-tice. The origin of medicine was built upon biological sciences. For years, medicine's goal was to diagnose, treat, and cure objective, verifiable signs of disease. To achieve such goals, providers cared for patients based on a *biomedical model of medicine*. This model focuses on the pathophysiology of a patient's disease through evidence-based scientific inquiry (Fortin, Dwamena, Smith, & Frankel, 2012; Sparks & Villagran, 2010). Thus, care from a biomedical perspective means identifying a patient's symp-toms and then isolating the biological abnormal causes of those symptoms in order to diagnose and treat them (Fortin et al., 2012).

However, in the last few decades, scholarship has questioned the effectiveness of this model, citing several limitations. For one, the biomedical model does not account for factors other than biological or anatomical causes for a patient's diseases and abnor-malities. In other words, it ignores the ways in which a patient's disease or illness may be influenced by psychological (e.g., emotions and feelings) and social (e.g., family, socio-economic status, and culture) factors. Moreover, its dependence on "'science' in effect is at the expense of the humanity of the patient" (Engel, 1980, p. 536). But the most problematic flaw of the model is that it does not take into account the patient as a person and the patient's attributes as an individual. That is, the biomedical model of medicine views a "patient as a cell rather than a human being" (Sparks & Villagran, 2010, p. 8).

To address the biomedical model's limitations, psychiatrist George Engel (1977) proposed a shift from objective biomedical explanations of illness to subjective biopsychosocial explanations for patients' health and illness experiences—coining the term *biopsychosocial model of medicine*. The biopsychosocial model takes into account what is missing in the biomedical model—the ways in which social factors (e.g., demographics, socioeconomic status, and home life), psychological factors (e.g., mental and emotional states such as stress), and behavioral factors (e.g., diet and exercise) may influence a patient's illness and overall health experience (Engel, 1980; Fortin et al., 2012). So, providers who adhere to this model acknowledge that in addition to patients' symptoms it is also important to consider their emotions, feelings, and concerns (Dean & Street, 2016).

More specifically, the biopsychosocial model of medicine is based on systems theory (Engel, 1980). Systems theory states "nature is ordered as hierarchically arranged continuums, with its more complex, larger units super-ordinate to the less complex, smaller units" (p. 536). Each system within the hierarchy is influenced by others and thus has implications. For instance, in healthcare, a patient's relationship with family, providers, and the environment is just as important as the patient's physical manifestations of a disease or illness (Fortin et al., 2012). Because of this interconnectedness, the best way for providers to care for their patients is by understanding how the patient fits into the system and how the patient and provider influence each other (Engel, 1980).

In short, a core difference between the biomedical and biopsychosocial models of medicine is the distinction between *disease* and *illness* (Fortin et al., 2012; Kleinman, 1980). The term "disease" is highlighted in the biomedical model as biological and therefore objective; the implication of this meaning of disease is that through observation and testing, providers can identify the abnormality, isolate the cause, and present a solution. On the other hand, "illness" is highlighted in the biopsychosocial model with the idea that a health experience is subjective—meaning that one patient's experience may be different than another's with the same disease. These distinctions are especially relevant in the PPI because patients may come to providers with their illness *experiences*, while the providers may be concerned only with the nature of the disease. Therefore, in this next section, I elaborate on this distinction by discussing relationship-centered and patient-centered communication in care. First, consider the patient-centered approach to interviewing, which is associated with biopsychosocial medicine, in Theorizing Practice 3.1.

Theorizing Practice 3.1
Biomedical Medicine vs. Biopsychosocial Medicine

One of healthcare providers' key fundamental skills is medical interviewing. *Medical interviewing* is defined as "the process of gathering and sharing information in the context of a trustworthy relationship that takes into account both disease, if present, and illness" (Fortin et al., 2012, p. 3). Interviewing is necessary in order to determine what is going on with the patient's body, to make an appropriate diagnosis, and to decide on the right course of treatment. Dr. Robert Smith and his colleagues (Fortin et al., 2012) developed one approach to medical interviewing, called the *patient-centered approach to interviewing*. The authors break down the interviewing process into two segments: (1) clinician-centered interviewing and (2) patient-centered interviewing. Clinician-centered interviewing is derived from the biomedical model, thus centering on extracting a disease's symptoms. In contrast, patient-centered interviewing is associated with the biopsychosocial model of medicine, as it recognizes patients' symptoms but also their emotions and feelings.

The following 11 steps represent Dr. Smith's *patient-centered approach to interviewing*. In your opinion, which of the following steps lend themselves to being more patient-centered in nature and which steps would be more effective from a clinician-centered approach?

1. Set the stage for interview
2. Elicit chief concern and set agenda
3. Begin interview with nonfocusing skills that help patient express
4. Use focusing skills to learn symptom story, personal context, and emotional context
5. Transition to clinician-centered interviewing
6. Obtain chronological description of history of present illness
7. Past medical history
8. Social history
9. Family history
10. Review systems of body
11. End interview

Is there anything you might add to this list? In other words, based on your own experiences, do you have any suggestions for other patient-centered or clinician-centered steps for the medical interviewing process?

Relationship-Centered and Patient-Centered Care and Communication

Because of the healthcare interaction with Dr. Thompson, Hannah decided to seek a second opinion—focusing specifically on finding a physician who will listen to her and then work with her to achieve her goal of preventative surgeries. After seeing several physicians, Hannah finally finds the physician for her, a breast surgeon based in Washington, D.C. named Dr. Austen.

Dr. Austen is very different from Dr. Thompson. Starting with the first interaction where she asks Hannah to share her story, to holding Hannah's hand as she is rolled into the operating room, Dr. Austen works to build a strong and trusting relationship with her patients. For example, during each interaction, Dr. Austen spends time with Hannah, asks about her opinions, provides lots of information, checks for understanding, listens to her feelings and concerns, and demonstrates empathy. Additionally, while Hannah makes her final decisions about surgery, Dr. Austen connects her with a former patient around Hannah's age and in a similar family situation not only to help her make an informed decision, but also to provide social support. Overall, Dr. Austen's commitment to meeting Hannah's health goals as well as working as her partner reassures Hannah that she made the right decision for her.

Relationship-centered or patient-centered care is rooted in the fundamental belief of shared power between providers and patients (Duggan, 2014). In the *Routledge Handbook of Health Communication*, Duggan and Thompson (2011) report that the term "patient-centered" moves beyond paternalistic model of providers as the primary source of influence (Barr, 2008). Patient-centered care and patient-centered communication are more commonly used in the literature, highlighting a "goal-oriented interaction" (Duggan & Thompson, 2011, p. 418), while relationship-centered care is a more recent term that recognizes the "mutual interaction" between patients and providers (Duggan, 2014). This section discusses both terms, but a more in-depth discussion is provided for patient-centered care and communication.

Relationship-centered care centers on the belief that both the provider and the patient bring a unique set of goals, emotions, and experiences to the health encounter (Roter, Frankel, Hall, & Sluyter, 2006). Additionally, a relationship-centered care model assumes that the PPI is co-created by both parties, meaning the provider must reach a shared understanding of the patient's health or illness experience (Duggan, 2014). In this way, relationship-centered care acknowledges that the nature and quality of the PPI is essential to diagnosis and overall care (Duggan, 2014; Sparks & Villagran, 2010).

Relationship-centered care: (1) recognizes the "personhood" of the provider and patient; (2) acknowledges emotions as part of the medical encounter; (3) values reciprocal influence in all healthcare relationships; and (4) understands "moral value" as essential to forming and maintaining relationships (Beach, Roter, Wang, Duggan, & Cooper, 2006). On the whole, to effectively engage in relationship-centered care, the provider must remove any judgment toward the patient, display empathy, and be open and create trust (Duggan, 2014), while the patient must describe her health experience, including important emotions and necessary information.

HCIA 3.2

"Hey Doc! What Do You Think about Acupuncture?": Talking about CAM

Evelyn Y. Ho

Numerous national studies find that more than 40% of the U.S. adult population uses some form of complementary or alternative medicine (CAM). Usually defined as that which is not conventional biomedicine, CAM encompasses everything from whole systems of medicine like traditional Chinese medicine or Ayurveda from India, to nutritional supplements like glucosamine chondroitin, to mind-body practices like meditation or Reiki. Although many people use some form of CAM, most studies find that most people do NOT talk to their biomedical providers about their CAM use. Why is that?

There are many reasons, but the main one is a simple one: Doctors don't ask! Most patients feel that if the doctor isn't going to ask, then why bring it up? The other reasons patients don't talk about CAM include: (a) the patient didn't think about it, (b) there wasn't enough time, (c) the patient didn't think the doctor knew about CAM or would approve, (d) the patient didn't want the doctor to know, and (e) the patient didn't think it is the doctor's business to know. When doctors are asked why they don't bring up the issue, they report similar things: (a) CAM is irrelevant to the visit, (b) they don't have enough background knowledge to talk about CAM, (c) there isn't enough scientific research about CAM, or (d) CAM is not readily available for patients.

Our research study assumes that talking about CAM is a good thing. As part of the study, we created a patient education class that focused on how patients could improve their communication about CAM. We wanted to teach patients—instead of providers—for a couple reasons. First, patients are very interested in developing their communication skills but aren't provided many opportunities to do so. Second, and perhaps most importantly, we believe that if you teach patients communication skills, they will have more control over what they say and do and therefore are more likely to have a positive communicative encounter. We worked closely with the National Center for Complementary and Alternative Medicine (NCCAM), which was promoting a public health campaign called *Time to Talk*. The campaign encouraged providers to "ASK" their patients about CAM and encouraged patients to "TELL" their providers about CAM.

The class that we designed taught patients four skills.: (1) Prepare—prepare in advance for conversations, including making a list of CAM treatments used or questions to ask; (2) Be Proactive—initiate the conversation even if providers do not; (3) Tell—disclose any and all CAM use; and (4) Ask—ask questions about current or future CAM use, especially related to any possible drug/CAM interactions. Participants watched fictionalized videos of providers and patients using these skills. The videos depicted both a positive provider response such as "Oh, that's great, keep doing that," and more negative responses like "Research shows that's a total waste of money." In the negative cases, the patient's response is helpful for patients to know what to do if providers are dismissive. For example, in the above case, the patient says something like, "Well, it may be a waste of money, but I'm asking you if you know if it's safe." The provider then responds, "Yes, it's safe," letting the patient decide whether or not to continue taking the supplement in question.

After the class, we asked participants to tell us whether they talked about CAM in their next two biomedical visits. Fifty-six percent of the participants discussed CAM in either their next one or two visits. We also asked patients to detail the conversation. From that, we were able to determine that 83% of patients were proactive and initiated the conversation; 76% used the "tell" skill of disclosing their current CAM use; and only 35% of patients "asked" a question about CAM. For those that did not discuss CAM, they reported that their provider did not ask about CAM or that CAM was not relevant to their visit.

This is a first attempt at teaching patients how to improve their communication skills about CAM. From the results, you can see that patients may still have a hard time bringing up the subject if there is a sense that it is irrelevant to the visit. From a patient-centered perspective, we believe that using CAM is an important part of a patient's history and preferences for treatment. It tells the provider that you may prefer certain forms of treatment to others. Talking about CAM gives you an opportunity to discuss those preferences.

QUESTIONS TO PONDER

1. Do you use any complementary and alternative medicine/treatments?

2. Does your biomedical provider know about your CAM use? Why or why not?

3. What questions would you like to ask your provider about CAM?

4. What advantages or disadvantages do you think there are in talking about CAM with your provider?

Source: Ho, E. Y., D'Agostino, T. A., Yadegar, V., Burke, A., & Bylund, C. L. (2012). Teaching patients how to talk with biomedical providers about their complementary and alternative medicine use. *Patient Education and Counseling, 89*, 405-410.

In addition to relationship-centered care, health communication and medical researchers also use the term patient-centered care. Patient-centered care was originally coined in 1969 by Balint as an attempt to understand the patient as a unique person and since has been conceptualized in a variety of ways. Dean and Street (2016) specify three important dimensions of patient-centeredness. The first dimension evident in the different definitions of patient-centeredness is that medical care does not focus solely on disease but also on other important "dysfunctional states" (Silverman, 1987) such as psychological, emotional, and social aspects of health and illness. The second dimension of patient-centeredness is that providers are responsible for these nonmedical issues because such issues can influence health conditions (Mead & Bower, 2000; Stewart et al., 1995). Finally, in order to enact patient-centered care, the provider must seek to view and understand the patient's condition from her perspective. So overall, patient-centered care includes four behaviors: (1) incorporating the patient's perspective through exploration of the illness experience; (2) acknowledging the importance of the psychosocial aspects of illness; (3) encouraging mutual understanding; and (4) sharing power and responsibility (Epstein et al., 2005).

Yet despite the numerous definitions and iterations of patient-centered care and communication, this chapter advocates for Epstein and Street's (2007) definition of *patient-centered care*:

- Eliciting, understanding, and validating the patient's perspective (e.g., concerns, feelings, expectations)
- Understanding the patient within his or her own psychological and social context
- Reaching a shared understanding of the patient's problem and its treatment
- Helping a patient share power by offering him or her meaningful involvement in choices relating to his or her health (p. 2).

More specifically, Epstein and Street (2007) articulate the following six key functions of patient-centered communication for patients and providers: (1) fostering healing relationships, (2) providing and receiving information, (3) responding to emotions, (4) managing uncertainty, (5) making decisions, and (6) enabling patient self-management. Figure 3.2 illustrates these six functions. Though they independently represent important communication tasks for achieving patient-centered care, in the performance of such care, these functions often overlap. Additionally, even though the provider is responsible for caregiving, the patient, the family, and the provider should work together to accomplish these functions (Dean & Street, 2016). I now describe each of these functions.

The first function of patient-centered care is *fostering healing relationships* (Epstein & Street, 2007). An effective relationship between the patient and the provider is contingent upon building rapport, developing trust and respect for each party, and having mutual understanding of roles and responsibilities (Krupat, Yeager, & Putnam, 2000; Street & De Haes, 2013; Teno, Fisher, Hamel, Coppola, & Dawson, 2002). Trust between the patient and provider is especially important to fostering a healing relationship because it affects two other patient-centered communication functions—information exchange and decision making (Gordon, Street, Sharf, Kelly, & Souchek, 2006; Salkeld, Solomon, Short, & Butow, 2004). If a patient does not trust the provider, he may not disclose vital health information or believe the provider's course of action is the

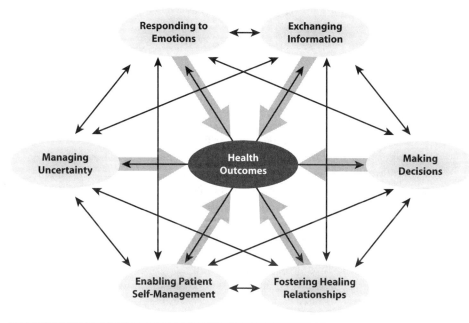

Figure 3.2   Patient-Centered Communication Functions

best option. Indeed, feeling connected to providers increases the likelihood the patient will be satisfied and therefore more likely to adhere to treatment recommendations and medical advice (Tickle-Degnen & Rosenthal, 1990). To foster a healing relationship, both the patient and the provider should build partnerships, actively listen, enact affirming verbal and nonverbal behaviors, and engage in agenda setting (i.e., crafting a plan for the future with the patient) (Street, Gordon, Ward, Krupat, & Kravitz, 2005; Street, Voigt, Geyer, Manning, & Swanson, 1995; Williams & Deci, 2001).

The second function of patient-centered care, *information exchange,* is essential to the PPI (Epstein & Street, 2007). Information exchange includes seeking information, giving information, verifying information, checking for understanding, and reaching agreement on medical decisions and plans (Cegala, 1997; Cegala, Coleman, & Turner, 1998). On the whole, physicians do more information seeking than patients, while patients tend to provide more information than physicians, and physicians verify information more than patients (Cegala, 1997). Information exchange is particularly important because it increases satisfaction, encourages participation, and enhances coping abilities (e.g., managing uncertainty and emotional distress, thus enabling the patient to focus on the task at hand) (Arraras et al., 2004; Davidson & Mills, 2005). For example, patients who are satisfied with their health outcomes tend to rate themselves as high in information seeking and their physicians as highly competent in information giving. Similarly, physicians who report satisfied patients rate themselves higher in information giving (Cegala, Coleman, & Turner, 1998). In short, patients and providers must identify each other's informational needs, understand the associated health beliefs, and manage the health information (Epstein & Street, 2007).

The third function of patient-centered care is *responding to emotions* (Epstein & Street, 2007). Because the PPI often addresses sensitive and uncomfortable topics, negative emotions such as fear, anxiety, frustration, anger, and depression may arise. Unfortunately, healthcare providers have a difficult time identifying and addressing such emotions (Dean & Street, 2014). Some reasons for this behavior include the following: not having the skills to recognize or respond to the emotions, thinking it is someone else's responsibility, or worrying that talking about the emotions will cause further distress for the patient (Butow, Brown, Cogar, Tattersall, & Dunn, 2002; Ryan et al., 2005; Zimmermann, Del Piccolo, & Finset, 2007).

In order to overcome these challenges to addressing emotions, providers can use Dean and Street's (2014) three-stage patient-centered communication model. Though a detailed description of this model is beyond the scope of this chapter, briefly, providers can engage in (1) recognition (e.g., mindfulness, self-situational awareness, actively listening, and facilitative communication), (2) exploration (e.g., acknowledge and validate emotions as well as demonstrate empathy), and (3) therapeutic action (e.g., provide interventions or referrals to manage the emotions). Overall, by identifying negative emotions, validating those emotions, and ultimately responding in appropriate ways, providers can assist patients in managing their negative emotions (Dean & Street, 2014).

The fourth function of patient-centered care, *managing uncertainty,* is important because uncertainty is inevitable in all health interactions (Babrow & Kline, 2000; Epstein & Street, 2007). An individual may be uncertain when she perceives an illness or issue that is unknown, unclear, or unpredictable (Mishel et al., 2005). Uncertainty may relate to the likelihood of future health states, conflicting evidence (or the strength of the evidence) about risk information, or unusable or unavailable scientific data (Politi, Lewis, & Frosch, 2013).

Because uncertainty is an inevitable aspect of health experiences, it is not easily eliminated and therefore must be managed (Epstein & Street, 2007). To assist patients in managing uncertainty, together, providers and patients can acknowledge and categorize the uncertainty, frame information based on what the provider knows versus what she does not know, actively listen, be empathetic, and learn particular coping strategies for their daily lives (e.g., meditation, journaling, and positive imagery and thinking) (Dean, 2014; Epstein & Street, 2007; Ryan et al., 2005).

The fifth function of patient-centered care is *making decisions* (Epstein & Street, 2007). Effective decision making encompasses information exchange, deliberation, and a final decision (Charles, Gafni, & Whelan, 1999). In order to make a high-quality decision, providers must identify and understand the patients' preferences (Janz et al., 2004). To do so, providers should ask about the patients' preferences, and patients should state their preferences. Decision making can either be paternalistic (i.e., the provider decides for the patient), shared (i.e., the provider and patient decide together), or informed (i.e., the patient decides based on information from provider and other sources) (Charles et al., 1999). To enact patient-centered decision making, providers should encourage patients' involvement and participation, accommodate preferences, and check understanding, and both providers and patients should actively listen and set an agenda together (Epstein & Street, 2007).

The sixth and final patient-centered communication function is *enabling patient self-management.* Bodenheimer and his colleagues (2002) indicate that self-management is the perceived ability of individuals to manage their illness personally by being able to identify resources and navigate the healthcare system. That is, self-management is a task patients engage in but also one that providers assist in by eliminating barriers (e.g., coordinating care or arranging referrals) and performing strategies (e.g., engaging in advocacy and supporting patient autonomy) to help patients care for themselves outside the medical encounter.

In summary, while both patient-centered and relationship-centered care emphasize the communication between patients and providers, relationship-centered care stresses the importance of the patient–provider relationship, while patient-centered care underscores communication tasks that are essential to meeting health goals and needs (see Theorizing Practice 3.2). And despite the fact that there are differing assumptions between the two types of care, overall, both "[provide] a context for understanding the ways provider-patient communication predicts outcomes, and [pose] questions for the pathways linking process and outcomes" (Duggan & Thompson, 2011, p. 419), which is explored next.

Theorizing Practice 3.2
Patient-Centered Communication

Mrs. Myers is a 74-year-old, Caucasian patient who was diagnosed with Stage III colon cancer six years ago. She received treatment at the time and has been cancer free ever since. Yesterday, she presented to the ER with shortness of breath, chest pain, coughing up blood, dry cough, and weight loss. A CT scan and a lung needle biopsy are positive for colon cancer metastasized to the lungs. The five-year prognosis is poor (around 8%) even with chemotherapy. The ER provider must now go and deliver this bad news to her, keeping in mind Mrs. Myers simply thought she had a lung infection and was waiting for antibiotics to go home. Mrs. Myers is widowed with three children and four grandchildren; does not have any other medical conditions that might be complicated by this event; and does not have any preexisting psychological problems that might be complicated by this event.

Write a conversational dialogue between the patient (Mrs. Myers) and the ER provider (you) in which you break this news. Focus specifically on incorporating patient-centered communication functions. For instance, as you write, make sure to specify what verbal statements and nonverbal behaviors relate to each function (e.g., responding to emotions = actively listening, enacting empathy, etc.).

HCIA 3.3

Cross-Cultural Care:
When Providers and Patients Do Not Share the Same Language

Elaine Hsieh

During my early days as a healthcare interpreter, I took a patient who suffered from scoliosis to visit rehab services. His illness was so advanced that his spine was bent to an extent that he would look backward as he walked forward. Upon seeing the patient, a young resident could not contain his excitement and with a big smile, he said out loud, "That's the

(continued)

worst case I've ever seen!" The comment caught me by surprise. I didn't know how to interpret the young resident's greeting. I could have interpreted it like a linguistic machine that relays information from one language to another accurately and faithfully (with equal enthusiasm), like I was taught in my professional training (i.e., interpreter-as-conduit). Yet, it felt wrong to do so. My dilemma was not caused by my lack of linguistic skills but something else.

Successful interpreter-mediated provider–patient interactions require all participants to coordinate effectively and appropriately with one another. Through the funding from the National Institutes of Health, I interviewed and surveyed providers from five clinical specialties (i.e., emergency medicine, OB/GYN, oncology, mental health, and nursing) about their needs when working with language-discordant patients. Here are some key findings:

1. Providers across different specialties share certain expectations for interpreters. For example, providers generally envision a competent interpreter as a professional who assumes the linguistic and cultural broker roles (i.e., individuals who bridge linguistic and cultural differences) without interfering with the process or content of provider–patient interactions. Providers also view interpreters as their allies and expect them to be responsible for assisting them in achieving their therapeutic agenda. It is interesting that few providers recognize these two interpreter roles as potentially competing (and even conflicting) demands (e.g., how can interpreters be neutral if she/he is also expected to side with providers?). Rather than viewing professional interpreters as the only solution, providers also strategically utilize different types of interpreters (e.g., a patient's family members or a bilingual nurse) and interpreting modalities (e.g., face-to-face interpreting, telephone interpreting, and video remote interpreting) to maintain provider–patient trust, organizational ethics, and clinical complexities.

2. Providers may hold specific expectations that are unique to their clinical contexts. For example, although nurses value interpreters' abilities to provide emotional support, many mental health providers noted that an overly friendly or supportive interpreter can prohibit provider–patient bonding and thus compromise the quality of care. In fact, some mental health providers do not even want interpreters to greet their patients. They argued that while causal greetings may appear natural in everyday social interactions, asking a war refugee about where he/she is from or how many kids she/he has may trigger unanticipated outbursts of traumatizing memories, resulting in setbacks in the therapeutic processes.

3. Language barriers often entail deeper and greater differences in areas not limited to languages. For example, a Chinese patient may use the term *"shenxu"* to describe his illness, which in English literally means weak kidney. But for male patients, this term can be used to imply various symptoms, including bodily coldness, defective cognition, erectile dysfunction, urinary frequency, among others. Although humor is valuable to promote provider–patient relationship in the U.S., providers' joking or teasing in a medical encounter can be perceived to be insensitive or patronizing in Japanese or French culture. As a result, as interpreters assist in cross-cultural care, they inevitably need to tread in the boundaries of medicine as they bridge the blurry boundaries of medicine, language, and culture.

It is essential to recognize the lack of language services as social injustice and to emphasize the need to provide interpreter services for improving language-discordant patients' quality of care and experiences of health and illness. My recent fieldwork as a Fulbright U.S. Senior Scholar found that immigrant workers from Southeast Asian countries (e.g., Thailand and Vietnam) mostly rely on their employers to be their interpreters when they first arrive in Taiwan. Because severe illness is listed as a reason for termination of their employment contracts, they may underreport the severity of their illness, seek underground care, or become undocumented to avoid deportation. When patients do not share the same language with the host society, they often experience disparities and social injustice in areas not limited to language.

As we consider the needs of language-discordant patients and identify ways to reduce disparities and challenges they face in health services, we can develop practical guidelines for meeting these needs based on my research findings and other recent studies:

- All participants need to actively discuss their communicative goals and therapeutic priorities to facilitate shared decision making. If patients do not know what to ask, how to ask, or are unaware of their rights, they may not be able to make informed decisions. Providers and interpreters need to be vigilant in ensuring that patients have sufficient knowledge and skills to exercise their autonomy in the decision-making process.

- The meanings of quality of care are contextually dependent. Providers and interpreters need to be sensitive and adaptive to meet the emerging demands. What is meaningful and appropriate in one clinical setting for a particular patient may not be applicable to another. Successful cross-cultural care is dependent on participants' ability to identify and respond to the often changing needs and priorities in a medical encounter.

QUESTIONS TO PONDER

1. Imagine that you need to seek healthcare services when visiting another country, and you also do not share the same language with your healthcare providers. How would that influence your help-seeking behaviors? What kinds of concerns would you have?

2. What are the strengths and weaknesses when a family member serves as interpreter in a healthcare setting? How about a professional interpreter? Who would be better to assist providers to take a medical history? Why is that? How about getting consent for a complex surgery? Again, why?

3. Do you think a doctor and a patient may have different preferences about the type of interpreters to be used during a medical encounter? Why? Would the specific tasks to be accomplished (e.g., discussing end-of-life decision making versus getting a flu shot) influence their preferences? If they have different preferences, who should decide which type of interpreter to use? Why?

Source: Hsieh, E. (2016). *Bilingual health communication: Working with interpreters in cross-cultural care.* New York, NY: Routledge.

Health Outcomes

Dr. Austen's communication with Hannah demonstrates a pathway in which communication affects health outcomes. In particular, through Dr. Austen's provision (and framing) of information about Hannah's genetic risk as well as their decision-making partnership regarding the variety of health options, Hannah gained knowledge about the complexities of her genetic test results and managed her uncertainty about the future. She then made the informed health decision to undergo a preventative double mastectomy now but wait a few more years before undergoing a preventative oophorectomy. Moreover, Dr. Austen's active listening, empathetic communication, and validation of emotions made Hannah feel known and comforted as well as feel a greater sense of control, ultimately enhancing her emotional well-being. In short, Hannah was able to cope—engaging in the cognitive and behavioral ways to manage, reduce, and/or tolerate both internal and external demands of threatening experiences [Bussell & Naus, 2010].

It is important, though, to not forget about Alison. From Mrs. Stanley's family health experiences, it is clear there are different preferences when it comes to dealing with cancer risk and health in general. While Hannah took an active approach in dealing with her high cancer risk, Alison chose not to seek information and ultimately avoided her genetic makeup as her way of coping. Though a different pathway, Alison's avoidance enabled her to achieve her own health goal—forgetting her genetic test results for now.

Health outcomes from a biomedical perspective refer to survival (i.e., early detection, accurate diagnosis, and treatment), while health outcomes from a biopsychosocial perspective refer to health-related quality of life (i.e., physical, cognitive, social functioning, and emotional well-being) (Epstein & Street, 2007). There are two ways to think about the relationship between communication and health outcomes. First, communication has a *direct effect* on health outcomes. Indeed, it is commonly argued that there is a connection between patient–provider communication and health outcomes (see, for example, Arora, 2003; Epstein & Street, 2007; Jackson, 2005; Kaplan, Greenfield, & Ware, 1989; Stewart, 1995; Stewart et al., 2000). Previous research indicates that effective communication produces better outcomes for patients' emotional, psychological, and functional health (Duggan & Thompson, 2011); increases patients' compliance to medical decisions and treatment (Wagner, Lentz, & Heslop, 2002); and has implications for the quality of patient care (Roter & Hall, 2011). Certainly, one of the most commonly cited arguments for the importance of effective communication in health contexts is that communication failures are the main cause for medical errors in patient care (Leonard, Graham, & Bonacum, 2004; Patterson, Cook, Woods, & Render, 2004).

Research that suggests this direct connection between communication and better health outcomes, like the above examples, tends to fall into two main categories (Street, Makoul, Arora, & Epstein, 2009). The first is randomized controlled trials (RCTs), which examine interventions designed to improve communication and decision making between providers and patients. Unfortunately, despite such efforts, fewer than half of these interventions have improved health outcomes (see Griffin et al., 2004 for a review). Cross-sectional, descriptive research studies comprise the second group. Some of these studies argue for correlations between patient–provider communication and health outcomes, while others report no connection to conflicting results regarding this relationship. For example, one such study by Fogarty, Curbow, Wingard, McDonnell, and Sommerfield (1999) found that female breast cancer patients and survivors reported decreased anxiety when their providers communicated empathetic expressions. However, more often than not, researchers do not test hypotheses that explain how communication may impact patients' health outcomes. Rather, the association between communication and health outcomes is assumed rather than empirically supported (Street et al., 2009). This leads us to the second way to think about this relationship.

In an effort to address this discrepancy in medical and health communication research, Street and his colleagues (2009) argue that communication has an *indirect effect* on health outcomes, meaning there are proximal and intermediate factors that serve as the mediators between communication and health outcomes (see Figure 3.3). Particular communication behaviors include the six previously discussed patient-centered communication functions—fostering relationships, exchanging information, responding to emotions, managing uncertainty, making decisions, and enabling patient self-management. Patient–provider agreement, understanding, trust, rapport, "feeling known," patient involvement, and satisfaction are examples of proximal outcomes. Intermediate outcomes then encompass factors such as care access, quality decisions, emotional management, social support, self-care skills, and treatment commitment. Last, possible health outcomes include, but are not limited to, the following: survival or cure, reduction in suffering, pain management and functional ability, emotional well-being, and quality of life.

In addition to these foundational concepts, Street et al. (2009) propose the following specific pathways that link health outcomes and communication: "(1) access to needed care, (2) increased patient knowledge and shared understanding, (3) enhancing therapeutic alliances (among clinicians, patients, and family), (4) enhancing emotional self-management, (5) activating social support and advocacy resources, (6) increasing the quality of medical decisions (e.g., informed, clinically sound, concordant with patient values, and mutually endorsed), and (7) enabling patient agency (self-efficacy and empowerment)" (p. 297). These pathways serve as avenues for future research examining the relationship between patient-centered communication and overall health outcomes.

Following this call for research to test hypotheses between communication and health outcomes, two recent studies provide good examples of this indirect pathway. The first study analyzed providers' decision-making communication styles with cancer survivors and improving quality of life and mental health. Arora, Weaver, Clayman, Oakley-Girvan, and Potosky (2009) found that providers who engaged in a participatory decision-making style significantly increased cancer survivors' self-efficacy and personal control as well as enhanced trust and reduced uncertainty. There-

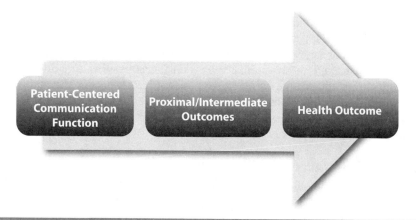

Figure 3.3   Communication's Indirect Effect on Health Outcomes

fore, they concluded that participatory decision-making communication facilitates patient empowerment and overall health-related quality of life. In the second example, Street, Cox, Kallen, and Suarez-Almazor (2012) tested the pathway of acupuncturists' optimistic communication regarding treatment effectiveness and satisfaction. The authors found patients experienced better health outcomes (e.g., pain and function management) and were more satisfied when their acupuncturists engaged in optimistic communication, thus supporting an indirect association between communication and health outcomes.

In short, the relationship between communication and health outcomes is essential to the PPI. Indeed, identifying desired health outcomes and then working backwards (e.g., intermediate factors, then proximal factors, and then patient-centered communication functions) may assist researchers and practitioners in better understanding this relationship in the hopes of improving health outcomes overall. Now, Theorizing Practice 3.3 invites you to explore indirect pathways between communication and patient health outcomes in a healthcare context of your choosing.

Theorizing Practice 3.3
Communication Pathways to Better Health Outcomes

Identify a particular healthcare context (e.g., cancer, end-of-life, ER, primary care) and hypothesize an *indirect pathway* between communication and patient health outcomes. Be able to explain why the pathway may be indirect versus direct.

■ Conclusion

Upon reflection on Mrs. Stanley's and her daughters' health experiences, it is clear that communication between herself, her daughters, and their providers will be essential to all family members' survival and emotional well-being. They will have to engage in verbal and nonverbal communication in order to create shared meaning about their health goals and needs, understand each others' unique situations, exchange information, make particular health decisions, respond to negative emotions, and engage in self-management. Furthermore, their providers should display relationship- and patient-centered care, rooted in the biopsychosocial model of medicine, to accomplish holistic, effective healthcare delivery for Mrs. Stanley and her family. Finally, all parties should pay particular attention to the ways in which communication has an impact on health outcomes.

Discussion Questions

1. Based on your own experiences with healthcare providers, why is communication so important to the patient–provider encounter? In contrast, can you think of a medical situation in which effective communication may be unnecessary?

2. Explain how the five contexts of the ecological model of health communication work together to influence patient–provider interactions. From your own experience, do you think there are any missing factors that influence patient–provider interactions in positive and negative ways?

3. Think back to a recent encounter you (or a family member) had with a healthcare provider. How would you characterize the interaction? In other words, did the provider demonstrate communication that fit within a biomedical model of medicine or a biopsychosocial model of medicine when practicing care?

4. Reflect on a personal health experience where your healthcare provider enacted patient-centered care. Can you identify and describe any specific patient-centered verbal and nonverbal communication behaviors of the provider? Also, how did you engage in patient-centered care for yourself?

5. Based on this chapter, what information can you take away to assist you in future health interactions? In other words, how can you be a proactive, empowered patient?

REFERENCES

Arora, N. K. (2003). Interacting with cancer patients: The significance of physicians' communication behavior. *Social Science & Medicine, 57*, 791–806.

Arora, N. K., Weaver, K. E., Clayman, M. L., Oakley-Girvan, I., & Potosky, A. L. (2009). Physicians' decision-making style and psychosocial outcomes among cancer survivors. *Patient Education and Counseling, 77,* 404–412.

Arraras, J. I., Wright, S., Greimel, E., Holzner, B., Kuljanic-Vlasic, K., Velikova, G., . . . Visser, A. (2004). Development of a questionnaire to evaluate the information needs of cancer patients: The EORTC questionnaire. *Patient Education and Counseling, 54,* 235–241.

Ashton, C. M., Haidet, P., Paterniti, D. A., Collins, T. C., Gordon, H. S., O'Malley, K., . . . Street, R. L., Jr. (2003). Racial and ethnic disparities in the use of health services. *Journal of General Internal Medicine, 18,* 146–152.

Ayantunde, A. A., Welch, N. T., & Parsons, S. L. (2007). A survey of patient satisfaction and use of the Internet for health information. *International Journal of Clinical Practice, 61,* 458–462.

Babrow, A. S., & Kline, K. N. (2000). From 'reducing' to 'coping with' uncertainty: Reconceptualizing the central challenge in breast self-exams. *Social Science and Medicine, 51,* 1805–1816.

Balint, E. (1969). The possibilities of patient-centered medicine. *British Journal of General Practice, 17,* 269–276.

Barbour, J., Gill, R., & Dean, M. (2016). Work space, gendered occupations, and the organization of health: Redesigning emergency department communication. In T. Harrison & E. Williams (Eds.), *Organizations, health, and communication* (pp. 101–118). New York, NY: Routledge.

Barr, M. S. (2008). The need to test the patient-centered medical home. *Journal of American Medical Association, 300,* 834–835.

Beach, M. C., Roter, D. L., Wang, N. Y., Duggan, P. S., & Cooper, L. A. (2006). Are physicians' attitudes of respect accurately perceived by patients and associated with more positive communication behaviors? *Patient Education and Counseling, 62,* 347–354.

Bodenheimer, T., Lorig, K., Holman, H., & Grumbach, K. (2002). Patient self-management of chronic disease in primary care. *Journal of the American Medical Association, 288,* 2469–2475.

Bussell, V. A., & Naus, M. J. (2010). A longitudinal investigation of coping and posttraumatic growth in breast cancer survivors. *Journal of Psychosocial Oncology, 28,* 61–78.

Butow, P. N., Brown, R. F., Cogar, S., Tattersall, M. H. N., & Dunn, S. M. (2002). Oncologists' reactions to cancer patients' verbal cues. *Psycho-Oncology, 11,* 47–58.

Bylund, C. L., Gueguen, J. A., Sabee, C. M., Imes, R. S., Li, Y., & Sanford, A. A. (2007). Provider-patient dialogue about Internet health information: An exploration of strategies to improve the provider-patient relationship. *Patient Education and Counseling, 66,* 346–352.

Caiata-Zufferey, M., & Schulz, P. J. (2012). Physicians' communicative strategies in interacting with Internet-informed patients: Results from a qualitative study. *Health Communication, 27,* 738–749.

Cegala, D. J. (1997). A study of doctors' and patients' communication during a primary care consultation: Implications. *Journal of Health Communication, 2,* 169–194.

Cegala, D. J., Coleman, M. T., & Turner, J. W. (1998). The development and partial assessment of the medical communication competence scale. *Health Communication, 10,* 261–288.

Charles, C., Gafni, A., & Whelan, T. (1999). Decision-making in the physician-patient encounter: Revisiting the shared treatment decision-making model. *Social Science and Medicine, 49,* 651–661.

Davidson, R., & Mills, M. E. (2005). Cancer patients' satisfaction with communication, information and quality of care in a UK region. *European Journal of Cancer Care, 14,* 83–90.

Dean, M. (2014). *"It's not if I get cancer, it's when": Exploring previvors' management of uncertainty for hereditary cancer in clinical encounters.* (Unpublished doctoral dissertation). Texas A&M University, College Station, TX.

Dean, M., & Oetzel, J. G. (2014). Physicians' perspectives of managing tensions around dimensions of effective communication in the emergency department. *Health Communication, 29,* 257–266.

Dean, M., Oetzel, J. G., & Sklar, D. P. (2014). Communication in acute ambulatory care. *Academic Medicine, 89,* 1617–1622.

Dean, M., & Street, R. L., Jr. (2014). A three-stage model of patient-centered communication for addressing cancer patients' emotional distress. *Patient Education and Counseling, 94,* 143–148.

Dean, M., & Street, R. L., Jr. (2016). Patient-centered communication. In E. Wittenberg, B. Ferrell, J. Goldsmith, T. Smith, S. Ragan, M. Glajchen, & G. Handzo (Eds.), *Textbook of palliative care communication* (pp. 238–245). New York, NY: Oxford University Press.

Duggan, A. (2014). Patient and relationship-centered communication and medicine. In T. Thompson (Ed.), *SAGE encyclopedia of health communication* (pp. 1029–1032). Thousand Oaks, CA: Sage.

Duggan, A. P., & Thompson, T. L. (2011). Provider–patient interaction and related outcomes. In T. L. Thompson, R. Parrott, & J. F. Nussbaum (Eds.), *The Routledge handbook of health communication* (2nd ed., pp. 414–427). New York, NY: Routledge.

du Pré, A. (2013). *Communicating about health: Current issues and perspectives* (4th ed.). New York, NY: Oxford University Press.

Engel, G. L. (1977). The need for a new medical model: A challenge for biomedicine. *Science, 196,* 129–136.

Engel, G. L. (1980). The clinical application of the biopsychosocial model. *The American Journal of Psychiatry, 13,* 535–544.

Epstein, R. M., Franks, P., Fiscella, K., Shields, C. G., Meldrum, S. C., Kravitz, R. L., & Duberstein, P. R. (2005). Measuring patient-centered communication in patient–physician consultations: theoretical and practical issues. *Social Science and Medicine, 61,* 1516–1528.

Epstein, R. M., & Street, R. L., Jr. (2007). *Patient-centered communication in cancer care: Promoting healing and reducing suffering.* Bethesda, MD: National Cancer Institute. [NIH Publication No. 07-6225].

Fadiman, A. (1997). *The spirit catches you and you fall down: A Hmong child, her American doctors, and the collision of two cultures.* New York, NY: The Noonday Press.

Fogarty, L. A., Curbow, B. A., Wingard, J. R., McDonnell, K., & Somerfield, M. R. (1999). Can 40s of compassion reduce patient anxiety? *Journal of Clinical Oncology, 17,* 371–379.

Fortin, A., Dwamena, F. C., Smith, R. C., & Frankel, R. M. (2012). *Smith's patient centered interviewing: An evidence-based method* (3rd ed.). New York, NY: McGraw Hill Professional.

Friedman, S., Sutphen, R., & Steligo, K. (2012). *Confronting hereditary breast and ovarian cancer: Identify your risk, understand your options, change your destiny.* Baltimore, MD: Johns Hopkins University Press.

Geist-Martin, P., Ray, E. B., & Sharf, B. (2011). *Communicating health: Personal, cultural, and political complexities.* Long Grove, IL: Waveland Press.

Gordon, H. S., Street, R. L., Jr., Sharf, B. F., Kelly, P. A., & Souchek, J. (2006). Racial differences in trust and lung cancer patients' perceptions of physician communication. *Journal of Clinical Oncology, 24,* 904–909.

Griffin, S. J., Kinmonth, A. L., Veltman, M. W., Gillard, S., Grant, J., & Stewart, M. (2004). Effect on health-related outcomes of interventions to alter the interaction between patients and practitioners: A systematic review of trials. *Annals of Family Medicine, 2,* 595–608.

Hall, E. T. (1976). *Beyond culture.* New York, NY: Doubleday.

Jackson, J. L. (2005). Communication about symptoms in primary care: Impact on patient outcomes. *Journal of Alternative and Complementary Medicine, 11,* S51–S60.

Janz, N. K., Wren, P. A., Copeland, L. A., Lowery, J. C., Goldfarb, S. L., & Wilkins, E. G. (2004). Patient-physician concordance: Preferences, perceptions, and factors influencing the breast cancer surgical decision. *Journal of Clinical Oncology, 22,* 3091–3098.

Kaplan, S. H., Greenfield, S., & Ware, J. E., Jr. (1989). Assessing the effects of physician-patient interactions on the outcomes of chronic disease. *Medical Care, 27,* S110–S127.

Kleinman, A. (1980). *Patients and healers in the context of culture: An exploration of the borderland between anthropology, medicine, and psychiatry* (Vol. 3). Los Angeles: University of California Press.

Kleinman, A. (1988). *The illness narratives: Suffering, healing, & the human condition.* New York, NY: Basic Books.

Krupat, E., Yeager, C. M., & Putnam, S. (2000). Patient role orientations, doctor-patient fit, and visit satisfaction. *Psychology and Health, 15,* 707–719.

Lare, K. M. (1997). Better health care legislation. *Michigan Medicine, 96,* 26–27.

Leonard, M., Graham, S., & Bonacum, D. (2004). The human factor: The critical importance of effective teamwork and communication in providing safe care. *Quality & Safety in Health Care, 13*(suppl 1), i85–i90.

Mead, N., & Bower, P. (2000). Patient-centredness: A conceptual framework and review of the empirical literature. *Social Science and Medicine, 51,* 1087–1110.

Mishel, M. H., Germino, B. B., Gil, K. M., Belyea, M., Laney, I. C., Stewart, J., . . . Clayton, M. (2005). Benefits from an uncertainty management intervention for African-American and Caucasian older long-term breast cancer survivors. *Psycho-Oncology, 14,* 962–978.

Oetzel, J. G. (2009). *Layers of intercultural communication.* New York, NY: Vango Books.

Patterson, E. S., Cook, R. I., Woods, D. D., & Render, M. L. (2004). Examining the complexity behind a medication error: Generic patterns in communication. *IEEE Transactions on Systems, Man, & Cyberenetics—Part A: Systems & Humans, 34,* 749–756.

Politi, M. C., Lewis, C. L., & Frosch, D. L. (2013). Supporting shared decisions when clinical evidence is low. *Medical Care Research and Review, 70,* 113S–128S.

Rider, E. A., & Keefer, C. H. (2006). Communication skills competencies: Definitions and a teaching toolbox. *Medical Education, 40,* 624–629.

Roter, D. L., & Hall, J. A. (2011). How medical interaction shapes and reflects the physician-patient relationship. In T. L. Thompson, R. Parrott, & J. F. Nussbaum (Eds.), *The Routledge handbook of health communication* (2nd ed., pp. 55–68). New York, NY: Routledge.

Roter, D. L., Frankel, R. M., Hall, J. A., & Sluyter, D. (2006). The expression of emotion through nonverbal behavior in medical visits. *Journal of General Internal Medicine, 21,* S28–S34.

Ryan, H., Schofield, P., Cockburn, J., Butow, P., Tattersall, M., Turner, J., . . . Bowman, D. (2005). How to recognize and manage psychological distress in cancer patients. *European Journal of Cancer Care, 14,* 7–15.

Salkeld, G., Solomon, M., Short, L., & Butow, P. N. (2004). A matter of trust—patient's views on decision-making in colorectal cancer. *Health Expectations, 7,* 104–114.

Silverman, D. (1987). *Communication and medical practice: Social relations in the clinic.* London, UK: Sage.

Sparks, L., & Villagran, M. (2010). *Patient and provider interaction: A global health communication perspective.* Malden, MA: Polity Press.

Stewart, M., Brown, J. B., Donner, A., McWhinney, I. R., Oates, J., Weston, W. W., & Jordan, J. (2000). The impact of patient-centered care on outcomes. *Journal of Family Practice, 49,* 796–804.

Stewart, M., Brown, J., Weston W., McWhinney, I., McWilliam, C., & Freeman, T. (1995). *Patient-centered medicine: Transforming the clinical method.* London, UK: Sage.

Stewart, M. A. (1995). Effective physician–patient communication and health outcomes: A review. *Canadian Medical Association Journal, 152,* 1423–33.

Street, R. L., Jr. (2003). Communication in medical encounters: An ecological perspective. In T. L. Thompson, A. Dorsey, K. I. Miller, & R. Parrott (Eds.), *Handbook of health communication* (1st ed., pp. 63–89). Mahwah, NJ: Lawrence Erlbaum.

Street, R. L., Jr., Cox, V., Kallen, M. A., & Suarez-Almazor, M. E. (2012). Exploring communication pathways to better health: Clinician communication of expectations for acupuncture effectiveness. *Patient Education and Counseling, 89,* 245–251.

Street, R. L., Jr., & De Haes, H. C. (2013). Designing a curriculum for communication skills training from a theory and evidence-based perspective. *Patient Education and Counseling, 93,* 27–33.

Street, R. L., Jr., Gordon, H. S., Ward, M. M., Krupat, E., & Kravitz, R. L. (2005). Patient participation in medical consultations: Why some patients are more involved than others. *Medical Care, 43,* 960–969.

Street, R. L., Jr., Makoul, G., Arora, N. K., & Epstein, R. M. (2009). How does communication heal? Pathways linking clinician-patient communication to health outcomes. *Patient Education and Counseling, 74,* 295–301.

Street, R. L., Jr., Voigt, B., Geyer, C., Jr., Manning, T., & Swanson, G. P. (1995). Increasing patient involvement in choosing treatment for early breast cancer. *Cancer, 76,* 2275–2285.

Teno, J. M., Fisher, E. S., Hamel, M. B., Coppola, K., & Dawson, N. V. (2002). Medical care inconsistent with patients' treatment goals: Association with 1-year Medicare resource use and survival. *Journal of American Geriatric Society, 50,* 496–500.

Tickle-Degnen, L., & Rosenthal, R. (1990). The nature of rapport and its nonverbal correlates. *Psychological Inquiry, 1,* 285–293.

Wagner, P. J., Lentz, L., & Heslop, S. D. (2002). Teaching communication skills: A skills-based approach. *Academic Medicine, 77,* 1164.

Williams, G. C., & Deci, E. L. (2001). Activating patients for smoking cessation through physician autonomy support. *Medical Care, 39,* 813–823.

Zimmermann, C., Del Piccolo, L., & Finset, A. (2007). Cues and concerns by patients in medical consultations: A literature review. *Psychology Bulletin, 133,* 438–463.

4

Communicating
Healthcare Teamwork

Laura L. Ellingson & Kristian G. E. Borofka

"Are you asleep?" Laura asked softly as she approached Mrs. Albright's chair. All dialysis patients sit in upholstered reclining chairs with their feet elevated during treatment to help maintain their blood pressure as their blood circulates through the filtering machines that approximate the function of kidneys for patients with end-stage renal disease. The middle-aged woman had her eyes closed, but Laura had learned that she often closed them without sleeping. Indeed, when Laura told Mrs. Albright that she hadn't talked to her during one previous research visit because she was afraid she would wake her, the patient had scolded Laura for assuming she'd rather sleep than chat.

At the sound of Laura's voice, Mrs. Albright's eyes popped open, and her lushly painted, hot-pink lips curved into a smile. "Hello!" she said. "You came to see me!" She blinked as she readjusted to the bright fluorescent lights and scanned the busy room full of dialysis patients, patient care technicians, and other healthcare providers.

"Yes, I always have time to chat on Tuesdays," Laura replied, pulling a rolling stool over and sitting down. "It's nice to see you," she added.

Mrs. Albright reached down into her tote bag and said, "You too. I had my husband pick you some lemons, after our conversation last week." Smiling, she held out a plastic grocery bag bulging with lemons from her prolific tree.

"Oh, that was so nice of you," said Laura, touched that the older woman had remembered. Laura set the bag on the floor by her feet. "Thank you so much. We'll enjoy those. I'll have to make lemonade or lemon curd. So what have you been up to?"

"Well, you know, my husband finally took me shopping, and I ordered a new outfit for Mother's Day. We're going to see my older son and his family, you know, and we'll all have dinner that day, so of course I need something new to wear." Mrs. Albright smiled impishly.

Laura laughed. "Well, naturally! Any excuse for a new outfit is a good one." At the moment, Mrs. Albright looked cheerful and comfortable in one of her many expensive but casual track suits, this one in a shade of pink that coordinated with her lipstick.

"We're going to The Hacienda. I can't wait," Mrs. Albright explained, proceeding to detail everything she expected to eat, not one item of which conformed to either the guidelines for man-

aging her diabetes or the dietary restrictions for dialysis. "Oh, there's Tim! Can you wait just a second, Laura?" Not waiting for a reply, Mrs. Albright waved to her patient care technician, Tim, watching him intently and trying to catch his eye. "Tim!" she called.

Tim nodded at Mrs. Albright and held up his index finger. "Just a minute," he replied, turning to press a series of buttons on the touch screen of a dialysis machine.

"Oh good," said Mrs. Albright. "I want to talk to him about having more weight taken off. I want to go up to four kilograms."

Laura was puzzled and asked, "Your doctor wants you to have more fluid removed during your treatments?"

Mrs. Albright shook her head. "Well, she didn't say. But I would really like to be able to fit into that new outfit. I'd like it if they took more weight off."

Laura was not sure how to respond. She knew that Peter, the unit social worker, had carefully explained how dialysis works before Mrs. Albright started treatment (as he did with all patients and their families), and while she was no expert on the technical details of dialysis, even Laura knew that fluid removal was monitored quite precisely to ensure that the patient's "dry weight" remained stable and only excess fluid was removed. "Um, they don't remove fat, you know. Just fluid and waste stuff, toxins in your blood, that kind of thing. Not your real weight, you know?" She hesitated, not wanting to offend.

Laura's favorite patient stopped smiling at her. "They remove weight every time I come here, three times a week."

"Ah, I think they have to have orders from your doctor on how much fluid to take off," Laura said tentatively. Surely she didn't think dialysis functioned as a weight loss method, or that the amount removed each time was arbitrarily determined by the patient's wishes? Mrs. Albright frowned at Laura steadily and with a shrug, Laura retreated in cowardice. "Well, I don't know how all that works, you know," she said. "You should talk to Tim."

Laura was rewarded with a nod and small smile. "Yes. I will, as soon as Tim gets over here. He's busy today, seems a little grumpy. Did I tell you Bob took me to the Rib Shack for dinner last night? We had baby back ribs and coleslaw and corn bread—it was delicious."

"Oh that sounds wonderful!" said Laura, thinking to herself, and non-adherent with your treatment regime. "I made fish last night, with zucchini. Not as exciting as what you had."

"But better for you," Mrs. Albright said, shrugging. Unable to walk more than a few yards at a time, fatigued by the symptoms of kidney failure, suffering from intense side effects of dialysis treatments, and left home alone much of the time while her husband worked, Mrs. Albright clearly felt eating was one of her few remaining pleasures. She had told Laura previously that she enjoyed coming to the dialysis unit since it got her out of the house and gave her a chance to talk to people. Her evident pleasure in Laura's visits as she conducted an ethnographic study in the dialysis unit was gratifying but also a poignant reminder of how little social interaction the woman had. Laura did not want to ruin their chat or denigrate Mrs. Albright's need for pleasurable eating by pushing her to conform to the dietary guidelines, but Laura felt guilty and worried about the patient's health.

"And how's your kitty doing?" Laura asked, changing the topic.

"Oh, Ginger is fine, sleeps with me every night," replied Mrs. Albright, smiling broadly, warming to her topic. "Yesterday she—Oh, Tim," she said as he approached. "I want you to increase the amount of weight you remove today."

Tim looked at her blankly and turned to check the display screen of her dialysis machine. "I can't change the amount. Got to have a doctor's order."

"My doctor said it would be okay," said Mrs. Albright. Laura looked at her, wondering if that was true.

"I'll ask Gabriella," Tim replied, referring to the registered nurse who was the charge nurse that day. He wandered off without another word.

"Humph," said Mrs. Albright. Laura saw Tim approach Gabriella and watched as they talked.

Mrs. Albright and Laura continued to discuss their cats until Gabriella came over and stood by Mrs. Albright's feet.

"I called and left a message," said Gabriella. Mrs. Albright nodded. "But I can't increase the amount of fluid we remove without an order. What did she say last time you saw her?"

Mrs. Albright set her mouth in a stubborn line. "I told her I wanted more taken off, and she said it would be fine."

"Well, I checked the faxes, and we didn't receive anything from her," said Gabriella, smiling but speaking firmly. "I'll let you know when I hear back from her, but I can't change anything until then. Okay?"

Mrs. Albright sighed, clearly displeased. "All right," she said begrudgingly.

"I have to go," said Gabriella, hurrying away as she was paged over the intercom to take a phone call. Mrs. Albright turned back to Laura and began describing Ginger's latest kitty antics, and Laura smiled sheepishly at Gabriella as the nurse moved off. Out of Mrs. Albright's sight, Gabriella caught Laura's eye and shook her head and shrugged, then smiled at Laura before moving to the nurse's station.

An hour later, Laura was stuffing her lab coat into the laundry bag in the dialysis unit's back hall as she did after each visit to her research site, when she saw Anne, the unit's registered dietician, walking down the hall with Peter, the social worker.

Laura joined them as Peter said, "Just had a nice chat with Mrs. Albright."

Anne rolled her eyes and asked, "You talked to her?"

"Yeah, we chat almost every week."

"Does she tell you about what she's eating? Her levels are really high; her labs [blood test results] are not good. And I tell her, 'You aren't watching what you eat.' Too much sodium, too much liquids." Anne shook her head, looking both annoyed and worried.

Laura flushed guiltily, remembering how quick she was to give up trying to persuade Mrs. Albright to be more reasonable in her eating. Peter nodded. "Yes, she tells me about all her meals out—really rich stuff, lots of sodium, alcohol, whatever."

Anne sighed. "She is clearly noncompliant."

Peter looked thoughtful. "It helps to remember that Mrs. Albright is proud of being in charge and in control. She would rather be in control than be compliant." As a social worker, Peter spent time talking with each patient about how they coped personally with kidney failure and dialysis, and how their friends and families handled their condition.

Anne shrugged. "Yeah. Well, she is very definite about making her own choices. I tried to suggest that this is not the best for her, explained again how nutrition relates to kidney failure and dialysis treatment, but she didn't want to hear it. She was in the hospital again last month. Complications," said Anne. Shaking her head, she added, "It's not up to me—I do what I can to explain."

"She wants the technicians to remove more weight so she can be thinner," added Peter with a smile.

Anne laughed. "Oh yes, she wants to lose more weight. She lost some weight last time she was in the hospital." Anne shook her head in dismay and then shrugged. "There is only so much I can do."

"Yeah, that makes sense," Peter said gently.

"I've to go run and pick up my kids. See you tomorrow," said Anne, nodding to Laura then heading into her office.

"See you later," Laura said to both of them.

In providing dialysis care, the patient care technicians, nurses, social worker, and dietitian work as a team. That is, they each utilize specialized skills acquired through their disparate educations and training programs to care for patients undergoing routine dialysis treatment. Healthcare providers pool their complementary perspectives in order to provide the most holistic, comprehensive care possible. Laura, the researcher in the story, was not formally part of the team or the organization. A communication professor at a local university, Laura had received permission from the management team to conduct ethnographic fieldwork (i.e., observation and informal interactions with patients and staff) to study collaboration among dialysis staff and its relationship to staff members' communication with patients (Ellingson, 2007, 2008, 2011, 2015). Collaboration and teamwork can be very challenging to accomplish. In this chapter, we will explore what makes a healthcare team, how healthcare providers are socialized into the norms and cultures of their professions, how teams made of up different types of professionals may collaborate, and how communication on teams can be improved.

■ What Is a Healthcare Team?

A *team* is three or more people working in "a group intended to achieve high levels of solidarity, purpose, and unity, whether or not it actually does so" (Poole & Real, 2003, p. 370). Healthcare teams may be made up of one type of professional—such as nurses—but more commonly are made up of providers from a variety of professions, including nurses, physicians, clinical social workers, dieticians, pharmacists, psychologists, as well as *paraprofessional* staff, including nursing assistants and technicians (Apker, 2012). Multidisciplinary and interdisciplinary teams are prevalent in areas such as geriatrics (older adults), neurology (brain injuries and degenerative diseases, such as multiple sclerosis), oncology (cancer), physical medicine and rehabilitation, and nephrology (kidney disease). In the opening narrative, the team includes registered nurses (one of whom is also the charge nurse for the clinic), patient care technicians, a clinical social worker, a registered dietician, and physicians (who conduct brief monthly visits with patients and are available to nurses via telephone).

Teamwork is challenging, in part because the professionals and paraprofessionals who collaborate on teams often have contrasting styles of caregiving and may differ significantly on the perceived goals of treatment. For example, a social worker who is concerned about patients' abilities to cope emotionally and to maintain supportive relationships with family and friends while undergoing treatment may think that honoring a patient's request for a treatment schedule change is important for emotional and relational reasons. At the same time, a physician, whose main concern is keeping regular and consistent removal of toxins in the patient's blood through dialysis, may resist changing a scheduled appointment to facilitate an important family event. How effectively do teams of different types of professionals function to deliver patient care?

Three areas of group performance that researchers measure to determine effectiveness are productivity, group maintenance, and member need satisfaction (Poole & Real, 2003). *Productivity* reflects the quantity, quality, and efficiency of the team's work (i.e., delivering patient treatment, as in the narrative). *Group maintenance* involves continual improvement and increased integration of team members into a coherent group that works well together. *Member need satisfaction* is the extent to which the team meets members' needs for work satisfaction in their individual roles and in their ability to make a contribution to the team's collective success, while minimizing unhealthy stress and burnout.

Barriers to teams' success in all three of these areas are complex and varied, and they are rooted in the fundamental differences in the ways in which healthcare providers are educated and socialized into their professional roles. Three key concepts help clarify what teams are intended to do structurally by bringing together members of different disciplines to collaborate (Poole & Real, 2003). *Boundedness* concerns the degree to which the team is administratively self-contained, with one or more supervisors to whom members report within the team, rather than members reporting primarily to the heads of each discipline's department. So, for example, the patient care technicians reported to the registered nurses who lead their dialysis teams, rather than to the unit's chief technician, an indicator of a higher degree of boundedness for the teams. *Centralization* of power reflects the concentration of decision-making authority within one or a few team members. With less centralization, power is more evenly spread in a more egalitarian manner among team members. Power was shared fairly equally among professionals in the dialysis unit, but that privilege was not extended to the paraprofessional staff. Patient care technicians, paraprofessional workers who attended certificate training programs, passed a licensing exam, and underwent extensive on-the-job training, enjoyed significantly less decision-making authority and autonomy than did the professionals, all of whom obtained significantly more formal higher education and earned degrees before training in dialysis. Registered nurses held supervisory power over patient care technicians, and the registered nurses, clinical social worker, registered dietitian, and head technician all reported directly to the unit's nurse manager. The nurse manager in turn reported to the physician-directors/franchisees who co-owned and operated the unit, one of a chain of freestanding dialysis units.

A third key team concept is *diversity*, or the degree of similarity among team members, including the variety of disciplines, status levels, and significant demographic categories such as gender and race (Poole & Real, 2003, pp. 374–375). Located in a diverse metropolitan area on the West Coast with a high cost of living, the dialysis unit employed people from a variety of ethnic and racial groups, primarily first- and second-generation Mexican, Portuguese, Chinese, Vietnamese, Filipino, and Japanese immigrants; the same groups were represented among their patients. At any one time, there were often seven or more languages being spoken in the unit. Women and men were represented roughly equally among the staff, although it is noteworthy that all of the registered nurses—and hence all supervisors—were women, and the two physician-directors were men. White, European Americans made up a minority of healthcare providers and patients. Many, but certainly not all, of the patients were from economically disadvantaged and working-class households.

Differences in power, ethnic and racial identity, gender, age, and level of educational attainment formed the context within which the dialysis healthcare providers created, sustained, resisted, and even transformed their unit's professional culture and communication norms and patterns. In addition to differences related to identity categories, team communication is also profoundly shaped by the theory and practice of professional fields in which they are trained. Now, consider your own perceptions of healthcare teams in Theorizing Practice 4.1.

Theorizing Practice 4.1
Patients' Perceptions of the Healthcare Team

Think back to a time when you have been a patient or have visited a friend or family member who was a patient in a hospital setting. In this context, many healthcare providers, some wearing uniforms or special attire (e.g., white coats or colored scrubs) or using specialized equipment, enter the patient's room for various purposes and functions.

1. Were you aware of the role each of these professionals or paraprofessionals played and the special expertise or functions each performed for you or your loved one or friend?

2. What did you observe about the way these health providers interacted with one another?

3. What assumptions did you make about which of these providers had the most authority about specific issues (such as obtaining medications, addressing pain or other worrisome symptoms, and arranging for discharge)? Based on what evidence?

4. Did you feel these individuals functioned as a team as has been discussed in this chapter? Why or why not? And if the answer is yes, what level of teamwork did you experience or observe?

■ Professional Socialization

People often take for granted that the way things currently are organized is how they should or must be organized. In understanding how different types of healthcare providers work together, it helps to keep in mind that the U.S. system of healthcare delivery is the culmination of a series of historical events, including adaptations that continue in light of changing state and federal laws and regulations—such as the implementation of the federal Affordable Care Act—and ongoing biotechnological innovation that makes possible new diagnostic procedures and treatments (Wear, 1997). All healthcare disciplines emphasize *professionalism*. While precise definitions of professionalism remain elusive (Beckett-Tharp & Schatell, 2001), they generally include civility or politeness, emotional control, confidence, and "an emphasis on rational appearances and technological displays of competency as appropriate behavior" (Morgan & Krone, 2001, p. 327). Yet how these norms manifest in communication varies widely among, for example, social workers and physicians.

Each healthcare discipline has a unique history and possesses its own culture, values, and language learned through years of education and socialization from peers and mentors in their field. Socialization can be understood as "attempts by organizations to help members transition from outsider to insider" (Apker, 2012, p. 48). Indoctrination into healthcare professions begins in the education of new members: one prime example is teaching medical students the virtues of medical professionalism. Although interdisciplinary in scope, medical education teaches students a doctor-specific language of ethics and professionalism (Buyx, Maxwell, & Schone-Seifert, 2008). After learning their professional culture, individuals carry their profession's goals and values. For example, the culture of physician training has focused on action and outcome more than on relationships (Hall, 2005). Traditionally, the physician–patient relationship tends to be authoritarian, whereas other professions, such as social work, place more value on patient self-determination. The main outcome valued by physicians is to save a patient's life, not a patient's quality of life (Hall, 2005). In comparison, clergy may have difficulty sharing information with a team, due to the tradition of confidentiality (Hall, 2005). Nurses and social workers also may value the patient's story and not rely on data from diagnostic tests as heavily as do physicians. Physicians will not easily listen to a patient's story from a nurse or social worker but will expect numerical data quickly to solve a patient's problem (Hall, 2005). Studies also demonstrate that healthcare professionals are socialized to understand what makes good quality medical care in very different ways, further complicating the process of collaboration (Geist & Hardesty, 1990).

Along with those differing professional cultures are differences in status and power. Physicians are held in higher esteem, typically receive higher salaries, hold more decision-making power, and bear more legal liability than other healthcare professionals (Wear, 1997). Further complicating this issue is the emergence of a class of paraprofessionals. As the cost of healthcare continues to rise, specialization continues to divide skill sets, and the need for skilled healthcare providers continues to increase, paraprofessionals have become essential, but often overlooked, members of healthcare teams. Paraprofessionals include those occupations in which workers "are relatively privileged, self-regulating, knowledge-based and service-oriented" (Evetts, 1999, p. 119). Increased reliance on paraprofessionals and "semiskilled" workers to provide the vast majority of direct care further complicates the enactment of professionalism in healthcare (Anderson et al., 2005).

Technicians are a relatively recent (post–World War II) workplace category, and the growth in technology since the 1970s led to a rapid increase of technicians: U.S. companies have long employed more than two technicians for each engineer, scientist, or physician (Barley, 1996). Technicians exist between traditional levels of expertise and "violate the alignment of those attributes that have long distinguished manual, blue-collar work from mental, white-collar work" (Barley, 1996, p. 412). Technicians resemble professionals in their socialized, analytic skills and artisans in their on-the-job training, manual skills, and operation of equipment. Their knowledge is contextual—specific to the dialysis clinic, patients, and equipment—rather than formal or abstract, as learned in college courses in anatomy, pharmacology, and biochemistry (Ellingson, 2008).

Patient care technicians, similar to those in the narrative that opened the chapter, resemble certified nursing assistants (CNAs) and other types of paraprofessionals in healthcare settings (Colon-Emeric et al., 2006). And like CNAs, technicians may find themselves marginalized within healthcare organizations. At the dialysis unit that Laura studied, the technicians were not invited to the monthly team meetings of physician-directors, nurse manager, registered nurse, social worker, and dietitian. They are not considered to have significant knowledge about patients, only to have acquired lots of practice operating dialysis machines, accessing patients' fistulas,[1] and conducting myriad other minor tasks necessary to safely treat dozens of dialysis patients each day. Ironically, none of the physicians who were in charge of patients' medical care could have operated the highly technical dialysis machines that were updated regularly and changed over time. Some of the physicians likely were not sufficiently proficient in accessing fistulas to be able to successfully access some of the trickier ones that technicians freely shared information about with each other.

At stake here is what counts as knowledge and expertise. Such dividing of tasks to grant more authority to professionals, while denying authority to and refusing to formally acknowledge the meaningful contributions of paraprofessionals, is not unique to physicians and technicians but is a regular practice among professionals and paraprofessionals in all types of workplaces (Cheney & Ashcraft, 2007).

Differences in professional cultures and hierarchies intersect in complex ways with gender, race, and class, making it difficult to comprehend and communicate effectively with members of other disciplines. Historically, the vast majority of physicians were men, and only in the past few decades have equal numbers of women and men entered the profession. While women are well represented in comparatively lower-paid fields such as pediatrics and family practice, specialty fields such as otolaryngology, orthopedic surgery, and neurological surgery, as well as medical school faculty, remain male-dominated (AAMC, 2014). For example, in the 2012 survey of medical schools, women represented only 18% of full-time faculty and 12% of medical school deans. In contrast, modern nursing continues to be a predominantly female field; today about 9% of all nurses are men (HRSA, 2013). Likewise, the field of social work remains dominated by women. Other fields, such as pharmacy, have seen rapid increases in the percentage of women (Bureau of Labor Statistics, 2014). Race also plays an important role in professional cultures. Medicine and allied health professions in the U.S. also have been predominantly White. People of color were banned from most medical schools until the civil rights movement challenged discrimination, and even today roughly 4% of practicing physicians are Black, 4.4% are Latino, and 11.7% are Asian American (AAMC, 2016). Socioeconomic class also plays a significant role. Parents of medical students are more likely to have a graduate degree, meaning that most physicians come from the middle and upper classes (AAMC, 2010).

Differing cultural standards for patient care and for professional collaboration often prevent different types of healthcare providers from communicating effectively with each other. Because a major motivation for the use of interdisciplinary teams in healthcare settings is to enable close collaboration across disciplinary lines (e.g., Opie, 2000) and to provide high-quality care to patients (Poole & Real, 2003), the manner in which norms of hierarchy constrain team members' communication is critical to understanding teamwork effectiveness. Teams are usually intended to promote egalitarian interactions; however, they often maintain professional hierarchies far more than they subvert them (Ellingson, 2005).

Moreover, the challenge in understanding how to make teamwork more effective is not merely that power disparities exist among disciplines and their gendered and racial legacies:

> How the relations of (disciplinary) power exists in a particular team affect how the team as a team elicits and engages with information from its different disciplinary sites and how, as a result of including or marginalizing particular types of knowledge, a specific team inscribes the bodies of its clients/families and itself, a process with material outcomes for all of the three groups involved. (Opie, 2000, p. 255)

That is, power allows some voices to be heard and silences or diminishes others, heavily influencing what knowledge goes into the team's understanding of and treatment plan for each patient, as well as the patient's engagement (or lack thereof) with that plan.

In the dialysis clinic described in the opening narrative, physicians are not present during routine treatments to gather patient information directly. Patient care technicians provide the vast majority of hands-on care and act as an intermediary between professionals—physicians and to a lesser extent registered nurses—and those about whom the professionals purportedly are most knowledgeable (i.e., patients). The mediating function of technicians reflects a partial decoupling of expertise and knowledge from authority (Barley, 1996). An underclass of technicians has emerged that occupies a paradoxical organizational position. They are experts in operating and maintaining technologically sophisticated dialysis machinery and are responsible for performing risky procedures upon which patients' lives depend, but physicians are skeptical of information gathered by technicians, and technicians hold little authority or autonomy within the organizations that employ them (Ellingson, 2008).

HCIA 4.1

Who, Me? Stressed?
Managing Role Tensions in Nurse–Team Interactions

Julie Apker

Experiencing job stress in some form seems to be an accepted part of work life. Many of us, including students, work in fast-paced organizations that demand multitasking and doing more with fewer resources. We also strive to meet different—and sometimes conflicting—role expectations from coworkers, customers, supervisors, and subordinates that contribute to chronic job stress. Such stress can wear us down and negatively influence our health and well-being, work relationships, and job performance. Certain occupations, however, encounter more job strain and associated negative effects on a persistent basis. According to a 2007 report by the U.S. Health Resources and Services Administration, healthcare workers experience greater stress, burnout, and turnover than people employed in most other professions.

Stress and burnout in healthcare is perhaps most problematic in hospital nursing, as nurses provide round-the-clock bedside care to patients and their families, coordinate care delivery with multiple and often-disparate health team members, and do so in busy environments with little down time or support resources. The nursing role is also full of discursive pressures that create adverse *communication load*. Nurses frequently communicate with multiple groups (e.g., health team members, patients and family members, nurse/hospital leaders) about challenging, complex, and/or highly sensitive topics. Further, nurses are often "caught in the middle" of the hierarchical healthcare team and must constantly negotiate and balance varied—and sometimes conflicting—team member needs. Over time, such

(continued)

context and communication pressures can drain nurses of emotional, cognitive, and physical energy. Some nurses leave their hospital jobs or the profession to avoid job strain, even though they care a great deal about patient care.

As we investigated nurse communication with health team members such as physicians, nurse assistants, and allied health professionals, we discovered a great deal about how communication with other team members not only contributes to nurses' stress but also how nurses communicatively manage stressors in team interactions. Nurses commonly experience stress when they encounter varied and often oppositional expectations of nursing roles. We found three overarching *role tensions* existing in nurse–team communication that guide how nurses alter their roles to best meet team expectations and deliver optimal patient care. We also identified different communication behaviors that nurses use to manage these role tensions with varying degrees of success.

First, the *equal-subordinate role tension* involves the contradiction of nurses attempting to be regarded as competent professionals and physician peers, while at the same time conforming to the traditional hierarchical structure that relegates nurses to a lower status position within the physician–nurse relationship. Nurse participants reported feeling stressed out or frustrated by this role tension, especially when physicians resisted their attempts to establish professional independence. Our findings show that nurses managed this role tension in two ways. First, they *accommodate the hierarchy*—using indirect forms of communication such as diplomacy when interacting with physicians. Said one nurse, "We have learned how to make excellent, brilliant ideas seem to be someone else's idea so the job can get done." Second, nurses *deny the hierarchy*—advocating for patients although doing so challenges physicians' authority. "If they [physicians] are on call, I am not apologizing for calling them," said another nurse. "I am calling them because I have a legitimate concern about their patient. There is no apologizing."

Second, the *superior-equal role tension* refers to the relationships between nurses with lower-status team members. We discovered that nurse assistants, unit clerks, and other subordinate personnel desire a democratic team in which all members contribute as equals. This ideal is counter to the realities of healthcare hierarchy, where nurses supervise subordinate staff, and educational differences put in them in authority roles. For instance, we learned that lower-status team members tend to create conflict—a known job stressor for nurses—when they believed nurses asserted authority unfairly. Nurses in our study used *softening the hierarchy* communication techniques to make them appear as equals to their subordinates. For instance, nurses make requests of subordinates (e.g., "Would you restock supplies?") rather than give orders. Softening also is displayed when nurses show politeness by praising and thanking lower-status team members for doing their jobs. A nurse provided this example: "I said, 'Hey guys, thanks a ton. That was very nice of you to do that.' And, immediately they perked up a little bit and I think, I hope, I communicated effectively with them."

Third, the *detached-attached role tension* is produced when team members expect nurses to build and nurture team attachments while simultaneously demonstrating the detachment necessary to make clinical decisions. Team members, especially those in lower-status positions, desire nurses to be caring and compassionate beyond the patient bedside, whereas physicians expect nurses to gather and interpret all clinical facts objectively, with little if any emotion. To manage this tension, nurses *segment expectations* by assessing distinct role expectations of team members and changing their communication behaviors. Nurses talked about conveying optimism, humor, and praise to lower-status team members. For example, a nurse described a colleague attending to such team member attachment needs: "She'd be swamped and she'd be like, 'How you guys doing?' Just so cheery and it totally changed the mood for the better. . . . Every time I work with the positive nurse, things will get done, people will pitch in." Nurses also tailor their communication to meet the needs of physicians, who have very different expectations than subordinate team members. Nurses told us that physicians want detached professionalism. To meet this expectation, nurses reported speaking "calmly," "directly, "accurately" and "in a timely manner" when interacting with physicians. One nurse explained that her communication style when calling physicians is "this is what I need and I need you to get it."

Constantly meeting contradictory expectations and associated role tensions exacerbates nurses' stress and burnout, especially in light of nurses' challenging working conditions. However, despite the multiple sources of stress, most nurses in this study adapted in ways that helped them effectively manage stressors inherent in team interactions. Ultimately, these techniques enabled nurses to reduce and even avoid job pressures so they could continue to provide patient care.

QUESTIONS TO PONDER

1. What are communication sources of stress in your work life? Personal life?

2. How do you manage your work and/or life stressors? Consider communication techniques as well as lifestyle strategies.

3. What other professions may encounter role tensions similar to nursing? Why do you think so?

Reference:
U.S. Health Resources and Services Administration. (2007, March). *Community health worker national workforce study*. Retrieved from http://bhpr.hrsa.gov/healthworkforce/reports/chwstudy2007.pdf

Source: Apker, J., Propp, K. M., & Ford, W. S. Z. (2005). Negotiating status and identity tensions in healthcare team interactions: An exploration of nurse role dialectics. *Journal of Applied Communication Research, 33,* 93–115.

■ Continuum of Collaboration and Teamwork

Healthcare professionals and researchers of healthcare teams generally use terms such as multidisciplinary, interdisciplinary, and transdisciplinary to designate the type and degree of collaboration among team members. These terms, when used in research, are often left undefined and used interchangeably, creating ambiguity. Lack of clarity in the use of this terminology may create difficulty in trying to communicate valid comparisons across studies of teams. We find it most useful to conceive of these terms not as distinct concepts but as existing along a continuum from loose (or no) coordination, through interdependency, to boundary/role blurring and synergistic teamwork (Miller et al., 2009; Stokols, Hall, Taylor, & Moser, 2008).

At one far end of the continuum of cross-disciplinary teamwork in Figure 4.1 is the *unidisciplinary* team. Unidisciplinary teams are organized around a single discipline and employ individuals from the same field to work on common goals (Poole & Real, 2003; Stokols et al., 2008). An example of a unidisciplinary group is a group of nurses working to coordinate the care of a patient in an intensive care unit of a hospi-

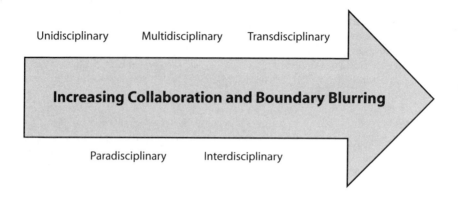

Figure 4.1   A Continuum of Teamwork

tal. Of course, these nurses also work with physicians and other staff, but the team goal of daily patient care and monitoring is one that the group of nurses carries out together. The simplest type of team with multiple disciplines is the *paradisciplinary* team, which includes awareness and courtesy between members of different disciplines, but no coordination of efforts or joint planning takes place among members (Satin, 1994).

Unlike paradisciplinary teams, *multidisciplinary* teams endeavor to promote cross-discipline work to a limited degree. A multidisciplinary team is a group of professionals from two or more disciplines working together on a focal problem. No integration of professional perspectives takes place, but an additive effect of different methods and ideas enhances the outcome of teamwork (Hall et al., 2012). Participants in multidisciplinary teams remain "anchored in the concept and methods of their respective fields" (Stokols et al., 2008, p. S78) yet learn to respect and work with the methods and values of other disciplines (Nash, 2008). Multidisciplinary, like paradisciplinary, teams include formal interactions between disciplines within a structured team environment, and little or no informal or spontaneous communication occurs among team members from different disciplines (Lawrence & Despres, 2004).

A more interdependent form of team includes *interdisciplinary* teams. These are groups of professionals that "mix" professional disciplines together to achieve a systematic outcome (Lawrence & Despres, 2004). These team members possess a "working knowledge of different disciplinary conceptual frameworks and methodological tools" and use them to create a more robust environment for collaboration (Nash, 2008, p. S134). Interdisciplinary team members ultimately achieve a significant degree of coordination and integration of their services and assessments of patients, due to their ability to share more information and collaborate on problem solving across discipline lines (Poole & Real, 2003). Some role shifting and evolution may occur over time as teams gain more experience working together (Hall et al., 2012; Poole & Real, 2003; Stokols et al., 2008).

In some cases, interdisciplinary teams evolve into *transdisciplinary* teams, in which "members have developed sufficient trust and mutual confidence to engage in teaching and learning across disciplinary boundaries" (Wieland, Kramer, Waite, & Ruben-stein, 1996, p. 656). These teams are able to synthesize theoretical and methodological perspectives of different disciplines. Disciplinary boundaries are very flexible in this model of teamwork, transcending professional boundary lines (Nash, 2008). Ideally, this form of deep collaboration across disciplines promotes synergistic teamwork in which the quality of the whole far exceeds the sum of its parts.

Transdisciplinary teams are achieved over time after overcoming these obstacles. Nash (2008) notes three individual characteristics that encourage transdisciplinary team formation: trust, clear communication, and a transdisciplinary ethic (e.g., open-ness and respect for different disciplinary approaches, broad-gauged contextual think-ing, and tolerance for uncertainty). Stable membership on the team and mentorship between new members and older members generally is a prerequisite to developing such a deep level of trust. External, or institutional, characteristics that encourage transdisciplinary work include funding for work and training within transdisciplinary teams (Nash, 2008).

Boundary-blurring, synergistic, interdisciplinary, or transdisciplinary teamwork is often the most difficult to achieve for many reasons. One important reason is shared language; within each discipline, a language of specialized terminology is created between experts and is perpetuated over time. However, within transdisciplinary teams, a common language needs to be formed from multiple different disciplinary languages (Nash, 2008). Moreover, working in the ambiguous areas between disci-plines can be frustrating; no one profession can claim the work as its own. Further, members must work with other disciplines despite personal dislike of certain method-ologies (Nash, 2008).

The dialysis team in the opening narrative collaborated in ways that likely would be described as falling somewhere between multidisciplinary and interdisciplinary teamwork. The work of the registered nurses overlapped significantly with that of the patient care technicians, and the social worker and dietitian both sought to encourage patients to adhere to a lengthy number of dietary and fluid restrictions in order to maintain their health as well as possible. All staff sought to ensure patient safety and to provide emotional support when patients were distressed. So role blurring did occur regularly, although certain tasks were exempt from this blurring and restricted to registered nurses, due to state and federal regulations. In addition to collaboration in providing hands-on treatments to dialysis patients who were treated three times each week at their unit, further collaboration occurred in formal monthly team meet-ings. Those meetings included the nurse manager, registered nurses, social worker, registered dietician, and nephrologists (physician-directors) but did not include the paraprofessional technicians (see Ellingson, 2008 for further discussion of power dynamics). These meetings, along with formal and informal staff meetings, took place outside of the treatment room, in "staff-only" areas of the building that included offices, storage rooms, equipment areas, and a break room. Patients seldom are granted access to such "backstage" spaces, making them ideal locations for healthcare providers to discuss patients without fear of being overheard by patients and visitors.

HCIA 4.2

Trailblazing Healthcare

Barbara F. Sharf ■ Patricia Geist-Martin

Most of us find that there are times when we just don't know what is wrong with us. We may feel stressed, can't sleep, struggle with pains in our bodies that just won't go away, or simply lack the energy to fully enjoy life. Some people consult with a doctor but end up with no diagnosis that identifies what is wrong. Sometimes the medicine that a conventional physician prescribes doesn't resolve the symptoms. In addition to following the advice of a medical doctor, another strategy that may address our concerns is the use of integrative medicine (IM), defined by the National Center on Complementary and Alternative Medicine as a combination of biomedicine and complementary modalities that are typically outside the conventional regimens used by physicians. Complementary or holistic healing modalities, such as acupuncture, massage, yoga, or meditation, treat the whole person (mind, body, and spirit), not just their bodies or physical health, as biomedicine tends to do.

We have been studying centers of integrative medicine for more than five years, and we have learned a great deal about the ways that such centers are structured. In one of our studies, we interviewed administrators and providers in three different IM centers, as well as spent time observing and participating in selected activities in order to understand the communication surrounding each center's evolution, mission, and internal and external interactions.

The three centers were very different in size and mission. Brazos Healing Center is a small community-based organization established in 2011 by two women, one a licensed holistic nurse, and both credentialed in yoga and energy healing. They describe the center's mission as providing a central place for people to (1) access complementary therapies and holistic health consulting, (2) learn about enhancing personal development, and (3) exchange ideas for balancing and strengthening the mind-body-spirit connection. The center offers services such as energy and massage therapies, yoga, pilates, tai chi, and holistic practitioner consultations.

A second community-based facility, Center for Well-Being, has been in operation since 1998. A medical doctor cofounded and directs the center, leading the team of 17 specialty providers, including a chiropractor, a naturopath, and marital counselors, in taking a "whole-person approach."

Finally, the third and largest center, Integrative Medicine Program (IMP), also started in 1998 and is now led by a research psychologist and a medical oncologist. It is both a treatment and a research facility located within a large nationally known cancer institute. Its integrative services include meditation, music therapy, nutrition, acupuncture, massage, expressive arts, yoga, and other movement-based therapies. Additionally, IMP distributes evidence-based information about complementary and alternative therapies to help patients and healthcare professionals decide how best to integrate such therapies into patients' care.

As we analyzed both the transcripts of interviews with directors from each of the three centers and the many pages of participant-observation field notes each team member had written, we were looking for overarching patterns of commonalities that construct meanings of the multilayered term "integrative," particularly in terms of organizational communicative functions. As is typically the process with team approaches to qualitative studies, there was much discussion among all four investigators in order to derive an agreed upon set of patterns and implications for clinical practice. We settled on the notion of "trailblazing" as a way of thinking about these three centers, as well as other U.S. IM facilities, both community-based and academic, striving to find new ways of helping patients, and educating the medical community and public alike.

The first pattern we identified is *integration of complementary and conventional medicine.* The key to accomplishing this goal in all three centers was the inclusion of a biomedically trained, licensed practitioner who had also developed expertise in one or more complementary modalities and was distinguished by a broad vision and strong motivation to find as many viable options as possible to help clients optimize health, quality of life, and clinical outcomes.

The second pattern is *communicating integration internally through team interaction.* All centers employed a variety of trained staff, each contributing expertise in one or more types of clinical therapies complementary to a biomedical perspective. Sharing the contributions and results of multidisciplinary care among the team is very important but difficult to achieve given spatial, scheduling, and economic constraints.

The third pattern is *communicating the concept of integration externally,* since each center operates within a cultural and geographic community and deals with the tasks of communicating its character and attracting a client/patient base. While challenges and tactics vary, there is one central issue—how to communicate each organization's identity, both symbolically and materially, including name, space, mission, and community outreach. A problem common to all three centers was difficulties with insurance reimbursement.

QUESTIONS TO PONDER

1. Have you ever heard of integrative medicine?
2. Have you ever utilized integrative medicine? What forms of healing did you use? Do you know anyone else who has tried an integrative medicine?
3. What motivated you to try something in addition to conventional medicine?
4. Did you tell your physician about using integrative medicine? Why or why not?

Source: Sharf, B. F., Geist-Martin, P., Cosgriff-Hernández, K., & Moore, J. (2012). Trailblazing healthcare: Institutionalizing and integrating complementary medicine. *Patient Education and Counseling, 89,* 434–438.

◾ Frontstage and Backstage of Healthcare Delivery

Later that week, the dialysis clinic team held its monthly case review meeting in the conference room. Stacks of bright blue and black three-ring binders surrounded Charley, the nurse manager, who sat next to Peter, his social work notes spread out before him. The physician-directors, Dr. Cheng and Dr. Gupta, sat at either end of the table, while Gabriella, one of the nurses, and Anne, the dietitian, sat across from Charley and Peter.

"OK, who's next?" asked Dr. Cheng, a hint of impatience in his voice. The meeting had started more than two hours ago, and they had completed the monthly review of fewer than half of the patients.

"Mrs. Albright," replied Charley cheerfully. Papers shuffled, and all eyes turned to Dr. Gupta.

"She's a 63-year-old woman, ESRD [end stage renal disease, i.e., kidney failure] since 2003. Her last check up with me was two weeks ago, nothing to report, stable diagnosis. Any changes?"

Charley nodded at Anne who offered, "Her [blood] counts are a mess, just awful. She's totally noncompliant with dietary and fluid restrictions." Dr. Gupta looked thoughtful while Dr. Cheng scowled.

Peter added gently, "It's important to her to be the one in control. She resists following orders." He shrugged. "I've suggested that she tell you how she feels about the treatment regimen,

Dr. Gupta, but it doesn't seem like she has?" Peter gave Dr. Gupta a questioning glance, and the physician just shook his head.

"She's not been readmitted since her last crisis—four, no five weeks ago," stated Charley. "Anything else—Gabriella?"

"Just what we've always heard: she wants more weight taken off," said Gabriella.

Heads shook ruefully around the table. Although the team often disagreed with one another—at times strongly—about how to handle a particular patient's side effects, complications, or resistance, all had become resigned in this case. Mrs. Albright's unwillingness to consider changing her way of living to conform to the recommended (quite oppressive) restrictions on amounts and types of food and beverages had been well established in the more than two years she had been treated at this clinic, and no one felt the need to urge others on the team to try to compel, cajole, or otherwise convince Mrs. Albright to change her behavior.

Charley waited a beat, scanning faces, then nodded. "OK, who's next?" she asked.

As they began the discussion of another patient, Laura reflected on the difficulty in balancing respect for patients' autonomy, that is, their right to make their own decisions, with the professional imperative to encourage patients to behave in ways that the healthcare providers believed would be best for their patients' health.

Most people are accustomed to communicating directly with their physicians and other healthcare providers. It may not occur to patients to wonder about conversations among healthcare providers that take place outside of patients' hearing, like the one portrayed in the narrative above. Staff-only spaces are referred to as "backstage" areas, and they play a vital role in healthcare delivery.

Atkinson (1995) pointed out that researchers have focused the vast majority of research and theorizing of healthcare practice on the *frontstage* of medical care, that is, healthcare providers' communication with patients as care is provided and received. The predominance of this focus has led to certain limits in understanding how day-to-day healthcare delivery works. One shortcoming is the lack of understanding of communication among healthcare practitioners that occurs away from patients. Yet much teamwork among healthcare providers takes place in the *backstage* of the healthcare system. Goffman (1959) defines the backstage region as

> a place, relative to a given performance, where the impression fostered by the performance is knowingly contradicted. . . . It is here that the capacity of a performance to express something beyond itself may be painstakingly fabricated . . . illusion and impressions are openly constructed. Here stage props and items of personal front can be stored in a kind of compact collapsing of whole repertoires. (p. 112)

For healthcare providers, the frontstage in outpatient treatment areas includes the waiting room and the examination rooms; within a hospital inpatient (admitted patients) unit, patient rooms and adjacent hallways form the frontstage. The backstage generally consists of a nurses' station, office or computer area, chart room, break room, conference room, and sometimes hallways to which patients' (and their companions') access is blocked. Significant communication among healthcare providers goes on in these backstage areas and needs to be taken seriously when we try to improve healthcare teams (Wittenberg-Lyles, Gee, Oliver, & Demiris, 2009).

In addition to focusing on the frontstage of healthcare and largely ignoring the backstage, researchers and healthcare providers tend to understand healthcare delivery as made up of a series of individual interactions between healthcare providers and patients or among healthcare providers. Of all types of healthcare communication, physician–patient interactions are by far the most frequently studied, and these interactions have become a model for understanding all healthcare interactions. Physician–patient interactions are generally brief, take place in single, relatively private locations, are usually scheduled, and thus are easily documented (Atkinson, 1995). Yet the majority of interactions in hospitals and clinics are not structured like physician–patient interactions at all. Researchers and healthcare providers (and patients) may erroneously generalize to think of medical interactions as normally spatially (i.e., one place) and temporally bound (i.e., with an identifiable beginning, middle, and end), when in fact, *unbounded* interactions are equally, and in many other healthcare settings, far more numerous than bounded ones.

Most research on healthcare teams clearly reflects this tendency to think of bounded, convenient interactions as the only or at least most important aspect of backstage communication. Researchers and professionals seeking to improve teamwork thus focus on formal team meetings that take place on a regular schedule, usually weekly or monthly but in some settings daily or even at every staffing shift change. Meetings have agendas, leaders, systems of turn-taking, and other norms associated with public communication, fitting naturally within researchers' existing expectations for teamwork. Such beliefs and preconceptions reflect an unconscious bias toward public communication norms, which largely reflect white, middle-class, heterosexual, male perspectives (Wyatt, 2002). Moreover, studies of meetings traditionally focus on decision making as the crucial task of groups; topics such as cooperation, socialization, and connection have been marginalized. Because of these research biases, current conceptualizations of how communication operates in small groups (and teams) are partial and even misleading when generalized to all communication in healthcare (Ellingson, 2005; Meyers & Brashers, 1994).

Such research ignores frequent *embedded teamwork*, when two or three team members communicate while accomplishing one of many backstage tasks, such as reviewing records, entering patient notes, or even quick visits to the break room or restroom (Ellingson, 2003), also called joint work (Opie, 2000). This is part of what it means to do teamwork, even though it is not during a meeting where all the different professionals are sitting down talking to one another about patients. For example, in the dialysis narrative example that opened this chapter, the communication between the patient, patient care technician, and nurse happened in front of several other patients and staff members, started and stopped, and referred to communication with a physician that had happened earlier. Also, the social worker and dietician talked about this patient in the hallway in a chance meeting. This communication between team members does not involve the entire team, but it does help to accomplish the team's patient care goals.

Moreover, unbounded and backstage communication often results in a modification of the agenda for a team member's subsequent encounter with a patient (Ellingson, 2005). The dialysis dietician's remarks led directly to the social worker spending further time with their patient. Healthcare providers should consider both formal and informal talk in the backstage as opportunities to adapt their own and each other's agendas for communicating with patients in ways that enhance healthcare delivery.

Team members' backstage communication also provides practical facilitation of encounters. For example, being told that a patient was very hard-of-hearing could encourage team members to speak loudly and more slowly from the outset of their encounter and thus improve communication.

On a cautionary note, it is important to understand that teamwork communication—including unbounded and backstage—involves the use of power. Despite its potential for improving patient care, team communication increases healthcare providers' persuasive power over patients, potentially undermining patient autonomy. The power wielded by certain team members gives them further rhetorical advantage over patients who already face status and knowledge differences that privilege medical professionals in their interactions (Ellingson, 2008). Team members strategize (often extensively) out of patients' presence about how to persuade patients to adopt or discontinue specific behaviors. Of course, the team members have the patients' best interests at heart as they seek to influence patient choices and actions. However, as one medical ethicist put it, "*one cannot not manipulate when communicating* about health and disease" (original emphasis; Witte, 1994, p. 288). The need to balance paternalism, or the assumption that the healthcare providers know best and patients should comply with their orders, and patients' autonomy in the healthcare provider–patient relationship is certainly not unique to team care (e.g., Pelto-Piri, Engström, & Engström, 2013) and is always a significant concern. That is, the knowledge and good intentions of the healthcare providers must be balanced with respect for the patients' rights to make their own decisions (see Theorizing Practice 4.2).

The unbalance of power between patients and healthcare providers is particularly evident with patients from marginalized groups, such as older adults, people of color, people living in poverty, and people who do not identify as heterosexual or straight, that is, lesbian, gay, bisexual, transgender, queer, intersex, or asexual people (Johnson et al., 2004). Further, the exclusion of patients and family members from many team

---

Theorizing Practice 4.2
Balancing Provider Expertise with Patient Autonomy

Sometimes finding the correct balance between physicians' (and other healthcare providers') paternalism and patients' autonomy is not as straightforward as it might seem (Rodriguez-Osorio & Dominguez-Cherit, 2008). At stake here is the concept of *beneficence*, wherein the healthcare provider is doing her or his best, based on substantial education, training, experience, and a professional code of ethics, to help patients in dangerous circumstances, such as a life-threatening illness or accident. At the same time, *paternalistic* attitudes assume that because healthcare providers have medical expertise, they should be obeyed by patients, even if the patient disagrees with their treatment recommendations. As one can see in the opening narrative example, healthcare providers often talk to one another about how best to urge patients to be compliant with their orders.

How do you feel about healthcare providers trying to devise the best ways to convince you to comply with their orders? If your physician and physical therapist talked to one another in the backstage about how to convince you to consent to a knee operation that you do not feel is right for you, would that bother you? Why or why not?

meetings has been highly criticized by some scholars of teamwork who object to the marginalization of patients' and families' perspectives (Opie, 2000; Wittenberg-Lyles et al., 2013). A similar criticism could be made of backstage teamwork that involves strategizing among team members on how best to persuade patients toward a particular decision, like that practiced by the social worker and the dietitian in the opening narrative. This ethical challenge to patient autonomy warrants attention from healthcare providers and health communication researchers alike.

◼ Improving Team Communication

Effective communication among team members can be fostered in myriad ways. In this section, we will review systemic- or organizational-level changes that support teams, strategies for fostering collaborative team cultures, and necessary interpersonal communication skills for teamwork.

Systemic Level Changes

Medicine, nursing, and allied health disciplines should promote respect and collaboration with other disciplines as key components of their professional cultures. In order to do this, there must be changes in the education of health professionals. Further, healthcare professionals and paraprofessional staff (such as patient care technicians and certified nursing assistants) need to work together within existing teams, rather than limiting team membership to professionals.

First, healthcare providers should be taught to value interprofessionalism—that is, collaborating with members of other professions to provide patient care. Professionalism for healthcare providers traditionally has been taught with an emphasis on meeting the treatment or care goals specific to one's discipline; so nurses focused on their own work—monitoring patients' vital signs and symptoms and meeting the physical and emotional needs of patients in hospitals, for example. With increasing reliance on interdisciplinary teams in healthcare (e.g., Opie, 2000), the performance of professionalism increasingly includes skills in collaboration, negotiation, and problem solving across disciplines; for example, nurses and physicians communicating together to address patients' needs (Propp et al., 2010). Indeed, McNair (2005) called for a shift in definitions of professionalism away from "uni-professionalism," or "the pursuit of goals for single healthcare professional disciplines to the exclusion of other disciplines," toward one of "interprofessionalism" that takes seriously the differences in values, norms, status, and power among healthcare disciplines as barriers to collaboration (p. 458). Instilling the value of interprofessionalism in students will help prepare them to be better team members as professionals.

Second, graduate programs in healthcare professions should include interdisciplinary educational experiences as a component of their programs. To promote systematic change in cultures of collaboration, students need to work and train regularly with students from other disciplines (Hall, 2005). In such learning experiences, students are exposed to the terminology and practices of other disciplines. For example, clinical social workers might work with students in nurse practitioner programs or with students in clinical psychology programs to design care plans for patients' complex diagnoses who will need psychological services as well as home nursing and physical therapy. Opportunities to learn with other disciplines can foster understanding of and respect for the contributions of other professions to patient care, providing a solid foundation for later teamwork (Khalili, Orchard, Laschinger, & Farah, 2013).

Third, healthcare organizations need to change policies and practices that devalue the contributions of paraprofessionals (i.e., technicians and assistants) to patient care and instead embrace them as complementing professionals (Ellingson, 2008). The relative scarcity of research that takes seriously the role of paraprofessionals in patients' care reflects their low status in the field (see Anderson et al., 2005; Colon-Emeric et al., 2006; Morgan et al., 2008). Yet paraprofessionals in many organizations have significant expertise; they lack disciplinary prestige but possess a great deal of useful, contextual, hands-on knowledge of processes, equipment, and particular patients (Barley, 1996). Healthcare organizations typically exclude technicians and assistants from formal definitions and (meetings of) care teams (Stoner, 1999), as did the dialysis team in this chapter's narrative. Healthcare organizations disenfranchise paraprofessionals by not allowing them to attend patient care team meetings to which members of professional disciplines are invited, such as management, nursing, social work, nutrition, and medicine. When the voice of paraprofessionals is left out of discussions of patient care, vital insights may be omitted, and opportunities for improved quality of care missed (Kontos, Miller, & Mitchell, 2010). Inviting paraprofessionals to be official members of care teams may significantly improve patient outcomes (Morgan et al., 2008).

Creating Collaborative Team Cultures

Another way to foster effective teamwork is to facilitate the development of collaborative team cultures. Healthcare teams should "create an open and trusting environment characterized by equal status among group members; shared goal setting; cooperating toward common goals," within organizations that support teamwork through their policies and procedures (Khalili et al., 2013, p. 450.). Of course, developing an ideal collaborative team is easier said than done.

One way to help teams foster collaboration is to urge them to recognize and reflect on communication among team members *outside* of team meetings as part of the fluid process of teamwork, rather than ignoring or discounting such communication as apart from or preliminary to the "real" teamwork that occurs in formal meetings (Ellingson, 2003; Youngwerth & Twaddle, 2011). Recognition could include documenting dyadic or triadic interactions by briefly logging date, time, topic, and participants in a team member's daily planner or notebook. Compiled periodically, these data would support team members' requests to administrators for (re)allocation of time for teamwork. Periodically bringing such data into meetings for discussion also would enable identification of trends in topics that necessitate frequent out-of-meeting interactions—such knowledge could lead to anticipating and preventing some problems by implementing changes to meeting agendas or procedures to address recurring issues. By recognizing such fleeting, dyadic or triadic communication among team members as important to team relationships and processes, team members and administrators can value and reward this professional work, reinforcing this informal, yet vital, practice (Ellingson, 2005).

Further, teams should create opportunities to develop common language for discussing frequently occurring topics that would help them to communicate more effectively and efficiently and to develop better solutions to problems (McNair, 2005). For example, Milligan, Gilroy, Katz, Rodan, and Subramanian (1999) developed a model to assist teams of diverse healthcare professions in communicating about "professional, community, and institutional issues relevant to pregnant women and new mothers as infant caregivers" (p. 47). The model established a shared set of terms and concepts that helped the professionals to understand how different disciplines' expertise shed light on complex prenatal and neonatal diagnoses, symptoms, and treatment options. The model gave all team members something to refer to when seeking clarity. More informal collaboration by teams to develop local terminology for common, shared phenomena may help both to enhance clarity and to foster a sense of group identity and relational cohesion among team members (Ellingson, 2005).

Individual Communication Skills for Effective Teamwork

While organizational- and team-level changes are important to fostering good teamwork, team members also have the opportunity and responsibility to develop individual communication skills that can help them to communicate more effectively with team members. Interpersonal communication skills are vital to collaborating, particularly on teams with healthcare providers from a variety of professions (Ellingson, 2005; Nørgaard, Ammentorp, Kyvik, & Kofoed, 2012; Reader, Flin, & Cuthbertson, 2007). Research suggests that collaboration among team members is enhanced by communicative strategies such as the following:

- Really listen. Listening is not the same as waiting for a turn to speak.
- Be open to new ideas and approaches. Consider how they enhance people's existing knowledge base and avoid knee-jerk rejections.
- Articulate a goal or perspective clearly and concisely.
- Identify common ground among members. What do all agree on?
- Ask open-ended questions that invite others to explain their perspectives.
- Speak respectfully at all times. When angry or frustrated, take time to calm down before speaking. No matter how provoked, every person is always responsible for her or his response, and people can choose to communicate respect even to those who do not demonstrate respect in return.
- Focus on the team's overall purpose rather than just one individual's contribution.

Like any other skills, interpersonal interaction skills can be learned and practiced until one becomes more proficient. Theorizing Practice 4.3 invites you to consider your own and others' effective team communicative strategies.

Theorizing Practice 4.3
What Makes a Good Teammate?

Youngwerth and Twaddle (2011) reviewed research to determine what factors influence healthcare team effectiveness. They found that communication, interpersonal relationships, team composition and structure, and organizational factors all played crucial roles in helping healthcare teams perform better.

If you have ever played on a sports team, acted or painted sets for a play, or held a job where you worked closely with others, such as a restaurant server, you had to learn to work as a member of a team. While you may not be able to control the composition of your team or the rules imposed on it by your employer, school, or other organization, you can make choices about fostering open, frequent, clear communication, and about being friendly and respectful toward your teammates. The goal is to develop trust among team members so that you can maximize each member's diverse strengths and collaborate as smoothly as possible.

What do you believe makes an ideal team member for you? How do you communicate to put forth your best as a teammate?

■ Conclusion

This chapter has explored how teamwork functions as a critical component of healthcare delivery, how teamwork happens in healthcare delivery, and how team communication and collaboration can be improved on organizational, team, and individual levels. Some team members enjoy more authority and prestige than others, and it is challenging yet necessary to integrate professionals and paraprofessionals on teams in order to efficiently deliver healthcare. Healthcare providers communicate with one another as they care for patients in the "frontstage" of healthcare delivery and also away from patients in "backstage" areas, where they may strategize on how to persuade patients to adhere to particular treatment options or guidelines. As the opening narrative illustrated, teamwork is necessary to coordinate all aspects of patient care, but it can be challenging to accomplish effectively.

Discussion Questions

1. What is professional socialization, and how can it function as a barrier to effective teamwork?

2. Describe how the members of the dialysis care team in the opening narrative communicated with Mrs. Albright. How could they have communicated differently to convince her to follow the dialysis patient guidelines for healthy eating and drinking?

3. Describe the continuum of teamwork. Is more boundary blurring and role overlap among healthcare providers always better? Why or why not?

4. Should patients be incorporated as members of the healthcare team and participate in team discussions of their current health status and treatment options? What are the advantages of including patients? What disadvantages might there be to having a patient present when team members are discussing the patient's status and options?

NOTE

[1] A fistula allows a large enough access point that blood can flow freely through the needles during dialysis. Fistulas are created by surgically connecting a vein and an artery under the skin. Once connected, the vein increases in size, becoming stronger and larger; this process can take several weeks.

REFERENCES

AAMC (Association of American Medical Colleges). (2010). Diversity of U.S. medical students by parental education. *Analysis In Brief, 9*(10). Retrieved from https://www.aamc.org/download/142770/data/aibvol9_no10.pdf

AAMC (Association of American Medical Colleges). (2014). *The state of women in academic medicine: The pipeline and pathways to leadership, 2013–2014.* Retrieved from https://www.aamc.org/members/gwims/statistics/

AAMC (Association of American Medical Colleges). (2016). Section II: Current status of the U.S. physician workforce. *Diversity in the physician workforce: Facts and figures 2014.* Washington DC: Association of American Medical Colleges. Retrieved from http://aamcdiversityfactsandfigures.org/section-ii-current-status-of-us-physician-workforce/

Anderson, R. A., Ammarell, N., Bailey, D., Jr., Colon-Emeric, C., Corazzini, K. N., Lillie, M., . . . McDaniel, R. R., Jr. (2005). Nursing assistant mental models, sensemaking, care actions, and consequences for nursing home residents. *Qualitative Health Research, 15,* 1006–1021.

Apker, J. (2012). *Communication in health organizations.* Malden, MA: Polity.

Atkinson, P. (1995). *Medical talk and medical work.* Thousand Oaks, CA: Sage.

Barley, S. R. (1996). Technicians in the workplace: Ethnographic evidence for bringing work into organization studies. *Administrative Science Quarterly, 41,* 404–441.

Beckett-Tharp, D., & Schatell, D. (2001). Today's dialysis environment: An overview. In C. Latham & J. Curtis (Eds.), *Core curriculum for the dialysis technician* (2nd ed., Module I, pp. 1–26). Thousand Oaks, CA: Amgen.

Bureau of Labor Statistics. (2014). *Labor force statistics from the current population survey.* Retrieved from http://www.bls.gov/cps/cpsaat11.htm.

Buyx, A. M., Maxwell, B., & Schone-Seifert, B. (2008). Challenges of educating for medical professionalism: Who should step up to the line? *Medical Education, 42,* 758–764.

Cheney, G., & Ashcraft, K. L. (2007). Considering "the professional" in communication studies: Implications for theory and research within and beyond the boundaries of organizational communication. *Communication Theory, 17,* 146–175.

Colon-Emeric, C. S., Ammarell, N., Bailey, D., Corazzini, K., Lekan-Rutledge, D., Piven, M. L., Utley-Smith, Q., & Anderson, R. A. (2006). Patterns of medical and nursing staff communication in nursing homes: Implications and insights from complexity science. *Qualitative Health Research, 16,* 173–188.

Ellingson, L. L. (2003). Interdisciplinary health care teamwork in the clinic backstage. *Journal of Applied Communication Research, 31,* 93–117.

Ellingson, L. L. (2005). *Communicating in the clinic: Negotiating frontstage and backstage teamwork.* Cresskill, NJ: Hampton.

Ellingson, L. L. (2007). The performance of dialysis care: Routinization and adaptation on the floor. *Health Communication, 22,* 103–114.

Ellingson, L. L. (2008). Changing realities and entrenched norms in dialysis: A case study of power, knowledge, and communication in health care delivery. In M. Dutta & H. Zoller (Eds.), *Emerging perspectives in health communication: Meaning, culture, and power* (pp. 293–312). New York, NY: Routledge.

Ellingson, L. L. (2011). The poetics of professionalism among dialysis technicians. *Health Communication, 26,* 1–12.

Ellingson, L. L. (2015). Embodied practices of dialysis care. In B. Green & N. Hopwood (Eds.), *Body/practice: The body in professional practice, learning and education* (pp. 173–190). Cham, Switzerland: Springer.

Evetts, J. (1999). Professionalisation and professionalism: Issues for interprofessional care. *Journal of Interprofessional Care, 13*, 119–128.

Geist, P., & Hardesty, M. (1990). Ideological positioning in professionals' narratives of quality medical care. In N. Denzin (Ed.), *Studies in symbolic interaction: A research annual, volume 11* (pp. 255-281). Greenwich, CT: JAI Press.

Goffman, E. (1959). *The presentation of self in everyday life.* Garden City, NY: Doubleday.

Hall, K. L., Vogel, A. L., Stipelman, B. A., Stokols, D., Morgan, G., & Gehlert, A. (2012). A four-phase model of transdisciplinary team-based research: Goals, team processes, and strategies. *Translational Behavioral Medicine, 2*, 415–430.

Hall, P. (2005). Interprofessional teamwork: Professional cultures as barriers. *Journal of Interprofessional Care, Supplement 1*, 188–196.

HRSA (Health Resources and Services Administration). (2013). *The U.S. nursing workforce: Trends in supply and education.* Washington, DC: U.S. Government Printing Office. Retrieved from http://bhpr.hrsa.gov/healthworkforce/supplydemand/nursing/nursingworkforce/nursingworkforcefullreport.pdf

Johnson, J. L., Bottoroff, J. L., Browne, A. J., Grewal, S., Hilton, B. A., & Clarke, H. (2004). Othering and being othered in the context of health care services. *Health Communication, 16*, 253–271.

Khalili, H., Orchard, C., Laschinger, H. K. S., & Farah, R. (2013). An interprofessional socialization framework for developing an interprofessional identity among health professions students. *Journal of Interprofessional Care, 27*, 448–453.

Kontos, P. C., Miller, K. L., & Mitchell, G. J. (2010). Neglecting the importance of the decision making and care regimes of personal support workers: A critique of standardization of care planning through the RAI/MDS. *The Gerontologist, 50*, 352–362.

Lawrence, R. J., & Despres, C. (2004). Introduction: Future of transdisciplinarity. *Futures, 36*, 397–405.

McNair, R. P. (2005). The case for educating health students in professionalism as the core content of interprofessional education. *Medical Education, 39*, 456–464.

Meyers, R. A., & Brashers, D. E. (1994). Expanding the boundaries of small group communication research: Exploring a feminist perspective. *Communication Studies, 45*, 68–85.

Miller, A., Scheinkestel, C., Limpus, A., Joseph, M., Karnik, A., & Venkatesh, A. (2009). Uni- and interdisciplinary effects on round and handover content in intensive care units. *Human Factors, 51*, 339–353.

Milligan, R. A., Gilroy, J., Katz, K., Rodan, M., & Subramanian, S. (1999). Developing a shared language: Interdisciplinary communication among diverse health care professionals. *Holistic Nursing Practice, 13*(2), 47–53.

Morgan, D. G., Crossley, M. F., Stewart, N. J., D'Arcy, C., Forbes, D. A., Normand, S. A., & Cammer, A. L. (2008). Taking the hit: Focusing on caregiver "error" masks organizational-level risk factors for nursing aide assault. *Qualitative Health Research, 18*, 334–346.

Morgan, J. M., & Krone, K. J. (2001). Bending the rules of "professional" display: Emotional improvisation in caregiver performance. *Journal of Applied Communication Research, 29*, 317–340.

Nash, J. M. (2008). Transdisciplinary training: Key components and prerequisites for success. *American Journal of Preventative Medicine, 35*, S133–140.

National Kidney Foundation. (2014). Your dialysis care team. Retrieved from: http://www.kidney.org/atoz/content/dialcareteam.cfm

Nørgaard, B., Ammentorp, J., Kyvik, K. O., & Kofoed, P. E. (2012). Communication skills training increases self-efficacy of health care professionals. *Journal of Continuing Education in the Health Professions, 32,* 90–97.

Opie, A. (2000). *Thinking teams/thinking clients: Knowledge-based teamwork.* New York, NY: Columbia University Press.

Pelto-Piri, V., Engström, K., & Engström, I. (2013). Paternalism, autonomy, and reciprocity: ethical perspectives in encounters with patients in psychiatric in-patient care. *BMC Medical Ethics, 14,* 49. Retrieved from: http://www.biomedcentral.com/1472-6939/14/49

Poole, M. S., & Real, K. (2003). Groups and teams in health care: Communication and effectiveness. In T. L. Thompson, A. M. Dorsey, K. I. Miller, & R. Parrot (Eds.), *Handbook of health communication* (pp. 369–402). Mahwah, NJ: Erlbaum.

Propp, K. M., Apker, J., Ford, W. S. Z., Wallace, N., Serbenski, M., & Hofmeister, N. (2010). Meeting the complex needs of the healthcare team: Identifying nurse-team communication practices perceived to enhance patient outcomes. *Qualitative Health Research, 20,* 15–28.

Reader, T. W., Flin, R., & Cuthbertson, B. H. (2007). Communication skills and error in the intensive care unit. *Current Opinions in Critical Care, 13,* 732–736.

Rodriguez-Osorio, C. A., & Dominguez-Cherit, G. (2008). Medical decision making: paternalism versus patient-centered (autonomous) care. *Current Opinion in Critical Care, 14,* 708–713.

Satin, D. G. (1994). The interdisciplinary, integrated approach to professional practice with the aged. In D. G. Satin (Ed.), *The clinical care of the aged person: An interdisciplinary perspective* (pp. 391–403). New York, NY: Oxford University Press.

Stokols, D., Hall, K. L., Taylor, B. K., & Moser, R. P. (2008). The science of team science: Overview of the field and introduction to the supplement. *American Journal of Preventative Medicine, 35*(2S), S77–89.

Stoner, M. H. (1999). The hemodialysis team. In C. F. Gutch, M. H. Stoner, & A. L. Corea (Eds.), *Review of hemodialysis for nurses and dialysis personnel* (pp. 1–9). St. Louis, MO: Mosby.

Wear, D. (1997). *Privilege in the medical academy: A feminist examines gender, race, & power.* New York, NY: Teachers College Press.

Wieland, D., Kramer, B. J., Waite, M. S., & Rubenstein, L. Z. (1996). The interdisciplinary team in geriatric care. *American Behavioral Scientist, 39,* 655–664.

Witte, K. (1994). The manipulative nature of health communication research: Ethical issues and guidelines. *American Behavioral Scientist, 38,* 285–293.

Wittenberg-Lyles, E. M., Gee, G. C., Oliver, D. P., & Demiris, G. (2009). What patients and families don't hear: Backstage communication in hospice interdisciplinary team meetings. *Journal of Housing for the Elderly, 23*(1–2), 92–105.

Wittenberg-Lyles, E., Oliver, D. P., Kruse, R. L., Demiris, G., Gage, L. A., & Wagner, K. (2013). Family caregiver participation in hospice interdisciplinary team meetings: How does it affect the nature and content of communication? *Health Communication, 28,* 110–118.

Wyatt, N. (2002). Foregrounding feminist theory in group communication research. In L. R. Frey (Ed.), *New directions in group communication* (pp. 43–56). Thousand Oaks, CA: Sage.

Youngwerth, J., & Twaddle, M. (2011). Cultures of interdisciplinary teams: How to foster good dynamics. *Journal of Palliative Medicine, 14,* 650–654.

5

Communicating and Navigating Digitized Healthcare

Jeanine M. Mingé & Nicole Defenbaugh[1]

Jane reaches up to the stubble on Joe's cheek. She draws herself closer to his lips. They kiss; hold lips together with a soft force. He smiles and hums. She moves her fingers on his neck, up to his ear. She feels his neck protruding with heat where there shouldn't be heat. She stops. He looks at her worried face. And he says, "Feel this. I found it a while ago." She draws her fingers to the lip of his jawbone and his neck. He moves his fingers away so she can apply pressure. She pulls away again and looks at him with wide eyes.

Her tone is serious, "You need to get that checked out. It isn't normal. Soon, OK? Promise?"

He nods and says, "Of course. I will call the Veterans Hospital soon." She wraps her arms around him.

Joe, retired from the Navy, was diagnosed with stage IV squamous cell carcinoma of the tonsils, a neck cancer, in August of 2012. His partner, Jane, was immediately thrust into the caregiving role.[2]

In this chapter, we follow Joe and Jane's journey on the wellness trail as *digital patients*. Jane, as caregiver, is not the immediate patient, but caregivers are integral, too, because they are embedded both in the medical system and in the life of the patient. Cancer certainly affects the family members and caregivers as well as the patient, albeit differently (Kim & Given, 2008). Throughout Joe and Jane's experience, they rely upon the support of various forms of social media and constantly seek information to survive this difficult situation. Their experience also offers insight into what it means to participate in a *digitized healthcare system*. In order to provide a deeper understanding of the experience of *digitized doctors*, we intertwine Joe and Jane's story with stories collected from physicians who speak about the impact technology has on their medical practice and patient care, specifically how it has affected clinician–patient communication. The physicians' stories, told via email or face-to-face conversations with one of the authors, were included to offer insight into the personal experiences and stories from those who work within healthcare. Their stories are captured in the "Physicians' Stories" boxes throughout the chapter.

This chapter on technology and health communication will examine three main components of our healthcare system and current uses of technology: (1) digitized healthcare system, (2) digitized health practitioner, and (3) digitized patient. The three components are addressed at various points throughout the chapter and speak to one another just as physicians, patients, and the system communicate both directly and indirectly. Western medicine itself is not linear but shifting, vacillating, and unstable for those who pass through its doors or reside within its walls.

The first of these intertwined contexts is the *digitized healthcare system* in which we explore the technological advancements that have shifted the climate and practice of providing healthcare. From electronic medical records (EMRs) and medical imaging to tablet computers and telemedicine, the realm of digital healthcare has reinvented Western medicine. This shift has created life-saving practices and also introduced a myriad of ethical and sociopolitical concerns, such as patients' access to information sharing and privacy.

The second context we explore is the *digitized health practitioner*. Because of these technological advancements, the role of digitized health practitioners and their communicative practices have changed. Digitized health practitioners include physicians and other clinicians such as registered nurses (RNs), certified registered nurse practitioners (CRNPs), physician's assistants (PAs), and other providers. However, in this chapter we focus on primary physicians and their one-on-one interactions with patients just like Joe. Digital health practitioners navigate "digital health," defined as "the products and businesses that apply modern digital technologies—the web, mobile, the cloud, miniature sensors" (Hixon, 2014). The learning curve for these advancements is steep, and the rewards to healthcare professionals and patients do not always outweigh the risks and disadvantages.

The third context, the *digitized patient,* participates within the world of telemedicine, seeks information virtually, creates support communities, and communicates about health and healing using various methods/means such as social media—Facebook, Instagram, community blogs, and online forums. While each of these contexts is examined separately here, we recognize that they are deeply intertwined and reciprocally connected. There will be important points of overlap. We begin with the digital healthcare system because the system of healthcare is where patient and clinician stories reside and where our journey begins. As the physician's story below explains, the relationship between healthcare and technology has been growing for over two decades.

■ The Digital Healthcare System

Physicians' Stories: The Inseparable Relationship

For me, technology and healthcare have become inseparable over the past 20 years, and yet the two are very early in getting the most out of their "relationship." From the moment I first had an electronic medical record, I began sharing it with patients as a way of engaging them. Once we had Internet access in exam rooms, I began using it to research evidence and find patient education. Without a doubt, it has expanded my capabilities to work with patients. Just as this integration has been a benefit to me, it has the same potential for patients. Most patients I see have used it wisely, to gather information and generate questions that are important to them. (BS email)

The "Smart" Diagnosis

Joe looks at the ER nurse over a white counter. "We were told to come into the ER by someone on the phone. I'm not sure if it's the right place to be, but I have a lump on my neck. It doesn't hurt or anything."

Jane interrupts, "Don't downplay it, OK?"

The nurse laughs out loud and says, "Your girlfriend knows what is what. She will take care of you. All right Joe, go on in."

The next nurse asks him, "Can you step on the scale for me?" A third nurse shuffles them into the waiting room and they are scheduled to meet with an RN.

Joe comes back out and says, "She didn't seem to take me seriously, but she got me an appointment to get blood tests done. I guess I also have to get a same-day biopsy in the ENT (Ear, Nose and Throat) Department."

"Today?" Jane asks.

"Yes." Joe responds quickly.

Now part of the medical system, they move through the white-walled building like rats in a maze. They move from waiting room to waiting room, from test to test, from nurse to nurse, who look up from computer screen to computer screen. They move up and down different elevators to find different offices. They do not speak about the possibility of a cancer diagnosis, as if saying it out loud would make cancer appear.

Jane and Joe reluctantly moved into the digital healthcare system on a trail toward wellness. They did not know this trail was heavily digitized (electronic records, technological advancements, and web resources for information seeking) and all a major part of their imminent journey. The communicative practices on the wellness journey within the digitized medical care system have changed. For Joe and Jane, it all began with the cancer discovery.

Discovery: Technological Advancements and the Rapid Result

Joe and Jane find ENT and sit in the hard, waiting-room chairs. Dr. Lee, a tall man in a white coat with blue embroidered letters, saunters to the front. He pushes his thin-framed glasses up the bridge of his nose. He calls, "Mr. Silver?" followed by an awkward, bubbled laugh. "Hey, man. I'm Dr. Lee. I come in here every once in a while. Do a little work. Help you guys out. Follow me." He brings them to a back room, sits them down on two blue chairs propped against a wall.

"So what I am going to do here is to take a sample of the lump in your neck, rather than having to wait for the results, ya know like the typical long process that makes you wait; we are, my team and I, going to get the results right here. You see we have made some advancements here in obtaining results. Basically, we are a rolling lab—these test tubes on the rolling cart, the slides and our microscope—will get you the results right here. You OK with that? You served us, now let us serve you. Sound good?"

Jane looks at Joe sitting to her left. His jaw seems tight but in typical Joe fashion he connects with the doctors; he smiles, he laughs, he is loving and kind. His eyes shine, but a thin veil of fear covers his body.

Dr. Lee introduces his team. "This here is Betsy, the best at her job, and Mimult, my trusty sidekick." He puts on blue rubber gloves. He grabs a needle out of a package. "Now, you aren't afraid of needles are you?"

Joe shakes his head. "Nope. I have a high tolerance for pain."

"I am going to numb it with this swab. Now, I am not going to lie, this is going to hurt a bit."
Jane cringes as the needle sticks deep into his neck. He moves it around like he is swirling a caul-
dron. Jane grabs Joe's hand. Joe's eyes shut tight, tighter; he gulps and winces. He takes a deep
breath. He exhales slowly as the needle is taken out.

Dr. Lee takes the needle and hands it to his assistants. They put some of the cells on the slide,
some in the test tube. He claps his hands awkwardly together and says jovially, "OK, let's see
what we have here." They treat the slides. Push the slide underneath the microscope. Betsy swal-
lows hard. She moves away from the slide and locks eyes with the younger man with olive skin
and thin bones. He moves to take a look. He clears his throat. Dr. Lee moves to take a look. Jane
looks at Joe, then back at the biopsy team for any sign of an answer.

"Hmm. OK. Let me see here. OK." He moves away from the microscope and sits back in
front of them. He claps his hands together and says, "OK, let me just come right out and say it; I
see some bad cells in there. So I am so sorry but it looks like they are malignant."

Joe swallows hard and his face goes pale. He takes a breath and asks to use the bathroom. Jane
sits there with them. Numb and breathing slowly, she takes in the words, "bad cells, malignant."
Cancer.

Technological advancements and the digitization of the medical care system have shifted the ways we communicate about health and healthcare. For Joe and Jane, the discovery of the cancer was abrupt and startling. They did not know it was possible to get the test results of a needle biopsy so quickly. Technological advancements within the digitized medical system have changed the speed at which people are diagnosed, thereby also increasing the speed at which they receive answers and proper medical care. This immediacy changed the communicative relationship between the patient, caregiver, and provider.

iPhones and other "smart" mobile devices are increasing in popularity across the U.S. The appeal of these devices goes beyond the Candy Crush game and social networking to accessing virtually any information at any time. In healthcare, the use of smartphones has far-reaching uses and implications for patient care, having already influenced the world of medicine as an important tool for healthcare professionals (Choi et al., 2011) and as a teaching tool in medical education (Franko & Tirrell, 2012; Wallace, Clark, & White, 2012). Doctors are using devices on their phones to access medical knowledge and communicate with patients and other clinicians. In the past, doctors had to rely on medical books they carried in their lab coats or make a trip to the library for up-to-date medical information. Today, smartphones enable clinicians to not only make calls and communicate with others more efficiently but also send emails, search for the latest medical information using medical apps (Ozdalga, Ozdalga, & Ahuja, 2012), take photographs of injuries, examine radiological images (Choi et al., 2011), and diagnose and treat patients.

Medical applications or "apps" enable doctors to quickly find the most up-to-date information. Various studies (Hafner, 2012; Terry, 2010) have researched different types of apps used by healthcare professionals such as Epocrates, an app for checking drug interactions and improving electronic health record (EHR) efficiency (www.epocrates.com); MedCalc, an app that allows the user to calculate medical formulas and scales (http://medcalc.medserver.be/); Skyscape a "medical library" app that includes a calculator, drug guide, clinical news, and resources (www.skyscape.com); and Dr. SMART S, an app used in South Korea that allows doctors access to patients and their medical information (Choi et al., 2011). Researchers have found that doctors most often use drug guide apps (79%) (Franko & Tirrell, 2011), given the ever-changing guidelines for medication dosage and the continuous introduction of new medications.

The digitization of the medical system has changed the ways in which providers make diagnoses and communicate with patients and caregivers about these diagnoses and treatments. For the physician below, electronic resources have made the provider's information-seeking process faster, smoother, and more precise.

Physicians' Stories: Armed with Electronic Resources

One of our interns was armed with both a smartphone and online resources. A woman came in with multiple comorbidities. She had come in with chest pain, but she also had symptoms of what looked like TIA (transient ischemic attack), and she has had known coronary disease (CAD) and had bypass surgery. She also has had a stroke in the past. She has known cerebrovascular disease. Each of these conditions would have recommendations for what she would take as an antiplatelet agent (e.g., aspirin or clopidogrel). There are a variety of these agents around to reduce the risk of subsequent heart attack, subsequent stroke. In this case, she had both problems and had her symptoms while she was on a regimen that was designed to prevent them.

Our intern was able to connect quickly with some articles that talked about just the kind of patient we had in front of us and give guidance, weighing the pros and cons of different agents for what could do the job to prevent bad things from happening without raising the risk of excessive bleeding, which is one of the problems of being on these medications. He [the intern] was able to get that information confidently, present it to the patient, and didn't need to consult a neurologist and cardiologist because it was very clear in what he was able to read that the information was up-to-date and relevant. It saved time, two consultations, and actually took her off one of the medications she was taking! This is as an intern. This is a doctor with one year of experience. I stopped him and said, "I would not have been able to make that decision without 2 hours in the library . . . and had been much farther along in my training." I probably would have either gotten a consultation because we didn't have 2 or 3 hours to figure it out, or I would have gone by the seat of my pants and made an educated guess that wouldn't have been consistent with the latest evidence. (RM interview)

As with the advent of any new advancement, apps face challenges that have yet to be fully addressed. For example, there is no information security or protection of patient information (Choi et al., 2011). Unlike other medical information that is regulated *within* a healthcare system such as EHRs, apps do not currently have the same restrictions or regulations. As Franko and Tirrell (2011) state, "No organizations or governing bodies currently exist to review or validate the content contained within these apps" (p. 3138). In addition to unrestricted use, applications pose challenges to users such as identifying reputable apps, preventing internalization of knowledge, causing distractions, and blurring personal/professional boundaries (Wallace et al., 2012) along with a loss of one-on-one connection with patients (Hafner, 2012). In spite of the personal and ethical challenges, apps continue to offer clinicians the tools to increase their knowledge and their quality of patient care.

Although the information-seeking process for providers has improved with the advancements of technology, technologies—electronic resources, electronic medical records, and advancements in medical technologies—have changed the way doctors and patients communicate. As Joe and Jane get the prognosis from the head ENT physician, they realize the doctor and the patient are on different sides of the room and what stands between them is a computer screen.

Prognosis and Treatment Plan: Just a Computer Screen Away

Joe and Jane arrive at ENT, the head and neck clinic on the basement floor of the hospital. In the waiting room, they wait. Jane takes out her small black field note journal. They wait. Jane stares at her Visitor Pass and says, "I wonder about the relationships, the hours of time spent in these hospitals. You think he has someone to take him home?" She points to the man sleeping in the wheelchair in the middle of the hospital.

"Him?" Joe looks at the man she is pointing to and smiles at her kindness, "Let's hope so, babe." He grabs her knee and squeezes it gently. "Let's hope so."

Jane stares straight ahead and says, "I hope this doctor is one of the good ones. I hope he or she will speak to us clearly, like humans, like we have beating, fear-filled hearts."

Joe keeps his hand on her knee and says, "Me too. And if not, we have you to tell him or her to speak slower."

Dr. Samat, a young chief resident at the VA hospital, enters the room. He takes the computer mouse and clicks a few buttons to look up Joe's EHR. He squints his eyes and moves closer to the screen. "Let me just take a look at the notes here. Who was working on you last time? Oh yes, Sue. She is a new resident here. I hope she was good with you." After scrolling through the notes, he turns in the four-wheeled desk chair and faces Joe. He explains, "We found cancer in your neck. We aren't quite sure of the primary source. About 10% of carcinomas have an unknown primary. Knowing the primary source changes the way we treat the cancer. So let's find it OK?"

"And what if we don't find it?" Jane asks.

"Then we will keep looking," Dr. Samat says curtly. Jane scribbles a note in her journal to research unknown primaries in cancer treatments.

"I'm just gonna take a look here. Open wide." Dr. Samat stands and grabs his light. He clicks it on. Joe opens his mouth and the doctor sticks his fingers and the light down his throat. Joe gags hard. He kicks his legs up as his whole body convulses. He laughs and says, "I have a crazy gag reflex. So don't be mad if I throw up on you."

Jane giggles. "Don't turn this way, OK?"

Dr. Samat sits back down at the desk. He explains the next steps. "You will have a tonsillectomy and biopsy surgery to find the primary source. First, we have to have a PET scan [see Definition Box] and a CT (computerized tomography) scan to make sure the cancer isn't anywhere else in your body. The surgery will be in two weeks." He begins to type notes in the computer. He has turned his body from facing them to facing the computer.

A **PET scan** "uses radiation, or nuclear medicine imaging, to produce 3-dimensional, color images of the functional processes within the human body. PET stands for *positron emission tomography*. . . . PET scans can be used to diagnose a health condition, as well as to find out how an existing condition is developing. PET scans are often used to see how effective an ongoing treatment is" (http://www.medicalnewstoday.com/articles/154877.php).

Jane starts to panic, "It feels like too long of a wait. We want it out right now."

Dr. Samat stops typing and turns back around. "We have to get blood tests done, go to the pre-op clinic, take these precautionary steps to measure ten times and cut once. Let me just finish updating the chart here and I will see you out. The admin at the front desk can schedule the next steps with you."

He turns back to his computer. Joe and Jane exchange helpless glances.

As displayed in Joe and Jane's story, the use of EHRs changes the ways in which providers and patients communicate. EHRs—also frequently referred to as EMRs (electronic medical records)—"is the official document for patient management" (Polack & Avtgis, 2011, p. 322). EHRs have benefits, as du Pré (2013) explains:

> But because EMRs can be viewed and shared by a number of health professionals in different locations, they allow caregivers to more easily avoid treatment overlaps and drug interactions and to track patients' overall progress. EMRs are also invaluable in emergencies, when paper records might be unavailable or when waiting for them would waste precious time. As a result, EMRs save time, money, and lives. (p. 330)

Furthermore, EHRs allow for multiple clinicians to view and access a single patient's records. Healthcare professionals from different areas/departments (e.g., oncology, cardiology, and gastroenterology), for example, can look up information on a patient to find out previous tests, medications, or diagnoses to avoid ordering duplicate tests or prescribing new medications. EHRs have the potential to increase health professionals' communication resulting in improved patient care and safety. And yet, as demonstrated above, Joe and Jane have a difficult time understanding the medical jargon associated with the EHRs. And this changes the way doctors and patients communicate.

The question then becomes, does the use of EHRs *actually* improve the quality of patient care? In 2003 the use of EHRs was predicted to increase and be fully implemented in the United States by 2014 (Institute of Medicine, 2003). However, the U.S. has not achieved universal EHR adoption (Ford, Menachemi, & Phillips, 2006) and, compared to other industrialized nations, the U.S. has lagged behind its use of EHRs in ambulatory care by 24–28% (Jha, Doolan, Grandt, Scott, & Bates, 2008). Like any technological advancement, EHRs come with a myriad of problems. In some cases, EHRs were not found to improve quality of care (Linder, Ma, Bates, Middleton, & Stafford, 2007) for patients. In a study on hospitals without EHRs, reasons for not using them included inadequate funding and physician resistance, among others (Jha et al., 2008). Researchers have examined various challenges related to sharing EHRs with patients such as cost, security, rights, and patient comprehension of medical information (Beard, Schein, Morra, Wilson, & Keelan, 2012).

Allowing patients access to their medical records has the benefit of less wait time for results, but it also increases the risk of confusion or added stress if a patient is unable to interpret the results that are usually written in medical jargon. As the authors (Beard et al., 2012) state, "Physicians and health systems administrators have noted concerns about patients viewing new clinical data before they have been explained to them, particularly if the results are abnormal or have negative health" (p. 118). Medical records are written by clinicians in medical language because those who are most likely to view the information are other clinicians. These clinicians will likely shape the story of the patient into "an efficient, objective, problem- or disease-focused medical record, and, as a result, many of the patient's values and priorities are not documented" (Winkelman, Leonard & Rossos, 2005, p. 310). The medical record, therefore, is a document filled with medical-specific language not intended for patient viewing.

Although patients have the legal right to view their own health information, some healthcare providers worry about patients' ability to understand their records. Patients, however, are finding ways to take control of their illness and their health information by being more involved and taking a more proactive role, especially for those with a chronic illness (Winkelman et al., 2005). Researchers have found that when individuals have access to their own records, it enhances both their illness ownership as well as participation in management and decision making with their physicians (Winkelman et al., 2005). According to the following physician, there is the "good, bad, and ugly" of having to work with EHRs.

Physicians' Stories: The Good, the Bad, & the Ugly of EHRs

The good is there's no way I would go back to using a paper chart again. I believe in this day and age you need to use electronic health records, electronic resources. I think it makes things easier to find. The huge amount of information we have, there's no question in my mind that it is overall the pluses and minuses safety-wise, especially with prescription writing, legibility, that type of thing. The pluses outweigh the minuses.

The bad. Let me give you an anecdote of the bad. Two healthcare systems within shouting distance of each other use Next Gen (a type of electronic health record system) and do you think these two systems talk to each other? They don't talk to each other at all. So this patient comes in, and I need to get her printed records off her previous doctor's Next Gen system, which was the same electronic health record as our Next Gen system, but they didn't talk to each other. It was printed, which was better than hand-written records, but we had to do the work again and print it. The whole idea that these things (health records) should communicate and be universal like web browsers, is a national disgrace. There's no defacto [sic] or de jure system whereby the systems can communicate. This has set back things enormously. If you would have asked me 10 years ago if these (electronic health record) systems would not be talking to each other in 2014, I would have said, "No way." I can't say it's injured or killed people, but it's had a tremendous impact on patients' flow from one system to another, and we use more than one system in an area. It's had an impact on the patient and on good medical care. (LS interview)

Joe is asked to fill out living directives, to be carried out by his son and Jane, if by chance the surgery goes awry. They go over each question about life support, life-sustaining treatments, end-of-life care. All of this information is entered into the database.

Jane asks, "So when I call now, as his caregiver, will they give me information?"

The administrator says, "Depends on who answers, and if your information is in the system. But really, only Joe can get the information about his own health."

Jane holds his hand. She kisses his face. She speaks softer, kinder. She says, every hour, "I love you—with all of me."

▨ The Digital Doctor

Doctor–patient communication continues to evolve as the healthcare system and individuals who frequent it change. With the ever-evolving advancements in technology, the medical office visit has changed and impacted effective communication. Teutsch (2003) explains that doctor–patient communication is "sacrificed with the intrusion of business into the patient–doctor relationship, the pressures of limited time for office visits, the culture of medicalization, and the sometimes all-consuming focus on technology" (p. 1115).

Communicative Barriers in the Business of Medicine

Joe and Jane are back at the VA for the pre-op blood tests and scans. The nurse reads off the screen as Jane looks over her shoulder. "You will have a bilateral tonsillectomy and panendoscopy with biopsy" [see Definition Box].

Panendoscopy is an "examination, usually with the patient under general anesthesia, of the pharynx, larynx, upper trachea, and esophagus with rigid and flexible endoscopes" (http://medical-dictionary.thefreedictionary.com/panendoscopy). A **biopsy** is "removal and examination, usually microscopic, of tissue from the living body, performed to establish precise diagnosis" (http://medical-dictionary.thefreedictionary.com/biopsy).

He looks at her and straightens out his long legs, "What does that mean?"
She moves her wire rim glasses down her face. She looks back at the screen then back at him squarely. "They are going to remove both of your tonsils, look around and biopsy different parts of your throat, tongue, and mouth to find the primary cancer source. OK?" He nods. "Now, let's go over your history and your health regimen." The nurse faces the computer, looks up his previous data, and begins to ask him questions about his workout schedule, his daily routines, and other pertinent questions. Joe puffs out his chest a bit, the looming fear of surgery embedded in his answers. He wants to seem strong, to feel strong, to be well.
She asks, "Do you work out?"
"I surf every day." He smiles, shifts in his chair and says confidently, "I am probably the most fit person in this building."
She clicks a button and types on the keyboard.
"OK, then. What about when you bleed, does it take a while to heal?"
"I heal in five minutes."
She clicks a button and types on the keyboard.
"Do you ever feel numb in your appendages, like your feet, fingers, toes?"
He scoffs at the question, laughs and boasts, "Only when I cut off my own circulation."
She clicks a button and types on the keyboard.
She then asks, "What about your teeth? Do you have dentures?"
"Nope."
She clicks a button and types on the keyboard.

As demonstrated in Joe and Jane's story, not only is it vital for doctors to communicate effectively because of patient care and safety, the ability to do so has become more challenging with the inclusion of computers and other technology in the exam room. Placing computers in providers' offices has proven to be an especially difficult challenge in the encounter, affecting overall rapport with patients and leading some general practitioners to be so absorbed with the computer and its required tasks that they ignore their patients (Booth, Robinson, & Kohannejad, 2004). To solve the dilemmas with multitasking, clinicians can use signposting, signaling that they are changing the direction of the conversation. They can also use signposting to inform their patients that they are using the computer, indicate that they are ready to listen again, continue general conversation to indicate they are listening, and stop typing to look at the patient whenever responding (Booth et al., 2004).

The use of technology changes the physicality of communicative practices. Quite literally, hospitals and doctors' offices are changing the space to account for advancements in technology. Changing the space to change the encounter is also explored in the following physician's story.

Physicians' Stories: Changing the Space to Change the Encounter

Then comes along the computer, our first desktop, and there was a lot of glancing over at the patient. I got feedback from Press Ganey [a patient satisfaction measurement instrument] from patients saying, "My doctor doesn't look at me anymore." Then as we were designing our new office, we made intentional, physical changes to the exam rooms. The table (to place your laptop) was lower and the computer would be off to the side. And each physician had a laptop instead of a desktop so there were intentional decisions for the communication piece. I can look at the patient more easily and frequently. Since the changes, I never got that feedback again about the computer. People are now used to it (computer) and hopefully I'm doing a better job. Patients can see my face. They can tell by my body language that I'm engaged in what they're saying. So I'm not losing focus as I'm typing something on the computer. I'll even say to a patient, "Hold on a second. I need to look this (fact/information) up." So in short, we made conscious changes to the physical/structural environment of the office to increase physician–patient communication because of advancements. (JB interview)

For clinicians to be effective communicators in a patient encounter, essential communication techniques are important to increase the likelihood of a productive and collaborative visit. Nonverbal techniques such as increased eye contact, use of facial expressions and awareness of proxemics (use of physical space), for example, are especially important in patient–physician encounters (Teutsch, 2003) but difficult for clinicians to do when they are looking at a computer screen while entering patient information into the EHR. It is important, therefore, for clinicians to be cognizant of the physical space of the office and their physical placement within it to maximize effective communication with the patient. Although technology can create communication barriers, it also has positive aspects that can improve clinician–patient communication.

The Doctor Is Just a Text Away

Joe walks faster than Jane. She calls, "Babe, can you wait up?" His long legs slow their stride. He turns to his left and reaches his hand back for Jane to grab it.

"Watch out," he warns as they cross the street, to reach the entrance into the hospital. A car, a silver Honda Civic, pulls to the side and Dr. L. jumps out.

"Hey, Mr. Silver so good to see you." He jovially says and extends his hand for him to shake it. "So, good news in there. I'm not really supposed to be telling you out here in the middle of the crosswalk, but if it were me about to head in there, I would want to know right away. They discovered it's local. The CT scan didn't show cancer anywhere else in your body! Good news, indeed." Joe and Jane look at each other. "Now, listen. Here is my cell phone number. Text or call me if you have any questions or concerns. I know I'm not supposed to be giving my number out, but heck. I don't care. I want to make sure you feel cared for." Dr. L. hands them his business card. Joe shakes his hand again, and Dr. L. hops back into his car.

Jane pulls Joe closer to her as they cross the next crosswalk, with pep in their step. Joe warns, "Don't get too overzealous. We still have a long way to go."

"Yep," Jane says warmly, "On our wellness trail." She hugs the side of her face into his chest. He smiles and turns to speak to the security guard at the entrance of the hospital.

"You know what, babe?"

"What, love?" she asks and squeezes his hand.

"I've been treated like gold here."

"Good; we need to feel protected, taken care of, on this journey."

Clinicians have also found ways to stay connected to their patients through ever-advancing forms of technology. One physician describes what is gained with his patient and what is lost by using texting as a method of clinical care.

Physicians' Stories: Reaching the Physician "Faster" through Emailing and Texting (Benefits & Risks)

I have a patient who's a prior employee of our department, whose family I care for. She has had my cell number since before she became my patient and so I get text messages from her maybe once a month with a question or a picture of a rash of one of her children. I have shared with her that those may not be secure messages and some of the risks. There are risks that come with that, but it's really enriched our relationship. So there is some risk with that, too, about barriers. At what point do we stop being friends and start being a patient and doctor? That's a little bit of a challenge, but I think in almost all of the cases where I have let down that barrier to give someone additional access, it's enriched our relationship, and I've been successful in being able to set the boundaries with it. So if we take the (medical staff) team out of our communication (by texting), then we can lose some of that safety netting.

I have been pretty successful in choosing the right communication tool for the right messages. So I haven't had a patient that's been anxious or worried by something I sent them via email. Occasionally texts are a different thing. There's a huge risk of losing nonverbal content that connotes the critical message. (anonymous interview)

Tonsillectomy: What the System Says

Jane feels Joe's heart beating, draws her fingers in the shape of his heart on the edge of his skin, willing his heart to stay strong during the procedure. Then she draws her lips to his forehead, spilling all of her strength and love to take away the squamous cells multiplying in his tonsil.

"Mmmmm. That feels good," he says as he draws his eyes to meet hers. "Can you do that again?"

She smiles slightly. "Of course, my love." And she does it again, draw her lips lightly across his brow, she kisses him for each inhale and exhale. "I love you. It will all be ok."

Nurses enter. The one with gold lining her teeth, a straight black haircut bob style, and an accent checks his pulse. His heart rate is only 42 beats per minute (BPM). They input this information into their tablet. One nurse says, "Your heart rate is too low for surgery, at least that is what the system says. I'll ask the doctor to check the chart."

Joe explains, "I have a runner's heart."

She leaves to check to see if his low BPM is "acceptable" for the surgery. She is checking the numbers, checking the charts, checking to make sure Joe measures up to the required numbers implemented by the medical system.

The nurse comes back after 30 minutes of waiting.

Then he is wheeled away. Jane says, "I love you," as he is wheeled out. He does not look back.

Here, the nurse is confined to and defined by what the chart says on her medical device. And this "catch" could save Joe's life. The electronic resource is an important part of the medical process. As in the physician story below, the medical device is so much a part of the "hellos and good-byes," it is almost an appendage.

Physicians' Stories: Power Cord Grounding

I have the pleasure of working at a young FQCHC (federally qualified health center) in an urban setting with many patients being primarily Spanish speaking from a variety of places within the Caribbean, and Central and South America. Our ten or so part-time medical providers share the five or so portable electronic tablets for patient care, as all our work is based within an electronic record. The collective, we, are all responsible to turn off and plug in when done, so that the tablet will gain charge and be available for the next user. As is to be expected, there are times that a tablet is not placed into its charger and this leaves the next provider with an uncharged tablet. To use an uncharged tablet, one has to bring along the power cord and plug it into the wall socket in the patient care room.

Today I find myself in the situation of the provider with an uncharged tablet. As I move in and out of patient care rooms, my tablet's long tail of an electrical cord marks my path behind me. I am time-challenged and perennially running late during patient care sessions. Now I have this leash to remind me of my hurry and my frustration with the limited technology support services available within my medical home.

The cord becomes part of my hello and good-byes. I greet patients with a monologue that my tablet got up late and did not eat breakfast and so I must bring its plug into the room or we will be without its company and hence without its resources. A 4-year-old girl has recovered from her coxsackie virus and needs a note to return to school. We talk about how my tablet needs "juice" and how she and I are healthier with drinking water. Next, the plug gets wound around the stool on which I sit while having a conversation as to what to expect from labor and birth with an 18-year-old in her first pregnancy, due next week. Her aunt with whom she lives and who accompanies her today is wisely commenting on the natural process of birth while also unwinding the electric cord and placing it in a safe arrangement behind me. Her aunt will be a reliable and grounded resource for this new mom and newborn, and today I am appreciative of her care of me as well. I am thankful to have the ability to access the Internet in this moment and the electric cord is light as a feather. I am content. I just may use the cord as a jump rope to skip on to my next venture. (Garufi, 2014)

■ The Digital Patient

As U.S. society continues to advance, the modernization of patients and doctors, in response to these changes, has occurred. For patients, this advancement to a state of modernity is focused on their ability to analyze and engage in their care based on their level of involvement. Buetow, Jutel, & Hoare (2009) define the "modern patient":

> The "modern patient" is the more recent social actor who is disposed to learn and exercise critically and responsibly an informed capacity and entitlement to use, evaluate and influence health services (Hibbard, 2003). While the non-modern, or less modern, patient lacks these qualities, the modern patient can take an active or passive role in interactions with the doctor, as circumstances require. Committed and enabled to take increased control over their own health, the modern patient can also take a part of the role of the doctor, both by co-providing formal health care (Stacey, 1988) and by providing educated self-care, for example in chronic disease management (Wagner, 2000). That the modern patient also heavily depends on doctor expertise, to meet their own high expectations for health care, does not diminish these abilities to engage in more equal ways, as in shared decision-making. (pp. 98–99)

This definition of *modern patients* places them in control of their care, taking an interactive role alongside the physician in everything from disease management to self-care. As a result, patients have also taken a more consumerist or "expert" approach in their care leading to an increase in patient literacy (Buetow et al., 2009). The modern patient has had an impact on clinicians, resulting in a need to be more flexible and collaborative in patient care and, in some cases, has led to a loss in authority and autonomy (Buetow et al., 2009).

Information Seeking: "It's All Jargon to Me"

Weeks after the tonsillectomy and the biopsy of the tissue in his throat, Joe and Jane are back in the hospital to get the result and to find out where the primary source of the cancer is.

"So even after the biopsy, we couldn't find the source of the primary. Sometimes this happens. But the good news is, we have removed your tonsils. So we are on to the next phase of treatment."

"What do you mean you couldn't find it? I'm confused." Joe sounds a little panicked.

"Sometimes the biopsy doesn't show us everything. Or the primary source was very small so your body may have taken care of it." Dr. Samat turns back to the screen. Another resident pops her head in the door and Dr. Samat excuses himself to go help her with another patient. In his absence, Joe and Jane anxiously pore over the computer screen. Joe shakes his head, "What does he mean my body may have taken care of it?"

Jane says, "I can't read any of this. It's all jargon to me."

Joe shakes his head. "I just want it to make sense, to be clear. It's my life they are talking about here."

Jane smiles. "I know who to call! Cee Cee will know what this means. She is an oncology nurse in another state. I'm gonna take a picture and send it to her." Jane snaps a picture of the screen and hits send with a message that says, "Help! What does this mean? Please call us after you read through it. I love you!"

Joe and Jane arrive home from the VA. They feel helpless. Jane starts to Google the information on the screen. She types in the words, "Squamous cell carcinoma, poorly differentiated. Vascular-lymphatic invasion by tumor is present." She looks at Joe who is propped up in bed reading a Jack Kerouac book. "I don't really understand any of this. And look, they even typed in the note, 'All questions answered.'"

"Yeah right. I am more confused than ever. I mean, I know they answered questions, but it is so hard to take this in right now," said Joe, his glasses on the brim of his nose.

They wait for Cee Cee to call them back with straightforward information, clarity, and an interpretation of language they don't understand. Jane suggests, "Let's take control of our own care; let's be ready with questions for them." Joe dictates and she writes questions, for the next doctor, for their own research purposes, so they can take control.

"I want to talk to the person who reads the actual scan. Is that a possibility?"

"I want to ask my friend Dr. W. about options, get my second and third opinion."

"I want to bring up my headaches. What's going on there?"

"I want to know the duration of the actual surgery. How long will I be under?"

"Are they just going to keep digging around in there?"

"I also want a clearer picture of the recovery time."

"I want to know their thoughts about integrative oncology. Do they even care about nutrition?"

She looks at him and asks, "Will it affect your fertility?"

Then Jane jumps onto WebMD.

Although the doctor offered Joe and Jane some information about not finding the primary source of cancer after the tonsillectomy and biopsy, Joe and Jane were not satisfied with the information they were given. Moreover, this is a stressful situation so Jane wants answers now, not later. She wants to be able to feel safe, to feel like they have the answers. In this terribly uncertain situation, they use the Web to reduce this uncertainty. Technology is both helpful (at least they got answers quickly) and also harmful or problematic as they aren't medical practitioners themselves and interpreting information from the Internet sources may render them more confused or with the wrong information. Technology has left Joe and Jane at the mercy of the medical system.

Joe and Jane are not alone in this information-seeking process. It is estimated that 4.5% of all Internet searches are for health-related information (Morahan-Martin, 2004). This includes approximately 70 million Americans who participate in medical information seeking (Nielsen-Bohlman, Panzer, & Kindig, 2004). Researchers have studied the use of technology as a tool for consumers searching for online medical information (Beck, 2001; du Pré, 2013; Geist-Martin, Ray, & Sharf, 2003; Parker & Thorson, 2009; Polack & Avtgis, 2011). If you turn to technology for resources or social support to find information on a specific illness/disease, then you are known as an *e-patient* (Polack & Avtgis, 2011). From websites designed by medical organizations, insurance companies, clinicians, and the "average" (lay) individual, to evidence-based articles and scientific studies, there is both a breadth and depth of information available for those who have the means to access, locate, and interpret what is on the Internet. Both advantages and disadvantages result from Internet-based health communication, ranging from decreasing the power imbalance between doctors and patients to increasing difficulties for patients to comprehend received medical information (Jucks & Bromme, 2007).

In Theorizing Practice 5.1, we ask you to consider the discussion that occurs between physicians and patients who search for medical information online before an appointment. Physicians have different reactions to "educated" patients who conduct prior research on a health-related issue before their visit. In the story below, one physician describes what an "educated" patient looks like and the dialogic dance that frequently occurs.

Theorizing Practice 5.1
Do You Surf the Internet for Medical Information?

Having read the physician story about "educated" patients, consider the following questions:

1. Why might some physicians encourage patients to seek online resources?
2. Why might some physicians be frustrated with patients who search for health-related information online?
3. Have *you* ever searched the Internet for medical information? If so, how did you decide on the site(s) you chose?
4. Did you have a discussion about the online information with your healthcare provider? Why or why not?

Physicians' Stories: Talking to an "Educated" Patient

Typically unbiased information is something you have to pay for and people don't pay for things when they look up stuff on the Internet. I don't even think there's up-to-date information for lay people.... I want to have an "educated" patient but it's not the same. They're coming in with information, but they're not really educated about what it (illness) is. So it's piecemeal information that they've put together in their own way, which wouldn't be how, clinically, it should be put together. So I have to tear it [information they've collected] down and build it back up again, which I didn't need to do. I could have just given them the information in the first place.

Turns out there are a lot of people who want to be reassured and *know* they have a cold and *don't* want the antibiotics. Typically I'll describe why they don't need one and the patient will say, "Oh good. Because I didn't want one based on the stuff I know." Now whether that's stuff on the Internet or stuff they've been told for the last 10 years about not overusing antibiotics, I'm not sure. The more "educated" person will say, "Do I actually need that test?" or "Do I need that medicine because things I've read said _____." The people who have better questions to ask, those people I don't get frustrated with. "That's a great question," I'll say, "And here's my answer to it"—as opposed to people who look things up and come to an office visit with *the* answers. (JB interview)

Cee Cee calls to report what she understands from the pictures on the computer screen. She cries and gives his life a number of years, 5 at the most. According to other patients with this type of cancer, Joe's percentage of survival is slim. Jane holds back a wall of tears so Joe won't become alarmed. Cee Cee says, "I can't tell from the screen shot, but you need to ask if there is necrosis. If so, then it's growing fast. Call me once you know that."

Jane looks at Joe's neck, the swollen skin, the mass underneath. To the outsider, it would not be noticeable. But she can see it, the small centimeter of swollen skin, cancer cells dividing so quickly they can't get enough blood supply so the cells at the center of growth die. "What did she say?" Joe asks.

Jane says, "Well, she gave me the statistics about survival rate." Her eyes gleam with tears.

"I don't want to know that," says Joe.

Jane says, "OK. Because you aren't like other people." She smiles and kisses his face. "Well, Cee Cee also said to ask about the necrosis. We should want to know at what rate it is dividing.

If it is dividing quickly, then two to three weeks to wait to start treatment may jeopardize your health. And we will want to fight for a sooner treatment start date."

Because of their friend's ability to read the documents sent via text message, and their information-seeking over the Internet, Joe and Jane feel more confident in their understanding of the difficult medical language. The use of the Internet by patients for health information continues to climb. As Fox (2006) states, "Eighty percent of adult Internet users seek health information from the Internet, with about seven percent of Internet users searching for health information on each day" (as cited in Bylund et al., 2007, p. 346). Beck (2001) recalls the story of a student who would invest hours researching before a doctor's visit. The student told her, "By the time I walk in the door, I make darn sure that I know more than that doctor does" (p. 174). Beck wondered how the information the student researched was presented to the doctor and concludes, "For many, the Internet constitutes an invaluable vehicle for diverse sources of information, especially for those who deliberately weigh the validity of 'facts' and claims" (p. 174).

HCIA 5.1

Calling Dr. Google:
Health Literacy and Media Agency for At-Risk Urban Youth

Angela Cooke-Jackson

When I asked my health communication students where they got most of their health information they said, without hesitation, Google. I can still remember my puzzlement at their responses. To better understand this phenomenon, I developed a class lecture to see what they were doing in their searches and how they were being impacted by what they learned. I started the class discussion with a candid yet honest scenario: "You are 15 years old and you just learned that your sexual partner has chlamydia. Walk me through the steps you would take to find out what it is and how it might affect you." I asked them to be prepared to share their explanations of each step, and after the allotted time, I began a class discussion that produced some of the most insightful dialogues I have experienced in my classroom.

The term *health literacy* is typically understood as the capacity of individuals to procure and process information related to their health status and services; however, research has proven that teaching health literacy also means training young people to be critical consumers, creators, and disseminators of health media. Young people have a multitude of Internet resources at their fingertips with unrestricted access. Yet they possess little knowledge about how to make sense of and use that information to their benefit. So, while 12- to 22-year-olds are exemplary in their use of emerging technology and social media, they are not critical consumers of this information and often do not reflect on the impact this information has on their health decision making.

As I have learned from my health communication students, websites like DietDoc or WebMD offer an overwhelming amount of information. Websites commonly perceived as most beneficial, such as the Centers for Disease Control and Prevention (CDC), the National Institute of Health (NIH), or the World Health Organization (WHO), are not utilized by this age group because, as my students attested, these sites are "too wordy" and "not accessible."

Class discussions became the impetus for a community-based, participatory collaboration between a group of people: two faculty members from Emerson College, an individual with the Boston Public Health Commission, and two individuals from local, community, youth nonprofits. This collaborative initiative, now entitled the Emerson Literacy Education and Empowerment Project (eLEEP), invites a group of at-risk youth to a seven-week health and media literacy training program that straddles higher education and community enhancement to promote the development of healthy, informed, and empowered young adults. Over the past decade, reflective participatory studies have proven that youth who are immersed in active learning, whereby they function as creators and disseminators of health messages, demonstrate greater self-efficacy and agency. Using storytelling constructs that place youth at the center as creators of their learning is paramount in advancing their ability to mindfully reflect upon health information before they adopt and negotiate their health behaviors.

eLEEP serves youth in several high-risk urban communities in Boston. Together, adolescents and college student mentors address a range of topics, from sexual health and healthy dating relationships to healthy lifestyle behaviors. The primary objective for the youth is to learn about health and media literacy, while simultaneously developing media skills like storyboarding, editing, and video production focused on a range of health issues they confront in their communities.

Health-literate youth view digital media as a means of communication in order to share their stories and initiate important conversations around sexual health. Using media skills acquired through this participatory-learning model and the power of peer-to-peer mentoring and collaboration, eLEEP adolescents produce digital health vignettes. The youth articulate their training with the use of everyday technology by conducting mentoring workshops with middle schoolers who attend community after-school programs. Digital media becomes a tool for health education. Through this program, youth become knowledgeable, competent, and critical consumers of media; they also become mindful citizens able to challenge societal norms regarding sexual health and healthy relationships.

Two particularly compelling youth-created health vignettes used digital techniques to encapsulate today's media outlets with a health-driven spin. In "It's Not As Rare as You Think," a news team follows a young couple just having a good time. Promoting the normality of a healthy relationship, this fun faux news segment proves there's more to dating than the media portray. Another student-created vignette called "Teen Harmony" mimics an online dating website, promising that you'll find the love of your life. But, hold on; there's a

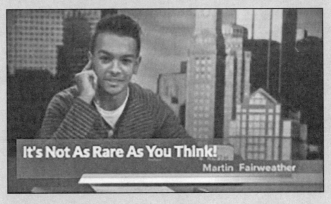

"It's Not As Rare As You Think," by eLEEP.

(continued)

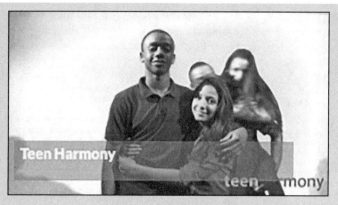

"Teen Harmony," by eLEEP.

disclaimer. People don't always portray themselves as they truly are on Internet dating sites, so you have to carefully take time to learn about your partner.

eLEEP's goal is to increase health literacy by empowering youth *agency*, the ability to act in a way that accomplishes your goals with purpose and understanding. Often, youth from at-risk, low-income communities think they don't have the means for agency; they often feel powerless given the overwhelming disparities they confront. After the health and media literacy training program, there is a shift in these youths' perspectives, as exemplified in the following quotes.

> I believe I do anything I can to accomplish my personal goals . . . when I set a goal and I want something done, I know exactly what I have to do to reach that goal.

> I have agency because I have a good understanding of what is good and what is bad. There is a time in life for everything, and I know what my main focuses are right now. I can prioritize and that helps me a lot in school to get the grades that I want, to reach the future I want.

This shift in perspective is what moves them to continue their critical consumption of health information on any website they encounter.

QUESTIONS TO PONDER

1. Name a couple examples of both positive and negative media portrayals about sexual health and relationships for youth and/or young adults (examples can include television shows, films, music videos, etc.). If you had to give a grade of A, B, C, D, or F to these examples, what grades would each receive and why? How do the media you consume help increase or decrease your health agency?

2. Hypothetically, if you were a peer mentor, what steps could you take to help youth initiate peer-to-peer messages and conversations that make it comfortable to talk about sexual health?

3. What other types of community-oriented collaborations with colleges/universities can be created for at-risk communities to promote positive health behaviors?

Sources: Cooke-Jackson, A. (2013). Harnessing collective social media engagement in a health communication course. *Communication Teacher, 27,* 165–171. Cooke-Jackson, A., & Barnes, K. (2013). Peer-to-peer mentoring among urban youth: The intersection of health communication, media literacy and digital health vignettes. *Journal of Digital and Media Literacy, 1,* 1–20.

Lost in Translation

On the basement floor of the hospital, Jane and Joe walk, their heads held high and their hands intertwined. He points to a sign that hangs from the ceiling. "You see that?"

She looks up and reads it, "Wellness Trail."

He grabs her hand a bit tighter and says, "Yep, we are on the Wellness Trail."

They enter radiation oncology to be fitted for his radiation mask. Dr. M. enters the room and turns to Jane and says, "You were right. There is necrosis."

"I knew it. So that means the cancer is growing quickly inside him. When can we start treatment?"

The doctor straightens his tie from underneath his white lab coat. "Jane, that's your name, isn't it? You need to just focus on the task at hand. Step-by-step. There is a process." He turns back to the computer.

Jane is frustrated. She looks at the doctor as he scans the record and makes more notes. She argues, "There are many processes. And no one has clearly told us what those processes are. We are going from here to oncology and you are saying different things. Asking us to do different things."

"If you listen to us both, it can save his life."

Joe adds, "I also have questions about nutrition, you know, the food I should be eating to help me stay alive."

Dr. M. says, "My biggest piece of advice is to eat. Just eat, get those calories in. Once you are through treatment, you can focus on the type of food you are eating. But believe me, you won't want to eat. So just focus on getting that food down." Dr. M. begins to dictate the treatment plan in what seems like several different languages, slowed tongues dripping out tales of caution for the caregiver.

"He will need radiation, five times a week, every day, for 7–8 weeks. During this process, he will need chemo, once every two weeks. Watch for fever, for nutrition. Keep him eating. Watch for nausea, constipation, fever. Make sure he does not miss an appointment, skipping a treatment changes everything. If he becomes too weak, too tired, sick in any form, bring him to the hospital. If his fever reaches 100.5, bring him immediately to the emergency room. Do not wait. He won't have an immune system to fight off any infection. The infection is what kills most people being treated with chemotherapy for cancer."

The issue here isn't the information-seeking process, but the ability for doctor, patient, and caregiver to come together. How clinicians talk to patients about the Internet is important for establishing and maintaining a trusted relationship. As Teutsch (2003) notes, "If clinicians want to remain a trusted source of information, how they react to patient-initiated information sharing is important in keeping open lines of communication" (p. 1138). In another study on the impact of patient Internet use, the results indicated the importance of doctors validating patients' efforts and taking the researched information seriously to improve the overall patient–physician relationship (Bylund et al., 2007, p. 350). For many physicians, like the one quoted on the following page, technology has its benefits when it comes to being a family physician.

How do physicians respond to patients who search the Internet for medical information? As predicted more than 15 years ago, the increase in Web-based material and email usage would change the landscape of medicine from doctors treating and diagnosing illness through email to patients seeking information on the Internet (Kassirer, 2000). In a study on the use of the Internet in patient care, 80% of physicians asked patients to bring in the information they found on the Web (Podichetty, Booher, Whitfield & Biscup,

Physicians' Stories: Supporting Relationships

Technology has its challenges, can add to obstacles, and it, too, needs to be nourished so that it can meet its potential. I am grateful when technology supports that which I value in family medicine: making connections with others, encouraging healthy choices, harnessing people's strengths, finding access to services, and even providing humor for healing. (anonymous email)

2006). Although physicians' responses to patients' use of computer-based information varies, researchers have found the Internet to be a positive and empowering experience for patients, impacting their sense of control and decision making (Broom, 2005c). In fact, some physicians view the Internet-informed encounter as one with more shared decision making. As a medical oncologist stated in an interview conducted by the author (Broom), "And they may, with that information, decide something that I don't agree with, but, that's fine, as long as it's an informed decision, and they are making it on the right basis, then they are entitled to do that and that's OK" (Broom, 2005a, p. 326).

But it's very important to keep in mind that not all individuals have the financial means to access professional healthcare. In fact, millions of people who live in the U.S. do not have insurance or enough government assistance to pay for medical coverage. As Theorizing Practice 5.2 reminds us, many Americans of different races and

Theorizing Practice 5.2
Barriers to Accessing Healthcare

Many Americans, including millions of immigrants, face multiple barriers to accessing healthcare, lack of insurance being the primary challenge.

- Out of the 46 million uninsured people in the U.S., 20% are noncitizens (Okie 2007).
- The U.S. Census Bureau (Smith & Medalia, 2015) examined the number of uninsured individuals by race: non-Hispanic Whites (7.6%), Blacks (11.8%) and Hispanics (19.9%).
- The U.S. Census Bureau (Smith & Medalia, 2015) reports that Americans of various socioeconomic status, including middle-income, are without health insurance. For example, 14.1% of people reporting a household income of $25,000–$74,000 are uninsured.

Without coverage, millions of U.S. citizens must decide how to seek medical advice and care.

1. Have you or someone you know not sought medical care because you could not afford the healthcare bill?

2. If you were (or are) without health insurance, where would or do you turn to for medical help?

3. Why do you think healthcare coverage is not equal? Upon entering the formal healthcare system, do you think healthcare workers treat individuals differently because of their background (e.g., racial, sexual) or insurance status?

4. In what ways and to what extent does access to health information on the Internet help to address inequities in the healthcare system? And just as importantly, to what extent do you think immigrants, people of color, or people with lesser economic means, for example, are able to access computer-assisted information and resources?

socioeconomic levels, including middle-income, are without health insurance, and thus may be forced to seek health information and assistance in alternate ways.

Social Support through Social Media

Jane and Joe navigate the cold hospital hallways to the fourth floor. There are men lined up sitting in brown, plastic, reclining chairs. Their skin is an acrid yellow. Each man is attached to an IV. The drip is slow. The TV is tuned to a bland talk show.

Joe is directed to the only open brown chair. Jane finds a stool and pulls it up next to him. A nurse walks over with a bag.

"This first bag is just saline to get you hydrated and Emend [see Definition Box] *to help the nausea. We need to get you hydrated for about an hour and a half. The second bag will be the Cisplatin* [see Definition Box]. *That will also take about two hours. Then we will move back to the saline. We need you to read through the precautions before you sign off for the treatment, OK?"*

Emend is used for the "prevention of acute and delayed nausea and vomiting associated with initial and repeat courses of highly emetogenic cancer chemotherapy (HEC)" (http://www.drugs.com/pro/emend.html).

Cisplatin is "called the 'penicillin of cancer' because it is used so widely and it was the first big chemotherapy drug" (http://cisplatin.org).

Jane frantically searches the Web for the definition of Cisplatin on her smartphone. It pops up on the screen that Cisplatin is one of the strongest chemotherapies on the market. It also warns of terrible nausea.

Joe turns to Jane, "Did you bring my glasses?" Jane grabs his broken reading glasses from her purse. He puts them on and reads through the precautions slowly.

Joe and Jane take a "selfie" in the chemotherapy chair. They are all smiles. Jane posts the photograph on Facebook. She captions the picture, "Kicking cancer's butt." After five minutes, there are more than 30 "likes" and comments. After an hour, more than 200 people have shown their support. Every time Jane reads Joe the next comment, he tears up. He feels the love that surrounds him.

Like Joe and Jane, those who face a new diagnosis may turn to online networks for social support. In recent years people have been seeking support for health-related issues on social media sites such as Facebook, Instagram, and Twitter (Bender, Jimenez-Marroquin & Jadad, 2011; Moorhead et al., 2013). Moreover, online groups for a specific illness or disease are quite common. Online support groups exist for thousands of medical conditions and diseases such as prostate cancer (Broom, 2005b), HIV/AIDS (Dutcher, 1998; Kalichman et al., 2003), breast cancer (Winzelberg et al., 2003), or rare diseases such as Creutzfeldt-Jakob, an incurable brain disease (as cited in Beck, 2001, p. 176). General websites such as MDJunction (http://www.mdjunction.com/support-groups) also allow people to find social support for a myriad of conditions and ailments. MDJunction alone has 26 categories for medical, psychological, and social support groups. These categories total 1,134 unique social support groups for people to write stories, ask questions, and leave comments. For those who want to communicate to a loved one during her/his hospital stay, websites such as CaringBridge (http://www.caringbridge.org/) allow them to send personal messages or photos through a protected site.

The use of social media by physicians is slowly, and cautiously, on the rise. Within the healthcare system, however, these advancements have not been embraced as quickly. As Hawn (2009) notes, "Although health care may be one of America's leading industries in terms of size and scope, it's been among the slowest to embrace advances in communications and information technology (IT) systems" (p. 363). Furthermore, some specialists view online support groups as a loss to their status and shared decision making (Broom, 2005b).

The reasons for not incorporating social media tools stem from lack of time and finances to support such a system. As Hawn (2009) states, "Many independent practitioners or small group practices don't appear to have the time or the money to adapt to the use of social media" (p. 363). Additionally, insurance companies do not currently reimburse for Internet "visits" with a doctor (Hawn, 2009). In short, until methods of reimbursement for medical treatment catch up with technology, healthcare is slow to embrace advancements that don't cover physician time and expenses.

Joe Is Cancer Free: Nasal Endoscopy and Laryngoscopy

After six months of cancer care for stage IV, squamous cell carcinoma, which included chemotherapy and five-day-a-week radiation treatments, this is Joe's first day back to the ENT clinic to get his post-treatment check-up. Surrounded by residents and the attending doctor, Joe laughs and then fidgets in his chair. The attending physician wheels over a cart with a nasal endoscopy machine on it. Jane sits in a hard plastic chair. She watches intently and takes out her iPhone camera to document the event.

The attending lets one of his residents attempt to put the long tube up Joe's nose to get it into his throat so they can look for any sign of recurring cancer. Joe squirms and he squints his eyes in pain. The resident doctor can't seem to get it past his blocked sinus. The attending doctor takes over and moves it through like a plumber with a snake in a drain.

And there it is, the pink flesh of his inner throat, the raw scars of a tonsillectomy, chemotherapy, and radiation. The doctors all turn to him with smiles. "We can deem you cancer free." Jane smiles but doesn't see what they are supposed to be looking for. Joe can't see. All he sees is the ceiling. He waits for them to pull out the long tube so he can swallow and bring his chin back down. Once they release the thin camera, he laughs and shakes their hands.

A month later they return for a check-up CT scan. A week later, a day after Jane's birthday, they receive the news that there isn't a trace of cancer in his body. Jane posts this on Facebook: "The best birthday gift to ever receive was the news that Joe's CT scan came back clean. We can officially say he is CANCER-FREE! Next scan in May. Let's pray and hope it stays that way!"

More than 200 people like it and 55 people make comments. As each "like" and message comes in, Joe's smile gets a little wider and relief washes over Jane's body. This softness and stillness has been a long time coming. They look at each other.

"I am so grateful for you," Joe says sweetly.

"And I'm so grateful for you." Jane grabs his hands and pulls them up to her face. She kisses the back of them. "I love you."

We followed Joe and Jane's journey on the wellness trail as *digital patients* participating in a *digitized healthcare system*. Throughout this journey it has become strikingly clear that technology has had a deep impact on *digitized doctors* in their medical practice and patient care. Many of Joe and Jane's experiences reflect the personal, cultural, and political complexities associated with the continued integration of information and communication technologies into healthcare.

HCIA 5.2

Uncertainty Management and Information Seeking in Cancer Survivorship

Laura E. Miller

As of 2014, the American Cancer Society approximates that 14.5 million cancer survivors were living in the United States. Thankfully, this number has been steadily rising as improved treatments have prolonged the life span and offered better quality survival for many cancer patients. As people transition from patient to survivor, uncertainty is a common experience, and many people will attempt to manage information in order to better cope. Cancer survivorship (beyond just the treatment period) is important because, even though cancer is out of the body, its challenges may linger long after successful treatment has been completed. Thus understanding how people manage such illness-related uncertainty throughout cancer survivorship has become an increasingly important topic of research.

To complicate matters, uncertainty among couples coping with cancer presents additional, unique challenges. A husband and wife, for example, may each have their own illness-related questions while simultaneously managing those of their partner. Because couples are interdependent, and one partner's uncertainty affects the other, couples provide a unique context in which to study the connections between uncertainty and information management.

To explore such issues, my study utilized one-on-one interviews with 35 cancer survivors and 25 partners. The participants were asked to describe their uncertainties throughout survivorship and the ways in which they tried to cope with an ambiguous prognosis and future.

An intriguing finding was that, in addition to seeking information as a response to uncertainty, many participants also discussed actively avoiding information in order to minimize ambiguities. Some participants, for instance, discontinued membership in support groups to avoid hearing about cancer, and others discussed decreased Internet usage to avoid reading about distressing experiences. One participant described her decision to stop searching the Internet for cancer-related information: "They give you everything, all possibilities, worst case scenario. Why do you need to be thinking about that?" For these individuals, avoiding information about cancer helped to manage their uncertainty by focusing on survivorship, not illness.

The participants in this study also discussed the challenges they experienced when trying to manage their uncertainty throughout cancer survivorship. One such challenge related to unanswered questions. Many participants felt frustrated and uncertain because of their physicians' unwillingness or inability to answer lingering questions. For some, it was difficult to manage questions about the cancer coming back. As one participant noted, "I wish they'd do a CT scan on me just to ease my mind. . . . Who's to say it couldn't come back six months from now?" Other participants described taking matters into their own hands to reduce uncertainty about a recurrence. As one wife of a colon cancer survivor said, "The doctor told him not to come back for two years. We don't like that. It's a long time. I said just go

(continued)

in August . . . tell them you are bleeding more. Tell a little white lie so you can have another colonoscopy." For these participants, unanswered questions about a recurrence created uncertainty, and some participants were even willing to lie to manage such questions.

In addition, some participants described uncertainty stemming from conversations with their medical team. Because many patients and partners wanted to seek information from physicians as a means of managing uncertainty, when such interactions did not go smoothly, uncertainty ensued. One participant described such uncertainty: "The emotional roller coaster comes after treatment is over. I wanted to talk to my doctor and nurses about how I was feeling, but all of a sudden, you don't see them for six months at a time. One guy told me that I would need to go talk with someone else because he didn't want to deal with my emotions. 'My job was to get the cancer out of your body. So my job is done. You will have to talk to someone else about that.' I felt lost and abandoned."

This study provides new insight into the uncertainty-related challenges couples face as they cope with survivorship. First, the data show that uncertainty lingers after the completion of cancer treatment. These insights may be useful for couples coping with cancer because it may help them understand their experience and make potentially confusing ambiguities seem less confusing or more normal. While surviving cancer is good news, looming uncertainties (for example, about the cancer coming back) may prevent survivors and families from returning back to their "normal" lives. One participant described the "emotional roller coaster" that ensues after treatment has been completed; preparing for this may be useful for couples who experience a cancer diagnosis as well as for others who interact with them. Second, these results have practical implications for healthcare providers and imply that continued care after treatment is complete would be beneficial for survivors and their families. As the individuals in this study demonstrate, access to continued contact with medical providers can reduce uncertainty, offering reassurance and information. Thus healthcare providers should strive to provide this type of informational provision, as failing to do so may only exacerbate cancer's lingering challenges.

QUESTIONS TO PONDER

1. Have you ever experienced illness-related uncertainty? If so, please describe the context and the emotions you experienced.

2. What uncertainties do you think you would have if you were diagnosed with cancer? What uncertainties do you think you would have if a loved one were diagnosed with cancer?

3. What information do you think would help you manage your cancer-related questions? What information do you think would distract you from managing your cancer-related information?

Source: Miller, L. E. (2014). Uncertainty management and information seeking in cancer survivorship. *Health Communication, 29,* 233–243.

▪ Considering the Complexities

As we followed Joe and Jane's journey, some of the many complexities related to a digitized world of healthcare became apparent. Some of these instances are specific to Joe and Jane's situation, while other elements of digitized healthcare apparent in their story are likely situations that many people experience. When considering how digitized healthcare might play into one's own healthcare experiences, it can be helpful to consider the personal, cultural, and political complexities. These complexities are best understood as interrelated intersections.

Joe is a U.S. veteran and his cancer journey takes place in a veteran's hospital and, subsequently, also involves the administrative and political infrastructure of the Veteran's Administration. One of the many cultural complexities within the veteran population is their health literacy and relationship to technology. As we see in Joe and Jane's story, their relationship to healthcare has been dramatically impacted by technology in varying ways. But Joe and Jane, like many patients, felt the digital divide. There are questions of access, literacy, and skills that impact the ways patients interact with ehealth interfaces. "Although more and more patients have broadband Internet access and are using smartphones, the digital divide may create connectivity barriers for low-income, minority, rural, and older adult patients. If up-to-date technologies are not available to certain populations, connectivity will be low (Fortney, Burgess, Bosworth, Booth, & Kaboli, 2011, p. 645). The VA, however, is working to improve access and close the potentially growing digital divide.

The Veteran's Administration is consistently building programs to try and remedy this disjunction.

> For example, VA's Connected Health program seeks to give veterans better access to medical care through smartphones, tablets and other mobile technology. The VA distributed over 10,000 tablets to clinicians across the country last year and launched a mobile app store with more than a dozen apps to provide veterans with access to health services. (http://www.washingtonpost.com/business/on-it/health-care-for-veterans-goes-high-tech/2015/03/07/168d74d0-c12e-11e4-9271-610273846239_story.html)

And yet, many of these programs fail because the population is not as digitally connected to health services as the VA may hope. This is one clear intersection where the desire to shift the culture of digitized healthcare in the VA has become a political issue. And this culture of healthcare impacts veterans on a very personal level.

A startling number of U.S. veterans who have access to computers or smartphones and report using the Internet on a daily basis do not use the Internet for medical purposes. The VA created MyHealth*e*Vet (MHV) in order to empower veterans as healthcare consumers. "The program is based on the core belief that knowledgeable patients are better able to make informed healthcare choices, stay healthy, and seek services when needed" (Nazi, 2010, p. 2). According to Tsai and Rosenheck (2012), "Yet despite outreach and promotional efforts, only 15% of veterans who receive VA care registered for MHV in 2008 and <20% registered for MHV up to 2010. The slow adoption of MHV by VA users parallels the slow adoption of similar online technologies in non-VA healthcare systems, despite their potential to improve services" (p. 1089). While these programs may be available, members of the population may not be comfortable with these programs or know how to use them, thereby impacting their access to personal healthcare information.

This low adoption of MHV may be fueled by the personal complexity of low ehealth literacy. Fortney et al. (2011) state, "Moreover, patients from some cultures, as well as those with lower education levels may have lower comfort levels with ehealth technologies, and experience greater usability problems if they lack the skills to engage digitally with their provider and to interface with computer health applications" (p. 645). As a cultural and political intersection, the VA has focused on creating programs to teach veterans how to use technology to improve their ehealth literacy.

Outside of the clinician's office, many patients, medical providers, and public health organizations are turning to social media to increase digital patient–provider interaction and ehealth literacy. This turn to social media has impacted the cultural, political, and personal complexities of digitized healthcare. Public health organizations believe that social media will increase a patient's connection and direct engagement with her/his own personal health. According to Heldman, Schindelar, & Weaver (2013), social media increases direct engagement, which increases trust and credibility. "Social media has been characterized as mutually beneficial for public health organizations and their audiences to connect to each other in ways that promote a "common good" (Heldman et al., 2013, p. 5). They argue that social media are multifaceted, interactive, and participatory. Social media increases conversations and interactions between public health organizations and its diverse audiences.

With an increase in community engagement reaching diverse audiences, public health organizations also face ethical and legal consequences. Use of social media is frowned upon by some healthcare organizations. New clinicians, for example, are likely to receive training about the ethical and legal ramifications of social media, specifically HIPAA violations. The American Medical Association has included a statement about professionalism and social media use citing the utmost importance of privacy and confidentiality (http://www.ama-assn.org/ama/pub/physician-resources/medical-ethics/code-medical-ethics.page?). Clinicians are also asked to maintain appropriate boundaries of the patient–physician relationship in accordance with professional ethical guidelines if they interact with their patients in a social media context.

Another political intersection that impacts patients personally is how medical providers, health organizations, and health administrations gather, share, and store very private medical information. How medical data are collected and stored is of upmost political concern. "Data moves at the speed of trust," said David Ross, Sc.D., director of the Public Health Informatics Institute and cochair of the Advisory Committee. "Those are the words we heard from people across the country. As a nation, we need to strike a balance between privacy and the free flow of information" (Robert Wood Johnson Foundation, 2014, p. 1). These recommendations include improving privacy and security safeguards, educating the public on the value of sharing personal health information and its importance, and investing in community data infrastructure. These concerns beg the political question of ownership. Who owns your very personal health information? Patients sign waivers about who can have access to their records and with whom providers can share their information. If you want your medical records, for example, you have the legal right to access them. But the question remains—who else has access to your records?

These concerns are embedded within a larger infrastructure that is currently under construction. Because of the massive shift toward ehealth and social media usage in digitized healthcare, the personal, cultural, and political complexities are being intersected, highlighted, and problematized. The culture of medicine is ever-changing for both patients and providers as we continue to face new challenges, become familiar with new technologies, and navigate the unchartered waters of digitized healthcare.

■ Epilogue

Two years later Joe goes into the VA for another CAT and PET scan. He will have to have a scan every year for the next 10 years of his life. Joe and Jane go through the doors they know well, pass through the hallways they don't want to remember. They sit in the waiting room chairs that seem to have their bodies' imprints on the plastic. They hold hands and breathe deeply. Joe walks out of the office with only a 6% chance of the cancer reoccurring. Joe is one of the lucky ones. Joe and Jane return home, beaming. Jane posts a happy message on Facebook to share the good news with their family and friends. "Joe is still cancer free!"

Discussion Questions

1. How does technology improve communication between doctors and patients? How might it hinder communication practices?
2. How do social media impact communication about health issues?
3. How do social media serve as social support and encouragement through the cancer journey?
4. What are the various ways to use technology to improve health communication practices? Give an example of each from your own experience.
5. How do you imagine new advancements in technology changing the digital doctor, digital patient, and digital medical system of the future?

NOTES

[1] Both authors contributed equally to this chapter. They would like to thank Jimmie Manning for reviewing their manuscript and adding valuable feedback and suggestions.
[2] This is a narrative account of Joe and Jane's real experience. While the story is true, all names have been changed to maintain confidentiality.

REFERENCES

Beard, L., Schein, R., Morra, D., Wilson, K., & Keelan, J. (2012). The challenges in making electronic health records accessible to patients. *Journal of the American Medical Informatics Association, 19,* 116–120.

Beck, C. S. (2001). *Communicating for better health: A guide through the medical mazes.* Boston, MA: Allyn & Bacon.

Bender, J. L., Jimenez-Marroquin, M-C., & Jadad, A. R. (2011). Seeking support on Facebook: A content analysis of breast cancer groups. *Journal of Medical Research, 13,* e16.

Booth, N., Robinson, P., & Kohannejad, J. (2004). Identification of high-quality consultation practice in primary care: The effects of computer use on doctor patient rapport. *Informatics in Primary Care, 12,* 75–83.

Broom, A. (2005a). Medical specialists' account of the impact of the Internet on the doctor/patient relationship. *Health: An Interdisciplinary Journal for the Social Study of Health, 9,* 319–338.

Broom, A. (2005b). The eMale: Prostate cancer, masculinity and online support as a challenge to medical expertise. *Journal of Sociology, 41,* 87–104.

Broom, A. (2005c). Virtually healthy: The impact of internet use on disease experience and the doctor-patient relationship. *Qualitative Health Research, 15,* 325–345.

Buetow, S., Jutel, A., & Hoare, K. (2009). Shrinking social space in the doctor–modern patient relationship: A review of forces for, and implications of, homologisation. *Patient Education and Counseling, 74,* 97–103.

Bylund, C. L., Gueguen, J. A., Sabee, C. M., Imes, R. S., Li, Y., & Sanford, A. A. (2007). Provider-patient dialogue about internet health information: An exploration of strategies to improve the provider–patient relationship. *Patient Education and Counseling, 66,* 346–52.

Choi, J. S., Yi, B., Park, J. H., Choi, K., Jung, J., Park, S. W., & Rhee, P. (2011). The uses of the Smartphone for doctors: An empirical study from Samsung Medical Center. *Healthcare Informatics Research, 17,* 131–138.

du Pré, A. (2013). *Communicating about health: Current issues and perspectives* (4th ed.). New York, NY: Oxford University Press.

Dutcher, G. A. (1998). HIV/AIDS information resources and services from the National Institute of Health. In J. T. Huber (Ed.), *HIV/AIDS internet information sources and resources* (pp. 91–98). New York, NY: Haworth Press.

Ford, E. W., Menachemi, M., & Phillips, M. T. (2006). Predicting the adoption of electronic health records by physicians: When will health care be paperless? *Journal of the American Medical Informatics Association, 13,* 106–112.

Fortney, J. C., Burgess, J. F., Bosworth, H. B., Booth, B. M., & Kaboli, P. J. (2011). A re-conceptualization of access for 21st century healthcare. *Journal of General Internal Medicine, 26*(Suppl 2), 639–647.

Fox, S. (2006). *Online health search 2006* (Report). Retrieved from Pew Research Internet Project website: http://www.pewinternet.org/2006/10/29/online-health-search 2006/

Franko, O. I., & Tirrell, T. F. (2012). Smartphone app use among medical providers in ACGME training programs. *Journal of Medical Systems, 36,* 3135–3139.

Garufi, L. (2014, May 15). Power cord grounding (Electronic list serve entitled *Thursday Morning Memo*). Retrieved August 26, 2014, from http://libraryguides.umassmed.edu/thursdaymemo

Geist-Martin, P., Ray, E. B., & Sharf, B. F. (2003). *Communicating health: Personal, cultural, and political complexities.* Long Grove, IL: Waveland Press.

Hafner, K. (2012, October 8). Redefining medicine with apps and iPads. *New York Times.* Retrieved May 22, 2014, from file:///C:/Users/Owner/Desktop/Book%20Chapter/Lit%20Search/Redefining%20Medicine%20With%20Apps%20and%20iPads%20-%20NYT.htm

Hawn, C. (2009). Take two aspirin and tweet me in the morning: How Twitter, Facebook, and other social media are reshaping health care. *Health Affairs, 28,* 361–368.

Heldman, A. B., Schindelar, J., & Weaver III, J. B. (2013). Social media engagement and public health communication: Implications for public health organizations being truly "social." *Public Health Reviews, 35,* 1-18.

Hibbard J. (2003). Engaging health care consumers to improve the quality of care. *Medical Care, 41,* 61–70.

Hixon, T. (2014). Why digital health will have huge impact. *Forbes.* Retrieved July 13, 2014, from http://www.forbes.com/sites/toddhixon/2014/02/03/why-digital-health-will-have huge-impact/

Institute of Medicine. (2003). *Priority areas for national action: Transforming health care quality.* Washington, DC: National Academy Press.

Jha, A. K., Doolan, D., Grandt, D., Scott, T., & Bates, D. W. (2008). The use of health information technology in seven nations. *International Journal of Medical Informatics, 77,* 848–854.

Jucks, R., & Bromme, R. (2007). Choice of words in doctor–patient communication: An analysis of health-related Internet sites. *Health Communication, 21,* 267–277.

Kassirer, J. P. (2000). Patients, physicians, and the Internet. *Health Affairs, 19,* 115–123.

Kalichman, S. C., Benotsch, E. G., Weinhardt, L., Austin, J., Luke, W., & Chauncey, C. (2003). Health-related Internet use, coping, social support, and health indicators in people living with HIV/AIDS. *Health Psychology, 22,* 111–116.

Kim, Y., & Given, B. A. (2008). Quality of life of family caregivers of cancer survivors. *Cancer, 112,* 2556–2568.

Linder, J. A., Ma, J., Bates, D. W., Middleton, B., & Stafford, R. S. (2007). Electronic health record use and the quality of ambulatory care in the United States. *Archives of Internal Medicine, 167,* 1400–1405.

Moorhead, S., Hazlett, D., Harrison, L., Carroll, J., Irwin, A., et al. (2013). A new dimension of health care: Systematic review of the uses, benefits, and limitations of social media for health communication. *Journal of Medical Internet Research, 15*(4), e85.

Morahan-Martin, J. M. (2004). How internet users find, evaluate, and use online health information: A cross-cultural review. *CyberPsychology & Behavior, 7,* 497–510.

Nazi, K. M. (2010). Veterans' voices: Use of the American Customer Satisfaction Index (ACSI) Survey to identify MyHealtheVet personal health record users' characteristics, needs, and preferences. *Journal of the American Medical Informatics Association, 17,* 203–211.

Nielsen-Bohlman, L., Panzer, A. M., & Kindig, D. A. (Eds.). (2004). *Health literacy: A prescription to end confusion.* Washington, DC: The National Academies Press.

Okie, S. (2007). Immigrants and health care—at the intersection of two broken systems. *New England Journal of Medicine, 357,* 525–529.

Ozdalga, E., Ozdalga, A., & Ahuja, N. (2012). The Smartphone in medicine: A review of current and potential use among physicians and students. *Journal of Medical Internet Research, 14,* Retrieved June 29, 2014, from http://www.jmir.org/issue/year/2012

Parker, J. C., & Thorson, E. (Eds.). (2009). *Health communication in the new media landscape.* New York, NY: Springer Publishing.

Podichetty, V. K., Booher, J., Whitfield, M., & Biscup, R. S. (2006). Assessment of internet use and effects among healthcare professionals: A cross sectional survey. *Postgraduate Medical Journal, 82,* 274–279.

Polack, E. P., & Avtgis, T. A. (2011). *Medical communication: Defining the discipline.* Dubuque, IA: Kendall Hunt.

Robert Wood Johnson Foundation. (2014). Retrieved from http://www.rwjf.org/en/library/articles-and-news/2015/04/report-highlights-publics-hopes-fears-about-using-data-to-improve-health.html

Smith, J. C., & Medalia, C. (2015). *Health insurance in the United States: 2014.* Washington, DC: U.S. Census Bureau. Retrieved from http://www.census.gov/content/dam/Census/library/publications/2015/demo/p60-253.pdf

Stacey, M. (1988). The sociology of health and healing: A textbook. New York, NY: Routledge.

Terry, M. (2010). Medical apps for Smartphones. *Telemedicine and e-health, 16,* 17–22.

Teutsch, C. (2003). Patient-doctor communication. *Medical Clinics of North America, 87,* 1115–1145.

Tsai, J., & Rosenheck, R. A. (2012). Use of the internet and an online personal health record system by US veterans: Comparison of Veterans Affairs mental health service users and other veterans nationally. *Journal of the American Medical Informatics Association, 19,* 1089–1094.

Wagner, E. (2000). The role of patient care teams in chronic disease management. *British Medical Journal, 320,* 569–572.

Wallace, S., Clark, M., & White, J. (2012). 'It's on my iPhone': Attitudes to the use of mobile computing devices in medical education, a mixed-methods study. *BMJ Open, 2,* 1–7.

Winkelman, W. R., Leonard, K. J., & Rossos, P. G. (2005). Patient-perceived usefulness of online electronic medical records: Employing grounded theory in the development of information and communication technologies for use by patients living with chronic illness. *Journal of the American Medical Informatics Association, 12,* 306–314.

Winzelberg, A. J., Classen, C., Alpers, G. W., Roberts, H., Koopman, C., Adams, R. E., Ernst, H., Dev, P., & Taylor, C. B. (2003). Evaluation of an internet support group for women with primary breast cancer. *Cancer, 97,* 1164–1173.

6

Communicating Health and Healing through Art

Lynn M. Harter, Michael Broderick,
Kristen Okamoto, Rebekah Crawford, & Sarah Parsloe

For the past decade, Courtney has done what millions of Americans do five days a week: she goes to work and earns a paycheck. Courtney's developmental disability has not stifled her desire to earn a living. Even so, Courtney has few choices other than employment at HighCo, a sheltered workshop where she earns below minimum wage and has little contact with community members other than supervising staff. Evan focuses the camera on Courtney's hands as she tears the newspaper into strips. For someone with limited manual dexterity, this is a cumbersome if not monotonous task with little room for creative expression. What is more troubling is that shredding paper is not necessary to fulfill HighCo's contract with Highland County Recycling. Courtney is one of many individuals paid to process materials to be recycled. Newspapers must be separated from magazines, cardboard flattened, lids discarded from jars. The organizing of paper and plastic products, however, does not provide enough employment for the individuals served by HighCo. Thus, like many other contemporary sheltered workshops, HighCo creates "simulated" work environments that offer time-consuming yet unnecessary and meaningless tasks. Shredding paper.

HighCo is a sheltered workshop populated with well-intended staff, individuals who coordinate self-care resources and employment opportunities for the people they serve. Several labels have developed over time to describe what we refer to as *sheltered workshops*. Example terms include industrial workshops, training workshops, vocational workshops, and rehabilitation centers (Dlouhy & Mitchell, 2015). We use the term *sheltered workshop* to refer to a wide range of vocational and non-vocational programs for individuals with developmental disabilities including facility-based employment (e.g., assembling pens) and, for higher functioning individuals, community-integrated employment (e.g. janitorial service, bagging groceries). Developmental disabilities are attributable to mental retardation or related conditions (e.g., neurological conditions, cerebral palsy) that impair the intellectual functioning of individuals (for a sound definition of developmental disability see http://www.ddrcco.com/resources-and-training/definition-of-developmental-disability.php). Beginning in the fall of 2014,

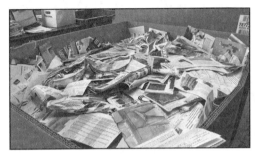 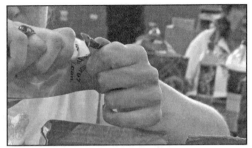

Shredding paper at HighCo (Lynn M. Harter).

the first author and several undergraduate and graduate students were granted access and approval to conduct ethnographic fieldwork at HighCo including both participant observations and in-depth interviews.

Like other sheltered workshops across the U.S., HighCo offers self-care, rehabilitative, and vocational services for individuals with developmental disabilities. Over the past 10 years, though, the supply of community-integrated employment has not kept pace with demand, and contracts for facility-based employment have dwindled (Butterworth et al., 2012). Meanwhile, disability activists have called into question the unintended consequences of the deficit-based model of care connected to Medicaid funding streams (e.g., Mackelprang & Salsgiver, 2009). Butterworth and colleagues challenged citizens to confront a pressing societal dilemma: the need to create expressive and vocational opportunities for people with developmental disabilities. Patty Mitchell, founder and director of Collaborative Art International (CAI), offers an aesthetic solution to revolutionize workshops (Dlouhy & Mitchell, 2015).

CAI facilitates art projects guided by the interests and talents of people with development disabilities. Patty and colleagues adopt an appreciative stance toward people, organizations, and communities. In her words, "we want to create positive environments where people are invited to explore and discover new ideas," later adding:

> If I only had a magic wand, then these people with disabilities could be creative, outgoing, inventive, individualistic beings. Oh wait! They already are those things. Individuals with perceived disabilities are often less fearful than typical people when responding to opportunities provided for creative exploration. Honestly, I have never come across a group of people more forgiving and patient than this population. They are just waiting for their support systems to get it together and provide the environment for investigation and creative exploration. It is as if they had been waiting all their lives for these opportunities.

Amidst discussions of "self-determination" and "think ability first," the provision of services in sheltered workshops generally continues to be organized around people's limitations (e.g., narrow range of motion). Deficit-oriented models focus on shortcomings (Singhal, Buscell, & Lindberg, 2010). As a result, programming can limit people by inadvertently positioning them as "bundles of pathologies" or problems to be fixed. Inspired by the Passion Works model (see Harter, Leeman, Norander, Young, & Rawlins, 2008; Harter & Rawlins, 2011; Harter, Scott, Novak, Leeman, & Morris, 2006), CAI focuses on people's interests and capacities. Patty recognizes fallibility and vulnerability as part of what it means to be human; however, she positions people's gifts as more powerful than their deficiencies or needs.

CAI envisions workshops as spaces for creative activity. An artistic mind-set is central to helping staff members break away from traditional ways of seeing things. Rather than correcting or curing perceived imperfections (e.g., limited mobility or obsessive compulsive behaviors), CAI staff help individuals identify and explore their capacities and interests. Staff members provide resources and support for individuals to develop previously untapped gifts. Whether the staff elevates a table to accommodate wheelchairs, engages in conversations about the mediums artists would like to work with, stirs paints or adjusts easels, they do so with the intent of helping others exercise their creative impulses. In short, participating artists are offered opportunities for self-discovery and expression. Importantly, artistic experiences provide a scaffold for the achievement of other goals, including the development of meaningful relationships and social change.

CAI and its efforts demonstrate the liberating power of the arts in health-related contexts. The State of the Field Committee (2009) for the Society for Arts in Healthcare, now known as the Global Alliance for Arts & Health, suggests diverse possibilities for arts-based programming with applications for a host of health challenges including post-traumatic stress disorder, autism, mental illness, child and adult oncology, and neurological disorders. Although arts-based programs differ in size, scope, and mission, most incorporate in practice John Dewey's (1980/1934) belief that art serves both *intrinsic* and *instrumental* purposes. For Dewey, a foundational educational philosopher whose work has greatly influenced U.S. educational practices, the experience of art is intrinsically valuable insofar as it fosters a heightened sensory absorption with present circumstances, attentiveness to relationships in which people are engaged, and a greater depth of insight that fosters new possibilities. Art forms represent crystallized moments in the creative process (e.g., a painting or a musical score). The process of aesthetic experience—including the creation and appreciation of art forms—in turn can serve instrumental purposes (e.g., pain relief, consciousness-raising, or employment opportunities).

In this chapter, we explore how people communicate about health and healing through the arts. The story of CAI is woven throughout the chapter, illustrating how arts-based programming offers participants (1) opportunities for *sensemaking* and *self-expression*, (2) moments of *solidarity* with others, and (3) rhetorical resources to enlarge the broader *social imaginary*. Following Taylor's (2007) lead, we understand the social imaginary to encompass

> the ways people imagine their social existence, how they fit together with others, how things go on between them and their fellows, the expectations that are normally met, and the deeper normative notions and images that underlie these expectations. (p. 23)

The social imaginary reflects *personal, cultural,* and *political complexities* that give rise to and are shaped by individuals' identities. The rhetorical power of art is revealed in its capacity to challenge cultural assumptions that otherwise remain taken for granted and unquestioned. In this way, art opens up inventional spaces (Hauser, 1999) in which personhood, health, and healthcare can be understood—by artists and contemplators alike—in novel and even transformative ways.

To begin, we advance an aesthetic view of communication as central to health-care systems, personal well-being, and public health efforts. Second, we explore relationships between aesthetic experiences and self-expression, solidarity, and the social imaginary. We advance arguments by moving between scholarly literature, our fieldwork experiences producing the documentary series entitled *The Courage of Creativity* that features the work of CAI (Harter & Shaw, 2013), and other exemplars of artistic efforts to (re)make meaning in the midst of profound vulnerability.

■ An Aesthetic Orientation to Health Communication

Scientific logics remain central to the practice of conventional medicine. In turn, scientific authorities legitimize technological interventions for urgent, acute, and chronic health conditions (van Dijck, 2005). The technological orientation is encapsulated in the metaphor of "body as machine," a way of defining illness as a malfunction of one of the "parts," and care as restoration of that part to "working order." The technological imperative is visually and verbally evident in hospitals, outpatient clinics, and long-term care facilities. Consider a typical scenario in an emergency room (ER). A patient is brought to the ER in the midst of a critical trauma. Providers immediately begin issuing commands such as "cross type and match," "ready an intubation tray," and "start an IV flow with normal saline." A patient is hooked up to machines, while the heart monitor in the background provides an auditory reminder of his or her status. Taken together, these images, sounds, and practices reflect the cultural dominance of science and technology. Such tools of the trade are equipped to address certain aspects of suffering but ultimately offer limited conceptualizations of what it means to care for others. We do not reject or abandon normative, scientific, logics of mainstream care; however, we join other practitioners and scholars who advocate for the adoption of diverse modalities that are different from but harmonious with conventional medical practices (Sharf, Geist-Martin, & Moore, 2013). In particular, we adopt an aesthetic orientation to healthcare that positions creativity as a form of reasoning worthy of consideration alongside scientific logics (see also Freeman, Epston, & Lobovits, 1997; Haidet, 2007; Kaplan, 2003; Shaughnessy, Slawson, & Becker, 1998).

Healthcare providers, patients, and families often relegate aesthetic experience to life spheres of consumption and leisure. This is not surprising given the culturally determined binaries that remain deeply rooted in modern Western cultures:

- science/art
- reason/emotion
- utility/beauty
- labor/leisure
- public/private
- ends/means
- ill/well
- intrinsic/instrumental

Although such paired terms are arbitrary and do not reflect inherent realities, their lingering presence is felt in contemporary personal and professional relationships (McKerrow, 1998). For example, the presupposition that medicine is a science is misleading to the extent that it fails to acknowledge other rationalities worthy of consideration alongside the patterned regularities valued by scientific and instrumental logics. We draw on the writings of John Dewey (1980/1934) to move past traditional notions that divide the world into polar opposites (i.e., dualisms). When we resist the science/art dichotomy, opportunities abound for sensemaking that enlarge the realm of possibilities for what it means to live well in the midst of illness, suffering, trauma, and chronic challenges. The power of an artistic or aesthetic approach in healthcare (and beyond) is that art—the single moment of aesthetic rapture—refuses habituated dualisms and creates room for personal fulfillment and effective long-term systematic change.

HCIA 6.1

The Human-Pet Connection

Jill Yamasaki

Anyone with a beloved pet knows the pleasure, relaxation, and joy animals can provide when we're well and the unconditional comfort, companionship, and support they give when we're ill. Given this intense human-animal bond, it's not surprising that many people value their pets as important members of the family. Even more, it's understandable they would want—and even need—their pet during long periods of hospitalization when they may be feeling especially scared, lonely, or critically ill. Some hospitals recognize this need and incorporate animal-assisted therapy programs as a way for patients to interact with companion pets. Doing so has been shown to reduce patient stress, blood pressure, and heart rate, as well as decrease anxiety and alleviate depression and loneliness. Other hospitals have gone even further and incorporated visitation programs for chronically, critically, or terminally ill patients and their personal pets from home.

I worked with PAWS (Pets Are Wonderful Support) Houston, a volunteer-driven nonprofit organization that facilitates personal pet visits to all patients, except those in bone marrow units, in all major hospitals within Houston's Texas Medical Center, the largest medical complex in the world. PAWS Houston volunteers facilitate approximately 30 personal pet hospital visits each month; more than 85 percent of these visits occur in critical care. Visits require a physician's order, are usually arranged within 24 hours (or in as little as 30 minutes in end-of-life situations), and typically last about an hour. All visiting pets (primarily dogs, but cats and rabbits are also permitted) are met in the hospital lobby by a PAWS Houston volunteer and escorted to the patient's room.

In critical care units, where patients are often unable to communicate and/or actively participate in care decisions, patient-centered care in a family-centered environment is especially important. Family members often have firsthand insight into patient preferences, can make important contributions to care decisions based on those preferences, and can assist care providers in getting to know the patient as an individual. My research focuses specifically on the novel ways personal pets can contribute to the meaningful communication comprising this care. To do so, I utilized a variety of ethnographic methods—including participant observation as a trained volunteer and interviews with healthcare providers, family members, and other PAWS Houston volunteers—and conducted thematic and narrative analyses of transcribed interviews, field notes, and organizational materials.

(continued)

In one study, my analysis revealed that personal pet visits prompt genuine interactions characterized by compassion, connection, and response between patients, providers, and family members. Personal pet visits enable providers to address the emotional needs of patients and their families by conveying empathy and offering support in nontraditional ways. Providers who are aware of the PAWS Houston program offer to make a visit possible when they recognize (e.g., through family conversations, photos, and other forms of communication) the importance of the pet to the patient or when they specifically ask the patient and/or family what could potentially help ease psychosocial burdens (e.g., depression, disorientation) of extended hospitalization or critical illness. Many providers characterize these visits as an additional tool to "give something extra to their patients." Relatedly, personal pet visits offer providers a glimpse into the lifeworld of their patients while connecting patients to this outside world and family. Providers understand the importance of their own pets and can connect to their patients through that mutual understanding and shared identity. Perhaps most importantly, personal pet visits elicit communicative responses that can contribute to personalized care. Despondent patients become more animated, and nonresponsive patients struggle to pet the dog they've loved for so long. Family members keeping vigil are often especially appreciative of these little responses, and providers can determine a patient's lucidity and abilities from them.

Personal pet hospital visits facilitate storied conversations, foster healing relationships, and offer alternative ways of knowing that can promote greater understandings of the patient's psychosocial context for more personalized care and improved well-being. Since patient-centered care requires meaningful consideration of a patient's health, well-being, and comfort, the deep personal bonds between patients and their pets should be acknowledged and provided as part of this care.

QUESTIONS TO PONDER

1. Think about the role your pet plays in your life. How has your pet influenced your health and well-being?

2. What are the different ways your pet's presence has (or could) help you interact and connect with others when you may not otherwise?

Source: Yamasaki, J. (in press). The communicative role of companion pets in patient-centered critical care. *Patient Education and Counseling.*

Central to our understanding of the importance of art is John Dewey's (1980/ 1934) philosophical analysis of art and aesthetic living. The term aesthetic derives from the Greek *aisthanomai*—to perceive and feel with the senses. Humans' experience of communal life is multisensory. Relationships, rituals, and routines enhance some of our perceptive and creative capacities at the experience of others. Writing at the turn of the 20th century, Dewey recognized dimensions of human experience constricted by the formalization and routinization that characterize the scientific method. Although he acknowledged the value of instrumental and goal-driven action, Dewey sought to develop individuals' creative capacities to enrich community life. Meanwhile, he traced the historical genealogy of Western dualisms and insisted that we typically undervalue the role of direct felt experience (i.e., the means) in favor of long-term instrumental goals (i.e., the ends).

The intrinsic/instrumental binary undergirds the deficit model of care in sheltered workshops where importance is given to goals such as job and social readiness, sometimes at the expense of intrinsic experiences such as personal fulfillment, happiness, and self-expression. One of the primary engines of sheltered workshops is the individual service plan (ISP). Within 30 days of intake and every year thereafter, ISPs are constructed for participants of sheltered workshops. ISPs typically cover several domains (e.g., mobility, personal care) and ensure that participants have access to rehabilitation opportunities. Funding streams for sheltered workshops such as Medicaid are instrumentally deficit-driven. In other words, monies are allocated in response to "fixing" the physical and social limits of participants. Dewey (1980/1934) insisted, however, that intrinsic experiences and instrumental goals are part of the same expression and we must expand our temporal frame to understand how individual intrinsic experiences are layered within long-term instrumental goals. If we are building a house, we must simultaneously pay attention to each individual brick placement as well as refer to the plans for the entire house. At CAI, Patty and her colleagues develop asset-based plans for participants that unite the intrinsic experience of art (e.g., enjoyment of the creation and/or appreciation of art) with instrumental goals (e.g., job opportunities, community integration).

It is important to note, however, that for Dewey (1980/1934) art is not found in an object but through a person's interaction with or experience of an object, event, or moment within an environment. It is the immediate experience in the present that is important, but this does not abandon us to hedonistic impulses—it is felt experience in the present with future goals in mind. Dewey refers to this notion as "ends-in-view." In this way, our present experiences (e.g., making and enjoying art) are not separate from our long-term instrumental goals (e.g., alleviation of suffering and generation of employment opportunities), but are part of the same dynamic expression. Drawing on Dewey, Stroud (2011) defined "ends-in-view" as "the label for consciously (reflectively) chosen values that guide action in the present" (p. 51). The orientation to the present moment is imperative, and experiencing art simultaneously tethers experience to the present moment and to potential futures. Or, as stated by Dewey (1980/1934), "Art celebrates with peculiar intensity the moments in which the past reinforces the present and in which the future is quickening of what now is" (p. 17). The deficit-based model of healthcare typically focuses its efforts toward instrumental goals over the emotive, intrinsic experience, and this has contributed to a host of existential, physical, and emotional problems including justification for harsh treatment, alienation, depression, isolation, and physical and emotional distress.

Well-being, from an artistic model, honors the everyday, felt, aesthetic experience of the creation and contemplation of art, but with full knowledge that individual experiences are hinged temporally to long-term instrumental goals. The problem arises when the intrinsic experiences (e.g., making art) and instrumental outcomes (e.g., a painting) are habitually separated instead of being seen as a unified expression through time. Stroud (2011), in his reading of Dewey, asserted that when we abandon the idea that objects intrinsically contain value, we can view *an* experience simultaneously as intrinsic (immediate) and instrumental (long-term) by a shift in orientation. Our aesthetic standpoint seeks to fully embrace the present emotive experience and couple these experiences with long-term instrumental goals including self-expression, the creation of social solidarity, and social change. Take a moment to engage with The ART of AUTISM in Theorizing Practice 6.1.

Theorizing Practice 6.1
The ART of AUTISM

The ART of AUTISM is a collaborative project linking more than 250 artists, poets, and authors on the autism spectrum (see http://the-art-of-autism.com). Founders Debra Musikar and Keri Bowers were inspired by the ways in which art gave their own children a chance to express an autistic perspective and engage in self-advocacy. Debra's son demonstrated gifts in oil painting. Keri's son, Taylor, dreamed of being a filmmaker. Together, they created a documentary film, *Normal People Scare Me,* produced by Joey Travolta. Invigorated by the success of their individual artistic projects, Debora and Kerry joined forces to develop The ART of AUTISM. This organization aims to enact "the autism shift"—changes in attitude and perception that "engage individuals and organizations at a higher level of dialogue, thought, and collective action steps to raise awareness, education, and opportunities in the global autism community" (The Autism Shift, http://the-art-of-autism.com/mission/the-autism-shift/, para. 1). The ART of AUTISM is driven by the key values of collectivity and collaboration:

> Through intentional collaborative efforts, we will vision for—and support others—at the same time we promote our individual goals to create sustainable programs, services, products, and possibilities on the world stage. Each member will contribute their time, talent and ideas to the collective—as the collective gives back to the individual members. (The Autism Shift, http://the-art-of-autism.com/mission/the-autism-shift/, para. 3)

To that end, a primary goal of The ART of AUTISM is to develop members' entrepreneurial capacities. The organization provides mentorship opportunities and work experience, assists with building resumes and portfolios, and locates venues for showcasing members' work. The organization's online gallery also showcases members' works (see http://the-art-of-autism.com/gallery/).

Given the above description, how does The ART of AUTISM disrupt the binary distinction between intrinsic/immediate and instrumental/long-term understandings of art's value? What purposes does art serve for this organization? How does The ART of AUTISM counteract a technological orientation towards disability?

■ Art Programming and Self-Expression

> Art gives them freedom . . . it's so wrapped around spreading your wings and being free from this person that they, you know, that they have always been. . . . You know, everybody sees the disability first and doesn't realize there's just this whole complex person working inside them just like everyone else. (Patty Mitchell, interview excerpt)

For artists at CAI, the experience of disability emerges, in part, from living in a body culturally marked as different. Physical variance is a focal point of attention, and this visibility typically works to exclude individuals with disabilities from fully participating in relational and communal life (Quinlan, 2010). Meanwhile, people with developmental disabilities are dismissed because they have not mastered the spoken word, a primary marker of achievement in our society. "Once you begin to present people with opportunities, particularly creative opportunities," stressed Susan Dlouhy, "their whole world begins to change. All of a sudden, they can express themselves in new ways. Art gives them a language. A voice. It's incredible to watch."

Susan is founder and director of Norwich Consulting Services, an organization that works to integrate the art programming of CAI into sheltered workshops across the U.S. "I think they are so grateful for that. To be able to communicate, and to be seen past their bodies," stressed Patty.

The expressive potential of art programming is life changing for the artists served by CAI. The communicative capacity of art is also significant for individuals whose lives have been changed by severe chronic conditions or acute disease (e.g., Borgman, 2002; Murrock & Higgins, 2009; Omar et al., 2011; Staricoff, Duncan, Wright, Loppert, & Scott, 2001). No one moves through this world without the stings and thorns of suffering. Life-changing illness represents a corporeal and social threat to people's previously imagined future. When the continuity of individuals' lives is disrupted by the uncertainty accompanying a life-changing experience, they must reevaluate life priorities, values, and goals in light of bodily changes. In short, they must imagine new normals (Harter, 2013). Individuals rely on rhetorical resources, including art, to make sense of expectations gone awry. Patients and family participation in art programming ranges from the role of artist to that of witness—someone who acknowledges the expression of another. Roles are shaped by the physical capacities of patients as well as modalities used by artists (e.g., painting, drumming, or drawing). Although artists in healthcare settings do not eliminate uncertainties surrounding illness and its treatments, they address suffering in ways that move beyond the traditional scope of science and the technological imperative (Harter, Quinlan, & Ruhl, 2013).

HCIA 6.2

A Story of Sixty-Five Roses

Amanda J. Young

Farrah, my niece, is a magnificent bodybuilder, with arms flexed and a gold medal hanging around her neck. She is smiling in sweet victory. Or at least that's how she is depicted in a colorful and complex collage that her best friend, Dannie, made for her as a wedding gift.

In reality, Farrah had cystic fibrosis (CF), a ravaging, life-limiting disease that affects about 30,000 people in the United States. The disease wreaks havoc in the body, affecting the digestive, reproductive, and respiratory systems and ultimately causing death from respiratory failure.

Farrah's first hospitalization was at age 12. It was then that she met Dannie, a CF compatriot who would be her best friend for the rest of her life. Often spending three or four weeks in the hospital at the same time, the girls shared plenty of shenanigans: holding a candy sale with a huge box of candy bars sent to Farrah by her great-aunt; leading a patient "rebellion" when the teenagers on 8 South were no longer allowed to go to the cafeteria by themselves; and routinely terrorizing the respiratory therapists. But they also held one another each time one of their friends died.

By the time she was 20, Farrah's respiratory function had become so compromised that she needed a double lung transplant. Even though it was grueling, she did well, and six months later she married her boyfriend, Cyrus. For her wedding gift, Dannie gave her "Breathe," a whirlwind of words and images on a background of wrapping paper patterned

(continued)

in red roses. (I've included two sections of the collage here.) "Breathe" tells the story of Farrah's and Dannie's life with cystic fibrosis, which bears the moniker of "Sixty-Five Roses" because of a young patient's mispronunciation of the term. Dannie did not use new technology to create the collage. Instead, she painstakingly cut out individual words, letters, and images, gluing them onto the rose-patterned wrapping paper to weave what appears to be, in Arthur Frank's terms, a chaotic narrative of a chaotic illness experience. But in the chaos, we see discrete details of stories that Farrah and Dannie, along with three other friends, created for themselves. The overarching story is about breathing, as signified in the top left corner: "Let's Talk About Your Future with Your Two

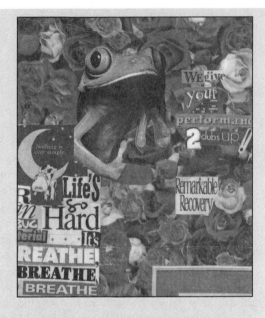

New Lungs," and the top right corner, where a sad cartoon cow hangs over the moon saying: "Life's So Hard, It's Breathe, Breathe, Breathe All the Time."

The collage is both a celebration and a memorial. In celebration of Farrah's successful transplant, we see a tree toad, with his clubbed "thumb" surrounded by the words, "We give your performance 2 clubs up." (CF insiders know that the toad's thumb is representative of the thickening and rounding of their fingertips, known as clubbing.) Near the toad are the words: "Congratulations on a Remarkable Recovery!"

Near the middle of the collage is a small picture of Rosie the Riveter, an icon of women's strength, saying, "We can do it!" The main celebration, however, is at the center of the collage, where we see Farrah, Dannie, and a third friend, Rachel. Their faces are superimposed onto photos of female bodybuilders, their bodies thickly muscled and glittering, their arms flexed. Farrah, in the center, wears a gold medal. To her left is Rachel, who at the time was doing well. She wears a superhero's cape. Dannie, who was sicker at the time than Rachel, is to the right, still sporting a mouthpiece that is part of a breathing treatment.

The collage is also a memorial. To the far right and the far left are Jim and Amy, again, with their faces superimposed on bodybuilders. Jim, clothed in a skimpy Speedo and looking ready to conquer the cartoon woman at his feet, had died a few years prior, after

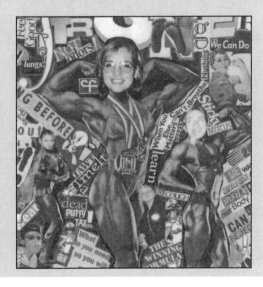

one year at college. Amy, too, had died; at 15, she was the first friend that Farrah had lost. She is sitting on a toilet, looking horrified and saying, "I tawt I tmelt a dead putty tat!" (reminiscent of Tweety Bird). This is another CF insider comment, referring to the digestive difficulties that the disease causes. We can almost hear the cacophony around Amy: "For the love of PETE! HOW LONG BEFORE **THEY** DO SOME THING About This digestive system!!!" Scattered in that area of the collage are the words "enzymes," "greasy," "diarrhea," "hot and fudgy," and "don't forget to wear your mask."

Dannie was a master storyteller, using her art to celebrate Farrah's new chance at life, and to memorialize their friends. She also used it to entertain, mollify, cajole, reminisce, and inquire. Sadly, Farrah's story ended too soon—six months after her wedding. Within the next five years, Dannie and Rachel also died. But thankfully and wonderfully, their stories are captured in Dannie's artwork, which continues to reveal new strands of the narrative every time I look at it.

QUESTIONS TO PONDER

1. Dannie was also a gifted writer. Why do you think she chose to tell Farrah's story using a collage?

2. Cystic fibrosis is not a common disease. Do you think it's easier to learn about an illness through graphics or through reading about it? Why?

3. Think about your own story. What would your collage look like?

Source: Young, A. J. (in press). Breathe. *Health Communication*.

What images of care emerge when guided by the expressive arts? The term "therapy" derives from the Greek word *therapeia*—to be attentive to another (Stuckley & Nobel, 2010, p. 254). Artists draw on a different toolkit than traditional care providers when attending to and joining with another who suffers. In therapeutic contexts, artists use various modalities (e.g., pencil and paper, music, or dance) toward various ends that include diagnostic, clinical, palliative, and vocational purposes. In some cases, artists have clearly defined goals that guide programming (e.g., strengthen eye-hand coordination or increase self-esteem) even as unintended benefits arise (e.g., anxiety reduction or pain relief). Initiatives differ in size, scope, location, and funding but most are united in their desire to empower participants through self-discovery and expression. Art making is a human act of creating meaning out of formless materials and, as such, is a powerful vehicle for self-expression, as demonstrated by The Awakenings Project in Theorizing Practice 6.2 (on the next page).

The arts offer a range of modalities for biographical performance. The visual arts, for example, foster nonverbal communication, bringing clarity to experiences that may be too difficult or too painful to put into words. In this way, visual narratives render experience "seeable" if not "sayable" (Riessman, 2008). Dancers negotiate identities through bodily movements (Quinlan & Harter, 2010). Human plight, vulnerability, and courage can be conveyed through music and its syncopated rhythms (Sellnow & Sellnow, 2001). The everyday sights and sounds and spaces of vulnerability come into fuller focus when expressed through multisensory art programming. Art programming offers meaningful opportunities for self-expression. Yet the trailer for our documentary series reveals a deeper understanding of how art can accomplish community—it

Theorizing Practice 6.2
The Awakenings Project

The Awakenings Project was founded to provide artists, writers, and musicians managing mental illnesses with opportunities for self-expression (see http://www.awakeningsproject.org/about.shtml). The organization has its own art studio, publishes *The Awakenings Review*, collaborates with musical conservatories, and partners with established theater groups. The Awakenings Project defines art as a "purposeful and optimistic activity," one that offers individuals with mental illnesses a grounding sense of identity forged through a gradual process of self-esteem building (About Us, 2009, para. 4). The Awakenings Project recognizes that, by joining a community of artists, members can overcome the sense of social isolation propagated by stigmatizing depictions of mental illness. Collaborative projects, like theater, forge friendships and encourage team building. In publishing their works and receiving positive feedback, artists with mental illnesses develop a sense of competence. The Awakenings Project nurtures this sense of purpose by providing their members with the opportunity to give back through charitable art projects at local nursing homes and hospitals.

The Awakenings Project provides several ways in which individuals with mental illness can engage in self-discovery and reimagine their identities. What avenues can you locate in this description? How does The Awakenings Project (re)envision therapy?

has the capacity to create relational connections (Harter & Shaw, 2013). In the next section, we discuss the role of creative programming in creating social solidarity.

■ Creating Social Solidarity

> Art can be a dusty thing on a shelf, or a live thing in a community. It basically allows for all of what we already have to bubble up and come together and to fuse into something we can have a shared experience around and see evidence of each other's beauty. (Patty Mitchell, interview excerpt)

The artistic practices of CAI foster the creation of social solidarity. Lives are made productive by social ties that facilitate cooperation for mutual benefit. Yet, political, economic, and cultural forces interlace to sustain the separation of people with disabilities from broader community life. Through art, CAI helps participants form relationships and confront their cultural isolation. "It [art] goes beyond expression," argued Susan, then interim director of HighCo, later stressing, "Participants are able to form bonds with one another" (interview excerpt). Organizations like CAI create what Putnam (2000) described as *social capital,* networks of trustworthiness and reciprocity that ultimately lead to the revitalization of civic life. Expanding upon Putnam, democratic theorist Allen (2004) urged readers to understand relational connections as *shared existence.* "Some live behind one veil, and others behind another," mused Allen, "but the air we all breathe carries the same gases and pollens through those veils" (p. xxii). The central purpose of organizations like CAI, from Allen's perspective, is to "prove oneself trustworthy to fellow citizens so that we are better able to ensure that we all breathe healthy air" (p. xxii). For Patty and her colleagues, trust is accomplished through artistic endeavors.

At its best, art making fosters solidarity among individuals, organizations, and communities. At the micro level, art connects individuals who may be experiencing similar situations. Although health crises represent an occasion for communion, illness and its treatment can be quite isolating. Depending on the nature of the condition, patients may be separated physically and geographically from their primary social networks. Meanwhile, stigmas that accompany some chronic conditions can contribute to stressful interactions or relational avoidance (Smith, 2011; Smith & Hipper, 2010). Art programming offers opportunities for individuals to connect with others and opens up conversations that might otherwise remain dormant. In doing so, aesthetic experiences can disrupt the physical and social isolation too often experienced by patients and families (Malchiodi, 2003; Riley & Malchiodi, 2003; Rollins, 2005).

Art making at CAI spurs dialogue and builds relationships among artists, staff, and community volunteers. From Patty's perspective, "art allows humans to connect with other humans. It's that simple." In reflecting on her life's work, she shared:

> I believe that people are included and excluded in lots of situations because of poverty, disease, different things. People with disabilities, it's just accepted that they are going to be separated from their own communities. Even the term "sheltered workshops" suggests that they are separate. They are sheltered. And that is just not OK.

A case in point: People with disabilities now constitute one of the world's largest minority groups facing poverty, unemployment, and cultural isolation (Butterworth et al., 2012). CAI disrupts the cultural isolation of people with disabilities with art programming. Through creative collaborations, participants confront their cultural alienation. Art emerges as a way of living in association with others, a means of cultivating and celebrating community.

Art programming in healthcare contexts realizes Dewey's (1980/1934) fundamental belief that art can be harnessed to develop fuller and richer relational life. In the Arts in Medicine Program at MD Anderson Cancer Center, art brings together similarly situated patients while also connecting patients and staff members. Various health scholars have critiqued biomedicine for not going far enough to understand the experience of being ill (Lupton, 2012; Sharf, Harter, Yamasaki, & Haidet, 2011). For Lupton (2012), Western medicine is "directed towards controlling the body, keeping it from subsiding into the chaos and disorder threatened by illness and disease" (p. 30). Being ill is a physical experience that affects various aspects of the body. Fever, vomiting, pain, and chills are all outward manifestations of physical experience. However, being ill also shifts patients' sense of self and their interpersonal relationships.

Socioemotional experiences may not be visibly evident or clearly captured by computerized axial tomography (CT) scans, blood pressure cuffs, or blood draws. Such procedures cannot capture the anxiousness felt by a parent caring for an ill child, the worry of a husband waiting for his wife's test results, or the confusion experienced by a family following a medical diagnosis of one of its members. The arts call upon care providers to connect with patients as people, disrupting the narrowing gaze of the biomedical model. The art produced by children serves as powerful evidence of their interests, inviting staff to understand children holistically. A child's painting, the singing out loud of a song, or the creation of a digital meme, all serve as tangible evidence that patients are people with a diverse array of life experiences that extend beyond their diagnosis and treatment plan. Meanwhile, art making can ease typical stressors that accompany patient and provider encounters (Staricoff et al., 2001). This may occur, for example, when a child sits and sketches a picture while a nurse inserts a new IV line. In this case, art works to assuage the child's sense of fear or anxiousness, making it easier for the nurse to perform his routine duties. In short, art programming offers opportunities for the development of social solidarity in contexts characterized by profound vulnerability. In so doing, art also has the capacity to enlarge the social imaginary.

■ Enlarging the Social Imaginary

> Artistic and cultural practices can offer spaces of resistance that undermine the social imaginary. (Mouffe, 2013, p. 88)

Art plays a vital role in creating, digesting, and ultimately reconstituting the ideas that any culture takes as common sense. Across generations, cultural values and practices are symbolically constructed, taken for granted as natural, and reified in ways that perpetuate the status quo as normal. The deficit model of care, for example, continues to shape how we understand and "do disability" in our personal interactions and in public domains. Art-based programming like CAI is especially adept at challenging normative assumptions. Consider Patty's testimony:

> Our goal is to use art to empower the peoples we serve and to educate our community. In many ways, I see this as civil rights work. Art ends up being a vehicle to express what goes on in people who don't have a good way to communicate. Art draws people in, and makes them step closer. And then they can witness what our artists of capable of. They have hopes, and dreams, and feelings, and aspirations. They can do more than screw in a nut or a bolt on an assembly line.

The aesthetic experiences facilitated by CAI function as a scaffold for the achievement of other goals including self-advocacy, consciousness-raising, and social change.

The art produced by participants of CAI is exhibited in galleries, sold in studios, and integrated in community-wide celebrations (e.g., homecoming parades). Through these efforts, CAI renders visible experiences that would otherwise remain obscured or distorted in public domains. The artists display alternative performances of disability, reinvent identities, and extend notions of societal inclusion. Importantly, artists capitalize on the power of emotion to motivate contemplators to reconsider what counts as normal. Mouffe (2013) argued:

> If artistic practices can play a decisive role in the construction of new forms of subjectivity, it is because, in using resources which induce emotional responses, they are able to reach human beings at the affective level. This is where art's great power lies—in its capacity to make us see things in a different way, to make us perceive new possibilities. (p. 96)

Creative encounters, in the case of CAI, enable consumers to comprehend, if only partially, what it means to live with a physical disability. By attuning us to one another, art fosters greater empathy for those living in the midst of chronic conditions or episodic illness.

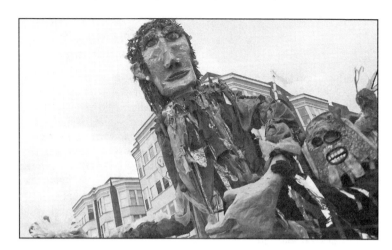

CAI participates in the Ohio University Homecoming Parade (Evan Shaw).

Healthcare systems recognize the power of art to transform their socio-spatial environments (e.g., waiting rooms). Hospitals and outpatient settings can be sources of distress to patients and visitors. Though the naming of health conditions can reduce uncertainty, medical environments often feel quite foreign. Treatment of life-changing and chronic conditions requires patients to survive in spatial domains that, by design, are sterile. Participating in art-making and witnessing art can transform individuals' sense of place. Not surprisingly, the exhibition of art is on the rise in U.S. hospitals and clinics (Landro, 2014). In fact, some scholars have argued that the success of art programs in healthcare settings rests in large part in their capacity to transform patients' and visitors' experience of space (Harter et al., 2013). For example, the Tree of Life installation featured in the photo is an exhibit at the University of Texas MD Anderson Children's Cancer Hospital in Houston, Texas. The exhibit was created by participants in the Arts in Medicine Program (see Theorizing Practice 6.3).

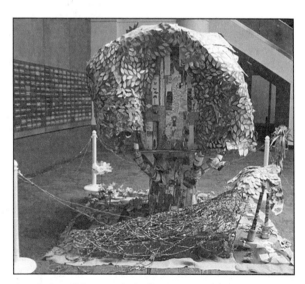

Art forms such as painting, music, sculpture, and photography feature central themes of tragedy and human suffering (Burke, 1968; Neill, 2013). Contemplators can be troubled by what the work depicts (e.g., the content) even as they appreciate the manner of its presentation (e.g., its form). Con-

Arts in Medicine Tree of Life Exhibit at MD Anderson Cancer Center (Lynn M. Harter).

Theorizing Practice 6.3
The Arts in Medicine Program

The Arts in Medicine (AIM) Program at the University of Texas MD Anderson Children's Cancer Hospital is directed by Artist in Residence Ian Cion (see http://www.mdanderson.org/patient-and-cancer-information/care-centers-and-clinics/childrens-cancer-hospital/support-programs/children-s-cancer-hospital-support-programs-arts-in-medicine.html.) Guided by Ian, AIM provides art programming to pediatric, adolescent, and young adult patients and their families. The programming is composed of personalized art sessions as well as collaborative large-scale projects. Through its programming, AIM helps to elevate patients' sense of well-being, reduce pain and anxiety, shift the nature of the hospital experience, connect patients with similarly situated individuals, and build a sense of community within the hospital.

What challenges might be faced by artists like Ian who work within hospital settings? What factors might prevent AIM from reaching its objectives? How could staff and administrators address such challenges?

---

sider, for example, the efforts of ArtWorks, one division of a social service organization located in Charlotte, North Carolina. On its website, ArtWorks (n.d.) describes its vision: "to restore voices and vitality to those who have so often been silenced and stifled" while at the same time "inspiring conversation around the larger issues of homelessness" (para. 2). Just as its exhibits can be beautiful, ArtWorks moves contemplators beyond their comfort zones. Bearing witness to once-silenced voices is difficult for some audience members. Viewing the AIDS Memorial Quilt, for example, can move some people to tears, even as it motivates others to seek information about treatment interventions (Knaus, Pinkleton, & Austin, 2000). Sponsored by The NAMES Project, the quilt consists of more than 48,000 individual 3- by 6-foot memorial panels commemorating the lives of individuals who died of AIDS. Images of the quilt can be viewed online and panels of the quilt itself are displayed in various community venues (see http://www.aidsquilt.org/about). Public art has been used to raise awareness about diverse experiences including mental illness (Bell, 2011), breast cancer (Dennett, 2011; Sharf, 1995), and brain injury (Lorenz, 2011). As argued by Sharf (1995), "Visual art, with its element of aesthetics, economy of statement, and individualized expression, conveys information and points of view in emphatic and convincing ways" (p. 72). In sum, communication about trauma through art can be a source of both delight and distress.

HCIA 6.3

When Cancer Calls . . .

Wayne A. Beach

Over the years, I have informally surveyed my undergraduate students by asking the following question: How many of your lives have been directly or indirectly impacted by cancer? It may be surprising that even with the average age of the students being 23, two thirds to three fourths of them claim personal cancer experiences. Yet three out of four U.S. families journey through cancer together. These undergraduates are family members who have somehow been involved in a wide variety of communication activities inherent to cancer diagnosis, treatment, and prognosis, including:

- waiting for and talking about biopsy results;
- delivering and receiving good and bad news;
- managing uncertainties, fears, and hopes;
- trying to remain stable in the midst of complex and confusing health circumstances;
- reporting on and assessing what doctors, nurses, and other healthcare providers have told patients and family members;
- updating others about a loved one's condition; and
- telling stories, joking, teasing, commiserating, and doing whatever families do to cope with possible dis-ease as time moves forward.

For some time we have been studying these, and many other social actions, occurring in the midst of communicating about cancer journeys. In my research, I have presented a longitudinal study, focusing on how family members talk and navigate their way through cancer on the telephone. The research closely examines 61 phone calls over 13 months, offering the first recorded and transcribed corpus of actual family phone calls, in the history of the social and medical sciences, from diagnosis through death of a wife/mother/sister. At once remarkable yet altogether normal and routine, these materials reveal the trials, tribulations, hopes, and triumphs of facing cancer together—as a family.

Scholars, healthcare professionals, and community members alike have heard these calls and participated in analyzing transcribed interactions. Consistent and strong encouragement has been offered to find a way to make these powerful materials available to all persons dealing with health challenges. Our response was to gradually develop a professional theatrical production, now entitled *When Cancer Calls . . .*, which relies on verbatim dialogue from real-time interactions between family members.

For example, in the second phone call, Mom informs Son about a serious cancer diagnosis. The moment below, following her delivery of bad news, begins as Son addresses how Mom's cancer might be treated:

SON   Whadda you do with this kind of thing. I mean . . .

MOM   Radiation, chemotherapy.

[pause]

SON   Oh boy.

MOM   Yeah.

[pause]

MOM   My only hope, I mean—[pause] my only choice.

The delicate and complex relationship between Mom's "hope" and "choice" is one of many topics raised and discussed by audience members following viewings. And with support from the American Cancer Society, the National Institutes of Health/National Cancer Institute, and philanthropists in San Diego, thousands of audience members (patients, family members, survivors, and healthcare professionals) have reported being significantly impacted by experiencing and talking about how *When Cancer Calls . . .* relates to their everyday experiences and social relationships.

(continued)

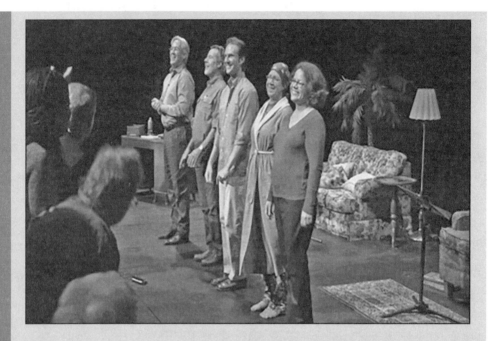

Live performances and DVD screenings in San Diego, and screenings in Denver, Salt Lake City, Lincoln, and Boston have confirmed the critical importance of family communication when facing cancer. Key insights have also emerged as healthcare professionals report being positively impacted by a closer look at what patients and family members actually go through, over time, in home as well as in cancer and other health clinics.

By integrating basic communication research in the social sciences with the power of the arts and mediated communication, we have been able to create a highly effective and sustainable educational tool that exposes ordinary family life while also making apparent often taken-for-granted conceptions of health and illness. Findings from our recent and highly successful national dissemination of *When Cancer Calls*... are currently being analyzed. A wide array of research, educational, and training possibilities are also being developed as plans are being refined to make *When Cancer Calls*... available to academic and healthcare professions nationally and globally.

QUESTIONS TO PONDER

1. Have you been to the theater? What emotions did you experience as an audience member?

2. How does a live performance evoke feelings in ways that other art forms might not?

3. What new understandings could these recorded phone calls offer health communication scholars? Healthcare providers? Patients and their family members?

Sources: Beach, W. A. (2009). A natural history of family cancer: Interactional resources for *managing illness*. New York, NY: Hampton. Beach, W. A., Buller, M. K., Dozier, D., Buller, D., & Gutzmer, K. (2014). Conversations about Cancer (CAC): Assessing feasibility and audience impacts from viewing *The Cancer Play*. *Health Communication, 29*, 462–472.

■ Epilogue

Patty facilitated a two-week art residency at HighCo in September 2013. Participants painted, sewed, and built objects out of discarded objects (e.g., CDs, driftwood). Over the following twelve months, HighCo established the Up and Beyond Studio, an art program that offers creative and vocational opportunities for individuals served by the county Board of Developmental Disabilities, including Courtney. In December 2014, the Up and Beyond Studio relocated its gallery to a storefront on West Main Street. Courtney's art is now for sale. Some of it contains shredded paper.

■ Conclusion

No biographical story is a straight line. The geometry of a life is too imperfect, too complex, too distorted by what rhetorical critic Kenneth Burke (1968) would term *Trouble* with a capital T. The making of art and the viewing of artistic performances show promise for helping participants make sense of and respond to life disruptions. In this chapter, we have featured the work of CAI, an organization that leverages creative acts to build social solidarity among people with and without developmental disabilities. In so doing, CAI is shifting the broader social imaginary from a deficit-oriented value system to an asset-based set of beliefs and practices. Participating artists are intrinsically rewarded by opportunities for self-expression. Importantly, though, creative practices provide a scaffold for the achievement of other goals including community integration and social change. CAI illustrates how sheltered workshops can embrace art as both intrinsically (i.e., process) and instrumentally (i.e., product) valuable, a vision articulated by Dewey (1934/1980).

Reaching beyond the work of CAI, we have illustrated the value of integrating an aesthetic orientation into healthcare systems dominated by scientific logics. Artists' creative use of various communicative modalities makes possible the affirmation of feelings and management of uncertainties inherent in the experience of patients, family members, and care providers. The recognition of ourselves in another is at the heart of artistic endeavors. Through art, we are more keenly attuned to others, our surrounding community, and ourselves. Art helps us to find beauty in the imperfect, and in turn, transform that imperfection into strength.

Discussion Questions

1. If you were speaking to a group of benefactors, what arguments would you use to convince them to support creative programming in healthcare settings?

2. Reflect upon a time that art helped you to cope with a difficult moment in your life. How did this process work, or not work, to help you understand the situation?

3. Brainstorm alternative ways we may think about art beyond traditional modalities such as painting, drawing, or sculpting.

4. Locate an organization within your local community that incorporates art into its programming. How does the organization utilize art? To what population is the organization speaking? Do you find their strategy to be effective or compelling?

5. How would you incorporate art into your regular community activities?

REFERENCES

Allen, D. S. (2004). *Talking to strangers: Anxieties of citizenship since* Brown v. Board of Education. Chicago, IL: University of Chicago Press.

ArtWorks. (n.d.). ArtWorks 945. Retrieved from http://www.urbanministrycenter.org/helping-the-homeless/community-works/

Bell, S. E. (2011). Claiming justice: Knowing mental illness in the public art of Anna Schuleit's "habeas corpus" and "bloom." *Health: An Interdisciplinary Journal for the Social Study of Health, Illness and Medicine, 15,* 313–334.

Borgman, E. (2002). Art therapy with three women diagnosed with cancer. *The Arts in Psychotherapy, 29,* 245–251.

Burke, K. (1968). *Counter-statement.* Berkeley: University of California Press. (Original work published in 1931)

Butterworth, J., Smith, F. A., Migliore, A., Winsor, J., Domin, D., & Timmons, J. C. (2012). *StateData: The national report on employment services and outcomes.* Boston: University of Massachusetts.

Dennett, T. (2011). Jo Spence's auto-therapeutic survival strategies. *Health, 15,* 223–229.

Dewey, J. (1980). *Art as experience.* New York, NY: Capricorn Books. (Original work published 1934)

Dlouhy, S., & Mitchell, P. (2015). *Upscaling sheltered workshops.* Athens: Ohio University Press.

Freeman, J. C., Epston, D., & Lobovits, D. (1997). *Playful approaches to serious problems: Narrative therapy with children and their families.* New York, NY: Norton.

Haidet, P. (2007). Jazz and the "art" of medicine: Improvisation in the medical encounter. *Annals of Family Medicine, 5,* 164–169.

Harter, L. M. (2013). The poetics and politics of storytelling in health contexts. In L. M. Harter & Associates, *Imagining new normals: A narrative framework for health communication* (pp. 3–28). Dubuque, IA: Kendall/Hunt.

Harter, L. M., Leeman, M., Norander, S., Young, S. L., & Rawlins, W. K. (2008). The intermingling of aesthetic sensibilities and instrumental rationalities in a collaborative arts studio. *Management Communication Quarterly, 21,* 423–453.

Harter, L. M., Quinlan, M. M., & Ruhl, S. (2013). The storytelling capacities of arts programming in healthcare contexts. In L. M. Harter & Associates, *Imagining new normals: A narrative framework for health communication* (pp. 29–50). Dubuque, IA: Kendall/Hunt.

Harter, L. M., & Rawlins, W. K. (2011). The worlding of possibilities in a collaborative art studio: Organizing embodied differences with aesthetic and dialogic sensibilities. In D. K. Mumby (Ed.), *Reframing difference in organizational communication studies: Research, pedagogy, practice* (pp. 267–289). Thousand Oaks, CA: Sage.

Harter, L. M., Scott, J. S., Novak, D. K., Leeman, M. A., & Morris, J. (2006). Freedom through flight: Performing a counter-narrative of disability. *Journal of Applied Communication Research, 4,* 3–29.

Harter, L. M., & Shaw, E. (Producers). (2013). *The courage of creativity.* USA: WOUB Center for Public Media. (http://woub.org/2013/12/17/documentary-series-explores-connections-between-art-and-well-being)

Hauser, G. A. (1999). *Vernacular voices: The rhetoric of publics and public spheres.* Columbia, SC: University of South Carolina Press.

Kaplan, F. K. (2003). Art-based assessments. In C. Malchiodi (Ed.), *Handbook of art therapy* (pp. 25–36). New York, NY: Guilford.

Knaus, C. S., Pinkleton, B. E., & Austin, E. W. (2000). The ability of the AIDS quilt to motivate information seeking, personal discussion, and preventive behavior as a health communication intervention. *Health Communication, 12,* 301–316.

Landro, L. (2014, August 18). More hospitals use the healing powers of public art. *The Wall Street Journal.* Retrieved from http://www.wsj.com

Lorenz, L. S. (2011). A way into empathy: A "case" of photo-elicitation in illness research. *Health: An Interdisciplinary Journal for the Social Study of Health, Illness and Medicine, 15,* 259–276.

Lupton, D. (2012). *Medicine as culture: Illness, disease and the body.* (3rd ed.). Thousand Oaks, CA: Sage.

Mackelprang, R., & Salsgiver, R. O. (2009). *Disability. A diversity model in human service practice* (2nd ed.). New York, NY: Lyceum.

Malchiodi, C. A. (2003). *Handbook of art therapy.* New York, NY: Guilford.

McKerrow, R. E. (1998). Corporeality and cultural rhetoric: A site for rhetoric's future. *Southern Communication Journal, 63,* 315–328.

Mouffe, C. (2013). *Agnostics: Thinking the world politically.* London, UK: Verso.

Murrock, C. J., & Higgins, P. A. (2009). The theory of music, mood and movement to improve health outcomes: Discussion paper. *Journal of Advanced Nursing, 65,* 2249–2257.

Neill, A. (2013). Tragedy. In B. Gaut & D. M. Lopes (Eds.), *The Routledge companion to aesthetics* (3rd ed., pp. 415–424). New York, NY: Routledge.

Omar, R., Henley, S., Bartlett, J. W., Hailston, J. C., Gordon, E., Sauter, D., Frost, C., Scott, S., & Warren, J. D. (2011). The structural neuroanatomy of music emotion recognition: Evidence from frontotemporal lobar degeneration. *NeuroImage, 56,* 1814–1821.

Putnam, R. D. (2000). *Bowling alone: The collapse and revival of the American community.* New York, NY: Simon and Schuster.

Quinlan, M. M. (2010). Fostering connections among diverse individuals through multi-sensorial storytelling. *Health Communication, 25,* 91–93.

Quinlan, M. M., & Harter, L. M. (2010). Meaning in motion: The embodied poetics and politics of Dancing Wheels. *Text & Performance Quarterly, 30,* 374-395.

Riessman, C. K. (2008). *Narrative methods for the human sciences.* Thousand Oaks, CA: Sage.

Riley, S., & Malchiodi, C. A. (2003). Solution-focused and narrative approaches. In A. C. Malchiodi (Ed.), *Handbook of art therapy* (pp. 82–92). New York, NY: Guilford.

Rollins, J. A. (2005). Tell me about it: Drawing as a communication tool for children with cancer. *Journal of Pediatric Oncology Nursing, 22,* 203–221.

Sellnow, D., & Sellnow, T. (2001). The "illusion of life" rhetorical perspective: An integrated approach to the study of music as communication. *Critical Studies in Media Communication, 18,* 395–415.

Sharf, B. F. (1995). Poster art as women's rhetoric: Raising awareness about breast cancer. *Literature & Medicine, 14,* 72–86.

Sharf, B. F., Geist-Martin, P., & Moore, J. (2013). Communicating healing in a third space: Real and imagined forms of integrative medicine. In L. M. Harter & Associates, *Imagining new normals: A narrative framework for health communication* (pp. 125–148). Dubuque, IA: Kendall/Hunt.

Sharf, B., Harter, L. M., Yamasaki, J., & Haidet, P. (2011). Narrative turns epic: Continuing developments in health narrative scholarship. In T. Thompson, R. Parrott, & J. Nussbaum (Eds.), *Handbook of health communication* (2nd ed., pp. 36–51). New York, NY: Routledge.

Shaughnessy, A. F., Slawson, D. C., & Becker, L. (1998). Clinical jazz: Harmonizing clinical experience and evidence-based medicine. *Journal of Family Practice, 47,* 425–428.

Singhal, A., Buscell, P., & Lindberg, C. (2010). *Inviting everyone: Healing healthcare through positive deviance.* New York, NY: CreateSpace.

Smith, R. (2011). Stigma, communication, and health. In T. Thompson, R. Parrott, & J. Nussbaum (Eds.), *Handbook of health communication* (2nd ed., pp. 455–468). New York, NY: Routledge.

Smith, R., & Hipper, T. (2010). Label management: Investigating how confidants encourage the use of communication strategies to avoid stigmatization. *Health Communication, 25,* 410–422.

Staricoff, R. L., Duncan, J., Wright, M., Loppert, S., & Scott, J. (2001). A study of the effects of visual and performing arts in healthcare. *Hospital Development, 32,* 25–28.

State of the Field Committee. (2009). *State of the field report: Arts in healthcare 2009.* Washington, DC: Society for the Arts in Healthcare.

Stroud, S. R. (2011). *John Dewey and the artful life. Pragmatism, aesthetics, and morality.* University Park: University of Pennsylvania Press.

Stuckley, H. L., & Nobel, J. (2010). The connection between art, healing, and public health: A review of current literature. *American Journal of Public Health, 100,* 254–263.

Taylor, C. (2007). *Modern social imaginaries.* Durham, NC: Duke University Press.

van Dijck, J. (2005). *The transparent body: A cultural analysis of medical imaging.* Seattle: University of Washington Press.

7

Communicating Workplace Wellness as Flourishing

Patricia Geist-Martin & Jennifer A. Scarduzio

I wasn't an undergrad when this started. I was a graduate student and a lot of factors come into play that wouldn't necessarily as an undergraduate. I was familiar with the department. I had grown up there as a kid. My mom had me when she was fifteen. So when she was getting her graduate degree there, I would hang out in the library. I had a strong affiliation before I even started. Further, I was older. I was returning after being in the business world. My son was two. I was married and I knew the faculty. So, you would think that I was going to be less susceptible. . . . My mom and all her friends teach at the community colleges here in town, so I knew that I didn't want to do that. I needed my own identity, so I was working and applying for a PhD program. Finishing my master's degree and getting letters were important to get into a PhD school.

In this opening narrative, Allyson reveals that she is not a typical graduate student and that she wants to establish her own identity apart from her mother. But at the same time, she has a strong affiliation with the university and clearly views professors as knowledgeable and respectable. The story she has to tell reveals how her experience at work as a graduate student assistant became extremely problematic and uncomfortable when her interactions with one professor changed the environment where she was thriving to a toxic environment that was impossible to work in and decreased her quality of life.

He asked if I would be interested, as he had funding for an assistantship. I said, of course. I called my mom and right away my mom said, "Beware of him" . . . but this is such an honored position. I took the position and I worked with him that fall as a research assistant. . . . And now that I look back, I can see where personality-wise, I'm very trusting. I had a little Beaver Cleaver kind of life in many respects, and I don't think I'm a really good judge of—how should I put it? I give people the benefit of the doubt.

Allyson continues her story by describing how working together closely, she and her professor got to know a lot about each other's families and life. He would talk about his marriage and why it broke up, and she would talk about her husband and son and some of the struggles of managing being a wife, mom, and student. She told him that she and her husband were seeing a counselor and how it helped them to remember how much in love they were. But in the midst of all of this talk, there were subtle but continuous ways that the professor's words and actions made Allyson feel uncomfortable at work.

For the first six months I worked with him, [he would say things like] "I love the cut of that dress on you. That looks really pretty." Or "Your legs are so shapely when you wear high heels." Or "Did you change your hair? It doesn't look as good pulled back as it does down." Always, in all honesty, I cannot imagine that there was one session, as far as grading papers or whatever the interaction, something was said about my physical appearance or a sexual innuendo. . . . I had worked in business and there were plenty of people and you'd just blah, blah, and kind of now pay attention. In that whole six months, I never said, "I don't like that." "Don't talk to me like that." It didn't really bug me. . . . However, when you look at it, the classical definition of sexual harassment.

Allyson later learned from other female students that the professor had a reputation as a "slime ball" with a long history of engaging inappropriately with women students, including directly saying "sleep with me" or else—no letter of recommendation, a lower grade, or other significant ramifications for their academic futures for not consenting.

Sexual harassment in the workplace is clearly abuse that keeps people, usually women, from flourishing at work. As professors of communication, we[1] have researched sexual harassment, not only because Patricia has been the victim of this toxic behavior, but also because her own students have come to her to disclose their own traumatic experience with sexual harassment.

It is ironic, really; as Patricia began to conduct interviews as part of her research on sexual harassment on college campuses and learn of others' stories, her own workplace began to feel toxic and stressful. While the stories that students and staff told her were mandated as confidential by her research protocol, it seemed that everywhere she traveled across campus, she would come into contact with alleged perpetrators and victims of this form of sexual violence. She interacted with them politely in committee meetings, at campus events, and at lunchtime in campus restaurants. Patricia experienced what feminists have termed "guilty knowledge" (Hughes, 1971) and realized that to feel healthy again and flourish at work she needed to discontinue her research on sexual harassment, which she did for 10 years. She and Jennifer returned to this data, not only because the stories haunted Patricia, but because both she and Jennifer felt responsible for becoming advocates for students like Allyson whose health was suffering greatly from being continuously impacted by this form of abuse in the workplace.

Good quality of life is something that most people struggle to achieve, both at home and at work. It is an elusive state of being that is constrained, compromised, and at times eliminated when people are ill, stressed, and facing the wide range of life's ups and downs and day-to-day challenges and abuses. At the same time, pursuing a quality of life at work can be joyful, inspiring, and even adventuresome as people meet new people, collaborate on projects, and devise new missions and goals. The meanings for work are communicated moment to moment and can contribute and detract from individuals' well-being and the quality of their lives.

Diverse academic disciplines have researched quality of life, including in this book in Chapter 2 in which Sharf first introduces this term in reference to aging, and in Chapter 4 in which Ellingson and Borofka explore how the functioning of work teams can impact health and quality of life. In fact, "the literature is rife with information that focuses on attributes, variables, and categories, and ways to measure and enhance physical, psychological, social, and spiritual well-being" (Parse, 2013, p. 111). Parse (2013) offers a reconceptualization of quality of life that focuses on *human becoming*, considering individuals' meanings from moment to moment. In her view, people live, construct, and change meanings, and we come to understand these meanings qualitatively in speech. "There is only the indivisible, unpredictable, ever changing, moment-to-moment, moving-initiating, anchoring-shifting, and pondering-shaping, co-creating living quality as the core whatness in the emerging now of everyday situations" (Parse, 2013, p. 111). Life quality, then, is something people strive for, but even when achieved, it is not a constant. What counts as life quality may change for individuals as they live through life challenges they may never have imagined they would face, let alone live beyond, including traumas such as the death of a family member, surviving a potentially terminal illness, or resisting/gaining support in the face of sexual harassment.

Many employees consider life quality as something they strive for outside of work, but since many employees spend most of every weekday working, it is important to include life quality at work. On average, individuals spend 7.94 hours a day at work each week, and for some, an additional 5.5 hours at home in the evening or on the weekend (U.S. Bureau of Labor Statistics, 2014), or what translates to one third of their life (Ahmad, 2013). So work, whatever and wherever that is for each employee, has the capacity to influence overall life quality in profound ways.

This chapter is designed to explore the meanings of life quality at work—what sustains it, what constrains it, and the ways people communicate to create work–life balance, to maintain workplace well-being, and to cope with the stress that work inevitably creates in their lives. We will also explore the five dimensions of communicating wellness at work (e.g., physical, psychological, social, spiritual, and eco). While organizations may offer opportunities that assist employees in achieving wellness at work, often the work itself and the organizational culture creates stress and thus constrains wellness at work.

■ Working Well: Quality Life at Work

Quality of Work Life (QWL) is a multifaceted construct that has been defined in many ways since it was first introduced in the 1960s and 1970s (Ahmad, 2013; Cherns & Davis, 1975; Davis & Taylor, 1972; Wild, 1975). Originally, QWL was defined as the ability to satisfy personal needs at work (Suttle, 1977) or job characteristics or work conditions that contribute to employees' well-being (Lawler, 1982). More recently, QWL is described as a construct with seven dimensions: (1) health and safety, (2) employment security, (3) job satisfaction, (4) occupational stress, (5) work environment, (6) work–life balance, and (7) human relations (Ahmad, 2013). Undoubtedly, communication is an essential ingredient in each of these dimensions of QWL.

QWL across the Life Span

Communication is essential as supervisors, subordinates, and customers interact in ways that contribute to QWL. In this sense, QWL is a shared responsibility that can enhance or constrain the health and happiness of employees (Ahmad, 2013), depending on the flexibility and adaptability of communication surrounding the dimensions. Even as people strive for work–life balance and a healthy, satisfying life, and as organizations attempt to construct an environment and work life for employees that contribute to their QWL, for many people, something more is essential. A life span perspective suggests that we place communication at the very heart of our consideration of the ways that people successfully negotiate and adapt to the challenges faced during different points of their lives (Nussbaum, 2007).

Taking the life span construct further, we can think about how people communicate to successfully negotiate the challenges they face at work and also consider QWL in terms of living lives where the goals people strive for and the tasks they perform at work are rewarding, fulfilling, and enriching, sometimes presenting the opportunity— or the risk—of living on the edge of possibilities. For some, this means that creativity and autonomy are encouraged and rewarded. For others, it may mean opportunities to integrate life with work through ecowellness (Reese & Myers, 2012), where natural environments are recognized as contributors to physical and mental health. And for still others, it may mean venturing forth when welcomed or unwelcomed changes occur in health and quality of life (PetersonLund, 2014). Allyson's story presents a real-life circumstance at work where what was once a rewarding career became an unwelcomed change that created both emotional and physical stress—clearly affecting her health.

The touching started more like he would take my arm and lead me somewhere. The more inappropriate stuff started after Christmas break. . . . So we were talking about dreams. And then before he left, he said, "I've been having a lot of dreams about you." And I said, "You have?" and he said something like "Yeah, but I'm a little bit uncomfortable because they always end with something sexual." And I said, "Oh I can see where that would make you uncomfortable." But I could tell the way he was saying it, he was looking at me to see how that was going to bother me. Immediately, I'm sick to my stomach, thinking, "Oh shit, please don't go there." The relationship has been borderline, all the sexual stuff. It's been like you haven't crossed the line. And I was really uncomfortable, because I thought once he crosses it, then the dynamics are going to change. I'm not going to be comfortable any more. So he was kind of testing me, and I said, "I can see where that would be really uncomfortable." He said, "Haven't you ever had dreams like that?" Obviously I've had sexual dreams in my life and I said, "You didn't do anything. It's just a dream," and we kind of laughed it off.

Throughout the 60 pages of her interview, Allyson constantly refers to the stress created through these interactions (e.g., "sick to her stomach," "really uncomfortable") and the difficulty of continuing her work as a research assistant. Her narrative also reveals the ways she rationalized coping with this stress and discomfort to justify remaining in this toxic environment in order to avoid risking any negative outcome for her grades, her master's degree, her PhD application, and her marriage, if her husband knew what she was enduring. She told us that she feared what her husband might do or how he might react if she told him about the professor's behavior. While she received support from other graduate students in the department that knew of the professor's reputation and witnessed his behavior around Allyson, this did not change her continual suffering and concern that everything in her life was at risk. She, like some other employees that suffer through sexual harassment, ventured forth with the hope that it would all be over soon and it would be worth it in the end when she reached the position, advancement, career, or quality of life she had dreamed of.

This venturing forth could be real or metaphoric frontiers, where risk, danger, trauma, or the unknown is present and what people value becomes clearer in the process. Well-being at work, therefore, may be dependent on some or all of these expanded notions of QWL.

HCIA 7.1

Quality Communication across the Life Span

Jon F. Nussbaum

I have always been fascinated by the way *things* change as time progresses. Some wines age very gracefully and taste better as time passes. Some baseball cards in pristine condition get more valuable with age. Human beings (all living things for that matter) progress through their lives with observable physical changes that are easily recognizable and are often looked upon as unwanted. Our hair turns grey, our skin wrinkles, we move slower, and all of our senses are not as sharp. Psychological and cognitive changes also occur. Although some of these changes may be quite detrimental (for instance, a reduction in memory or other cognitive processing abilities), positive change is also a part of the aging process (for instance, wisdom is associated with increasing age). Our communication behavior and our relationships that are constructed through the process of communication are in a constant state of change as time passes as well. For the past 35 years, I have actively researched the communication changes that occur as we age and have attempted to document how these changes are related to our overall quality of life.

Positive markers of communication change include the fact that our vocabulary grows as we age and that we often choose and have the ability to execute much more competent strategies as we confront various life crises across the life span. We also discover a much deeper appreciation of intimacy as we age. In addition, for the past few decades, communication technologies have erased some of the distance barriers that prohibited daily contact in the not so distant past. As a matter of fact, the fastest growing segment of the population who are now utilizing social media are those over the age of 70! In fact, the use of social media has dramatically changed the very nature of the grandparent–grandchild relationship.

Beyond good health and income, the best predictor of maintaining a high quality of life throughout the life span can be found in our ability to construct a network of positive relationships within our family, among our friends, and with various healthcare professionals who become more significant within our lives as we age. Those individuals who can learn and adapt their communication skills to enable the formation and maintenance of a positive social network at every phase of life have the best chance of maintaining a high level of quality within their life.

A primary focus of my research program is understanding how older adults living within assisted care and skilled care nursing facilities and the healthcare workers who provide the care within those facilities can optimize their quality of life within the facility. A significant

(continued)

challenge for organizations focused on providing quality within assisted living and skilled nursing facilities is how to maximize the quality of life for the older residents and, at the same time, create a work environment that reduces healthcare provider turnover and may even produce a high level of satisfaction with the workplace.

We have found that both the residents of assisted care and skilled nursing facilities and the healthcare workers within these facilities enjoy a higher quality of life/work-life when a moderate, "friendship type" of relationship can be constructed and maintained by the healthcare workers and the residents (Nussbaum, Robinson, & Grew, 1985). The healthcare workers are often much younger than the residents. Intergenerational communication in general, when enacted competently, can provide a wonderful context for the transmission of valuable information and life lessons between the generations.

Healthcare workers are often taught not to become close or to share personal information with their patients. We found that this "informal/formal code of appropriate workplace conduct" actually creates a poor work environment for healthcare staff within assisted care and skilled nursing facilities and leads to lower levels of life satisfaction for the residents who wish to interact with these healthcare workers in a more meaningful manner. A moderate sharing of personal life stories by both the residents and the healthcare staff creates a moderately close, trusting relationship and improves the quality of life for both the staff and the residents. Too much self-disclosure of personal issues by both residents and staff is just as inappropriate as too little sharing of their life stories. With some minimal communication training within the facility for both staff and residents, the organization becomes less institutional and more warm and inviting for both residents and staff leading to higher levels of life quality.

QUESTIONS TO PONDER

1. What changes in our relationships over the life span help to improve or help to limit our ability to maintain a quality life?

2. How can institutions that care for older adults be structured not only to maximize the well-being of the older residents but also to help improve the organizational climate for healthcare providers?

3. Why do you think our friendships are so important for us to maintain a high quality of life throughout the life span?

Source: Nussbaum, J. F., Robinson, J. D., & Grew, D. J. (1985). Communication behavior of the long-term health care employee: Implications for the elderly resident. *Communication Research Reports, 2*, 16–22.

Of course, most of us want to believe in and strive for quality of life, including at work. Often, we are not always clear about what it takes to make this happen. We continue this chapter by considering *flourishing* and positive organizational communication as concepts that offer insight into how people achieve a good quality of life. Then we turn to a discussion of some of the factors that may contribute to QWL.

Flourishing as Communicating Well-Being at Work

The concept of flourishing (*eudaimonia*) was developed by Aristotle (1566/1999) more than 2,000 years ago to describe a human ethic that involves both reason and virtue. While etymologically it consists of the words *eu* (good) and *daimōn* (spirit), it is often translated to mean flourishing, considered the highest good in human action

(Robinson, 1989). The best life, according to Aristotle, is one where flourishing, happiness, or well-being is valued for its own sake and becomes people's central aim, toward which all action is directed (Hursthouse, 1999).

More recently, flourishing is discussed as a concept in positive psychology (e.g., Seligman, 2011) but remains connected to the overall life well-being that is important to happiness (Dunn & Dougherty, 2008). To flourish is "to live within an optimal range of human functioning, one that connotes goodness, generativity, growth, and resilience" (Fredrickson & Losada, 2005, p. 678). Flourishing, or well-being, is affected by a number of quality-of-life factors, including health status, work and life balance, education and skills, social connections, civic engagement and governance, environmental quality, and personal security (Hall, Giovannini, Morrone, & Ranuzzi, 2010).

One example of how flourishing can be enacted by a company is the Grameen Bank Study (see Hashemi, Schuler, & Riley, 1996, for a full description). The Grameen Bank provided credit to poor women living in rural India. The program offered small loans ($75 and $100, for example) to women and allowed them to pay them off with manageable weekly payments. If the women took the money, they had to accept a small group of other women in their village who would help them make decisions. The women succeeded in the program with a return rate of 99%. Grameen Bank "increases women's mobility, their ability to make purchases and major household decisions, their ownership of productive assets, [and] their legal and political awareness and participation in public campaigns and protests" (Hashemi et al., 1996, p. 650). In sum, the program is an example of teamwork and flourishing because it helped to transform women's lives by helping them to feel empowered and work with other members of the community.

Within this chapter we will focus on those characteristics of flourishing that may be within our control as employees and employers in today's organizations and those that impact employee health and wellness. Additionally, we will learn that flourishing can have both positive and negative impacts on employees' QWL. For example, in Theorizing Practice 7.1 we explore the dark side of flourishing.

Theorizing Practice 7.1
The Dark Side of Flourishing

In recent years, scholars have started studying the positive aspects of organizational communication—such as compassion, happiness, and gratitude. Research on happiness describes it as either a pleasant feeling or a feeling that is related to virtuous behavior (Fisher, 2010). Gratitude is defined as an "emotion which occurs after people receive aid which is perceived as costly, valuable, and altruistic" (Wood, Froh, & Geraghty, 2010, p. 890). And finally, compassion has most recently been defined as a three-part process of recognizing, relating, and (re)acting to the experiences of others (Way & Tracy, 2012).

As discussed previously, to flourish is "to live within an optimal range of human functioning, one that connotes goodness, generativity, growth, and resilience" (Fredrickson & Losada, 2005, p. 678). Thus it seems to make sense that employees who display a pleasant disposition, are generally grateful and altruistic, and also compassionate towards their coworkers will flourish in the workplace. But is this always the case? Could there be situations where positive emotions stifle employee wellness?

(continued)

A critical perspective might propose that wellness programs and a strong focus on positivity by employers can also lead to micromanaging of employees' work *and* home lives. Research reveals that workplace wellness programs often place managers in a role like that of physicians, communicating incentives for healthy behaviors (May, 1998, 2015). This medicalization of work (Farrell & Geist-Martin, 2005) can "marginalize, stigmatize, and even silence employees with health concerns" (Ford & Scheinfeld, 2016). It is important to consider who benefits from the promotion of positive emotion and how the expression of manufactured emotion could create feelings of resentment and stress rather than wellness. In other words, in some cases, rather than helping us flourish, the communication of happiness, gratitude, and compassion could be used to control and discipline employees (Simpson, Clegg, & Pitsis, 2014).

A recent National Public Radio (NPR) program suggested that it's possible that there is a coercive element to some wellness programs (Noguchi, 2015). The programs may be designed to offer an incentive to engage in healthy behavior. However, they may become mandatory rather than voluntary, especially when organizations mandate health screenings as part of their programs.

Think about your own experience working in organizations and ask yourself these questions:

1. Have you been offered incentives to engage in healthy behaviors in any organization where you have been employed? Were you motivated to participate? Why or why not? If you did participate, do you believe that you experienced improvements in your health?

2. Have you ever felt pressured to participate in a wellness program at work? What forms of communication (formal or informal) suggested to you that your participation was not voluntary, but instead mandated?

3. If you were to design a wellness program for your place of work that would help you to flourish and be happier at work, what would it offer? In other words, what kinds of activities or programs could you see yourself participating in voluntarily?

Organizational communication scholar Sarah Tracy is a professor who has published research as part of Arizona State's Project for Wellness and Worklife, which is one prong of The Transformation Project. Through research, teaching, and training, The Transformation Project focuses on communicatively transforming lives and relationships at all levels of human interaction. Here is how they describe their mission:

> We are a consortium of faculty, students, and community members who seek to discover and promote creative change processes that encourage healthy communication patterns, collaborative group behavior, and equitable forms of social organization. Our work centers on harnessing the energy and urgency inherent in problematic situations and directing it toward empowering individuals, nurturing relationships, enriching organizations, and cultivating community. (The Transformation Project, n.d.)

They engage in activities with organizations to promote civil dialogue; facilitate peace building; create compassion, resilience, and generosity; and assist employees in constructing work–life balance and "an economy of gratitude."

In both her research and teaching, Tracy is working to facilitate employees' well-being and happiness. In fact, she teaches a course entitled Communication and The Art of Happiness, which focuses on the communication behaviors that are related to constructing happiness and well-being in groups and organizations, including gratitude, forgiveness, social support, appreciation, social networks, and communicative contagion of mood and humor. It would not be surprising at all if each of these behaviors contributed in some way to employees flourishing in their workplaces. In one study in particular, Way and Tracy (2012) found that communicating compassion was critical to staffs' performance of their roles in caring for patients in hospice and increasing their degree of comfort and wellness during their end-of-life experiences. In other research, scholars have explored how compassion is communicated during care at the end of life (Candrian, 2014; Foster 2007). For example, Candrian (2014) reveals how "providers who work every day in the face of life and death speak through voices, interactions, norms, stories, realities, and experiences that are rarely questioned and deeply misunderstood by many of us on the outside" (pp. 7–8). Some of these same behaviors are integral to the art of positive communication (Mirivel, 2014).

In his research and teaching, communication scholar Julien Mirivel focuses on how to improve communication practices in everyday and professional life. In his book, Mirivel (2014) offers a wealth of knowledge about the theory and practice of positive communication, including a Model of Positive Communication. He offers seven communication behaviors that represent the practice of positive communication, including greeting, asking, complimenting, disclosing, encouraging, listening, and inspiring. Mirivel (2014) suggests that positive communication can be learned, is rewarding, and can make a difference. Aristotle's notion of flourishing as a virtue fits well with Mirivel's (2014) view that "practicing positive communication cultivates the development of self, the quality of human relationships, and a healthy society" (p. 160). By practicing positive communication, employers and employees can create the kinds of relationships that allow each other to flourish in the workplace.

HCIA 7.2

Take This Job and Hug It: The Bright Side of Working

Pamela Lutgen-Sandvik

Notwithstanding our tendency to focus on the pitfalls and problems of our work lives, working sometimes brings about extraordinary, positive experiences.

When we feel like others appreciate our efforts, their appreciation can make our endeavors feel worthwhile and can open up our creativity in previously unexplored directions. When a coworker or boss voices a heartfelt thank you, that thank you can contribute to our overall sense of contentment, infuse a positive mood throughout our workday, and sometimes even color our conversations after work. If we receive an important award or promotion, this usually affirms a positive sense of who we are, builds confidence, and even uncovers sources of strength of which we were not previously aware.

Positive emotions are those pleasant feelings we experience, typically in response to commonplace events or circumstances but also to singularly outstanding events at work. Research is very clear that we reap numerous benefits from positive emotion. Feeling good can improve our health and extend our lives. When we feel good, we are usually more altruistic, courteous, and conscientiousness. Positive affect enhances our willingness to help others, opens our minds in new and creative directions, sharpens our intuition, and leads to impressive innovations in our work lives. Positive emotion can protect us from illness and undo some of the

(continued)

damaging aftereffects of physical trauma to our bodies. What is more, these benefits appear to be quite durable, outlasting the transient experiences that elicited the positive feeling.

As an organizational researcher who studies workplace communication, I wondered, *what happens at work that makes people feel good?* To answer this question, I asked people (more than 800 adults working in the U.S.), "What was your best job experience?" Here are some of the things they told me:

- *Being recognized:* "The highest honor I have ever received in my life is when, at the end of a company dinner held in his [her boss's] honor, he and his family all came up to me and each in turn performed 'namaste' [a reverential greeting] with the very low bow, which is done only for a mahatma, a 'great soul.' I felt I did not deserve that honor, but they insisted. I am truly lucky to have worked for such a wonderful, caring person."

- *Relationships:* "The last place I worked was like working with family; even my boss and I were very close." "Currently I work in an organization [where] we truly feel like we are part of one big happy family." "Everyone is like family, we may fight sometimes but we always make up."

- *Being appreciated:* "I was able to make a huge difference in day-to-day operations by creating a suite of tools that were outside of my job description. I did not receive any financial or professional recognition for this project (no raise, no promotion), although supervisors were well aware of this contribution and its effects, but my coworkers at the same level were very appreciative."

- *Having a great boss-mentor:* "I had a boss who took me under his wing when I was 18 and taught me the ethics of work. It's 30 years later, and we still see each other and admire each other just as much if not more than we did then. All because he treated me the way he wanted to be treated. I worked harder for him than anyone else ever. Money never mattered as long as I got to work alongside my mentor!"

- *Working with a team:* "Several times we were very busy with pressing deadlines and our entire team came together to get the job done by our deadline."

- *Receiving social support:* "When I worked for a large utility company, I was going through a divorce. Everyone, including my supervisors, supported me emotionally and with work schedules, so I could go to court and deal with other matters."

People told me about many wonderful work experiences, and two things struck me after analyzing these heartwarming stories. First, nearly all of the wonderful things people experience at work are interpersonal—someone notices my good work, someone appreciates me, someone surprises me with an award, someone donates their sick leave to me when I run out of leave, and so forth. Second, whether we're fully conscious of the belief, we expect work to be safe and secure in more ways than providing our paychecks. We want to feel physically safe certainly, but more than that, we want to feel emotionally and psychologically safe in the organizations in which we're embedded to earn a living.

QUESTIONS TO PONDER

1. Consider your own organizational life and those with whom you work. How can you contribute to others' positive emotional experiences at work?

2. What has someone said to you at work that made your day? How might you pay it forward, so to speak? That is, how might you return the favor to someone else?

3. Whom can you thank, recognize, or appreciate today in a way the person will "hear"?

Source: Lutgen-Sandvik, P., Riforgiate, S., & Fletcher, C. (2011). Work as a source of positive emotional experiences and the discourses informing positive assessment. *Western Journal of Communication, 75,* 2–27.

Organizations across the nation are taking steps to facilitate the quality of life in corporations and nonprofit groups. For example, The Heart and Stroke Foundation of New Brunswick partnered with the College of Psychologists and the New Brunswick Department of Wellness, Culture, and Sport to develop an award "recognizing businesses that are helping to build a stronger New Brunswick through workplace wellness." Here is how the website describes the award:

> One of the keys to shaping the future of health promotion is at the workplace. Workplace wellness is the one time we want you to bring your work home with you. . . . The "Wellness at Heart Award" was established to encourage all organizations, large and small, to stand up and be recognized as an employer who cares about the health of their employees. (Wellness at Heart, 2015)

In addition, there are several other practical examples of how companies are being helped to implement and sustain effective workplace wellness programs and healthy employee behavior.

For example, the Centers for Disease Control (CDC) Healthier Worksite Initiative provides a resource for state- and federally run workplace wellness programs. The Initiative provides web links, resources, and step-by-step toolkits to help organizations implement quality wellness programs (Healthier Worksite Initiative, 2015). Additionally, educational institutions can receive an award designed to recognize schools and school districts that are dedicated to improving employee health and wellness programs. The three awards they grant every year are listed on their website as honoring schools/school systems that: (1) Developed School Employee Wellness Program Plan, (2) Implemented School Employee Wellness Program, and (3) Evaluate and Adapt School Employee Wellness Program (School Employee Wellness Awards Program, n.d.). Some states even have award programs to recognize individual companies for their efforts to implement workplace wellness programs. For example, Wisconsin offers bronze, silver, gold, and platinum awards to companies based on their level of quality and excellence in workplace wellness (Wellness Council, n.d.). One final exemplar of organizational wellness awards includes the Loch Lomond Villa Nursing Home in Canada, which offers a quality of life award to individuals for their service. As the website states, the quality of life award "honors those who go beyond their job description to improve their patients' lives through their desire, creativity, and dedication. It is a celebration of the human spirit" (Loch Lomond Villa, 2013). What these awards collectively demonstrate is that there are precedents for organizations and employees to create opportunities to be recognized and celebrated at work for promoting healthy behavior, wellness, and quality of life. For many of these individuals and organizations, QWL is an ethic that is promoted and rewarded.

Improving the quality of life at work, as well as encouraging and rewarding behaviors that contribute to employees' flourishing, is undoubtedly a significant goal for many organizations. Flourishing at work requires organizations and individuals to prioritize ways that employers and employees communicate.

Flourishing was far from what Allyson was experiencing at her work as a research assistant. Clearly, the quality of Allyson's life deteriorated with the progression in severity of the sexual harassment she experienced. As a married graduate student, with a small child, she never imagined she would face a situation like this, or feel as powerless.

HCIA 7.3

Organizational Ethics and the Quality of Work Life

Steve May

A significant portion of people's lives will be spent at work. Yet, although most people recognize the importance of sleep, exercise, and eating well to improve their overall well-being, we sometimes tend to overlook the conditions at work that may negatively affect our physical and psychological health. For example, researchers have determined that a person's quality of work life is directly related to overall life satisfaction and happiness. That is, the quality of our work experiences will affect how we feel in other areas of our lives. As a result, it is important for us to consider the various ways that the quality of work life impacts employee well-being.

There are a number of factors that affect the quality of work life for employees in today's organizations. Some of these factors include basic elements of work, such as a safe work environment, equitable wages, equal employment opportunities, opportunities for advancement, opportunities to learn and grow, and protection of individual rights. Besides these basic factors, though, a positive work life is also associated with meaningful work, the variety and significance of job responsibilities, autonomy and participation, good relationships with coworkers, social support, and work–life balance, among others.

Not surprisingly, researchers have learned that stress and anxiety negatively affect quality of work life. Workers may experience stress because of ambiguity about their jobs, being overworked, having a lack of control over their work, or feeling like a boss is engaged in unfair or discriminatory behavior. One area, however, that has a significant impact on stress and quality of work life has been nearly completely overlooked—organizational ethics.

In one recent survey by the management consulting firm Deloitte, more than 50% of employees in the United States stated that they would leave their current employer if given an opportunity to do so. Some respondents mentioned their desire for better salary, benefits, and opportunities at work. But, nearly 25% of all respondents said they would leave because of unethical behavior that they have experienced at work. In short, the quality of work life for a quarter of the American workforce has been so negatively affected by ethical issues that they would leave their current company. Why would so many employees want to leave their current jobs because of ethics issues at work? Why wouldn't we know this information?

Over the last 15 years, I have sought to learn the answer to these questions, and others, related to organizational ethics. During that time, I have collected stories about ethical challenges from more than 700 employees in a range of jobs, ranks, and industries. I have learned that employees are willing to leave their current employer, when possible, because they are asked, if not required, to engage in behaviors that are inconsistent with their own values and, in some cases, even to act contrary to company values. For example, nearly every participant in my research study has been able to identify at least one ethical dilemma (and typically more than one) that s/he has faced in the last year at work. Approximately 83% of the employees I have studied state that they can recognize an ethical dilemma when confronted with one. Yet only 36% of them have acted on those same ethical dilemmas. So, a lot of employees in today's organizations see ethical challenges all around them, but very few do anything about them.

Further, when asked, employees report that less than 5% of them have had a face-to-face discussion about ethics with a boss or coworker in the last year. Many of them report doing ethics training modules (usually, computer-based) each year, but very few have had direct conversations about the ethical issues that they face at work. Today's workers are receiving little guidance or support when it comes to handling ethical dilemmas. Not surprisingly, then, nearly all of the employees in my study explained that their own ethical dilemmas have been a source of stress and anxiety. Frequently, employees talk about losing sleep over the issue or feeling a sense of dread going to work, as a result. Ultimately, a significant number of employees choose to quit or change jobs. When they do leave their jobs, though, they rarely, if ever, explain their reasoning—usually in hopes of maintaining good business relationships with prior employers. So, we also underestimate the frequency with which employees confront ethical dilemmas at work because they are discussed infrequently on the job or even when they become a factor related to leaving the company.

Over the course of my research, I have learned that the most challenging ethical dilemmas for employees are what can be described as "right/right" dilemmas, in which they face competing "goods" or values. Of all the ethical dilemmas that I have studied so far, 85% of them are truth vs. loyalty dilemmas, for example. During such dilemmas, employees struggle with the tension between telling the truth or remaining loyal to a coworker, a boss, or even the company. Perhaps the quality of a product or service is not as good as the company claims. Or, maybe an employee sees a coworker stealing or engaging in other inappropriate behavior. Finally, consider that a manager has been told that layoffs are immanent but asked not to tell her/his employees. In each of these cases—and others like them—approximately 75% of employees chose loyalty over telling the truth. We have, in effect, a loyalty problem in today's organizations that is minimizing the quality of work life for workers and, worse, producing a series of business scandals.

In order to strengthen ethics at both the individual and organizational levels, I have focused on "ethical engagement" in hopes that it will improve the quality of work life for employees who face ethical dilemmas. Ethical engagement involves the practice of ethical principles in the search for greater ethical awareness, the deliberate process of ethical decision making, and the aim for ethical behavior in organizations. Based on my research to date, I believe that five practices play a significant role in the creation of ethical engagement in organizations: (1) dialogic communication, (2) transparency, (3) participation, (4) courage, and (5) accountability. I argue that a low level of ethical engagement creates a culture where leaders and employees fear delivering bad news, fail to explain decisions, disregard stakeholders, dismiss ethical dilemmas, and hide mistakes. By contrast, a high level of ethical engagement creates a culture where leaders and employees speak up without fear of retribution, align policies and principles, account for stakeholders, integrate ethical concerns into decision making, and take action to uphold values.

QUESTIONS TO PONDER

1. In your opinion, what are some key ethical challenges for today's organizations and how are they likely to affect the quality of work life for employees?

2. What are some of the most common ethical dilemmas that employees are likely to confront at work?

3. What kinds of interventions are most likely to improve ethical awareness, judgment, and action in organizations?

Source: May, S. K. (Ed.). (2012). *Case studies in organizational communication: Ethical perspectives and practices* (2nd ed.). Thousand Oaks, CA: Sage.

It would get more physical, and then he would say, "Please, can I have a hug before you go?" . . . I realize now, I'm using him to get into a PhD program and he's using me. I think that's a part of what made me not ask him not to touch me again. . . . I didn't realize, so it just kept getting worse. He would hug me every time that I left. Then one time when we were hugging when I left, he kissed me on the neck. . . . I was sick to my stomach the whole time, and I would sit through the whole time of working with him, scared for the time when I had to hug him goodbye. I would set things up, and this is what really helped me in my case too, as far as getting other people involved. . . . I was always setting up with my friends in graduate school to come and get me because he wouldn't hug me if they were there. Then he started catching on and he'd say, "What time do you have to leave?" If I said 1:00, like at 10 minutes to 1:00, he's like, "You have to leave pretty soon, give me a hug." Then it was this cat-and-mouse game trying to get people to be there. He would go to open the door and he'd go, "Just a minute. Let us get our clothes on," or he'd go zip with his pants [here Allyson mimics the professor's action of pretending to zip up the front of his pants] or whatever, and my husband would be like sitting there and my heart would go like this [Allyson drops her hand from her heart to her abdomen], and all I wanted to do was to not get into a confrontation.

Allyson goes on to report that at this point, she continues to suffer through both the harassment and her effort not to tell her husband about the abuse. When an opportunity arose to tell her husband, Allyson was relieved that her husband saw the professor's action as harmless joking and that he seemed "clueless" to what she was experiencing. Allyson's story reveals that the quality of her life both at work and at home suffered greatly from this continuous, debilitating experience of being victimized by a perpetrator of sexual harassment. In the section that follows, we offer what we believe are some of the constraints on employees' quality of life and health that must be addressed if they are to communicate wellness at work, including sexual harassment.

■ Constraints on the Dimensions of Health and Quality of Life

There is a wide range of communicative phenomena within organizations, which constrain, suppress, or eliminate QWL and thus the dimensions of communicating wellness and health. We focus on absenteeism, presenteeism, workplace bullying, sexual harassment, and violence because they are phenomena uniquely influenced through communicative practices and behaviors that can adversely impact employee health. In the following paragraphs, we explain how these phenomena impact QWL and health through communication.

Absenteeism

Absenteeism is a phenomenon that significantly impacts employees' quality of life and their ability to thrive and be well at work. Absenteeism is defined as an "employee's time away from work typically consisting of illness-related scattered absences, short- and long-term disability, and workers' compensation" (Schultz, Chen, & Edington, 2009, p. 366). The causes of absenteeism may include depression, burnout, stress, low morale, disengagement, illness, or injuries, or focus on responsibilities outside the workplace, such as elder care, child care, or job hunting ("The Causes and Costs," 2013). People may feel uninspired at work—it could be the work they are required to do, the people they work with, the lack of effective leadership or supervision, or any number of issues that are not being addressed at work. Whatever the reason, this lack of inspiration or connectedness at work may end up in some way negatively influencing people's health via lowered morale for the individual and for the team of individuals he/she works with that must carry the extra workload, filling in for the absentee.

In past research, two types of absenteeism have been named—planned and unplanned (Belita, Mbindyo, & English, 2013). Planned absenteeism occurs when the employer and the employee are aware ahead of time that the employee will not be at work, such as taking off a few days to go to a family wedding. Unplanned absenteeism happens when the employee is not at work and the employer expects him/her to be there (Belita et al., 2013). For example, if an employee wakes up with a fever and has to call in sick that morning, this would be labeled as an unplanned absence. There are also specific factors that influence the level of employee absenteeism at a company.

First, absenteeism is more common in the public sector and especially in health-care settings, where employees may be facing higher levels of stress and burnout (Belita et al., 2013). Second, organizations with higher numbers of employees have been found to have more absenteeism because typically there is less group cohesiveness and more bureaucratic control in a larger organization. Third, a heavy workload has been found to have a strong relationship with high levels of absenteeism at work because typically a heavier workload equates to more stress and increased health consequences.

Communication plays a role in absenteeism because it may be through communicative practices that employees develop their desire to be absent from work. For example, when employees experience a controlling boss who communicates in a demeaning manner, they may decide to be absent more often from work (Vorell, Carmack, & Scarduzio, 2014). Thus, the specific communicative practices of his or her boss directly influence the employee's choice to be absent from work. However, the communication style of a boss does not account for every case of absenteeism. So many other factors may come into play including communication among employees, customers, or vendors, as well as the organizational culture, demanding work hours, or individual factors such as lack of motivation, chronic illness, or other life stressors that cause people to miss work. In addition to absenteeism, presenteeism describes employees who are at work but not fully present or productive because of various health issues.

Presenteeism

Presenteeism is measured in the research as the "decrease in productivity for the much larger group of employees whose health problems have not necessarily led to absenteeism and the decrease in productivity for the disabled group before and after the absence period" (Schultz et al., 2009, p. 366). Interestingly, many popular press articles discuss presenteeism as a factor that may interfere with productivity at work (e.g., child care or coworker distractions), but typically the research is focused on health-related issues. The most common reasons for presenteeism are psychological (e.g., depression), musculoskeletal (e.g., back pain), and respiratory (e.g., cold) (Schultz et al., 2009).

Presenteeism can occur because the employee has a chronic illness, such as arthritis. In this case, the employee's illness prevents him/her from working to full capacity;

however, it is not severe enough in most cases to warrant being absent from work (Schultz et al., 2009). But even then, the employee may not have a choice but instead must work through the pain of arthritis or other severe forms of chronic illness. Moreover, presenteeism due to an acute or chronic illness is frequently exacerbated by factors such as workplace stress and work–life balance challenges. When employees have a chronic condition, they frequently have to work when they feel impaired, which can impact their job satisfaction and stress (Schultz et al., 2009).

While presenteeism may be an issue for employers, it is equally an important issue for all individuals to consider about their work and workplace. Presenteeism may be a sign that action needs to be taken on the part of employees before it begins to have a detrimental effect on their health. Taking a holistic approach, individuals might reflect on the causes of stress in the work environment as well as the unique work–life and health issues they face. For example, individuals may be stressed by a range of workplace conditions, including vibration, low temperatures, impact stress, and improper equipment ("Overcoming Ergonomic Risks," 2012). Environmental stressors can include lighting, temperature, and noise. Psychological stressors can encompass high workloads, fast-paced jobs, little job variety, micromanagement, and a lack of control. By reflecting on the physical and psychological stressors employees face at work, they may begin to voice to their supervisors the factors that need to be addressed at the individual, dyadic, and organizational levels to help them address their specific presenteeism situation.

Communication plays a role in presenteeism because employees are influenced to be productive or unproductive at work based on their coworkers' and supervisors' responses to their particular health issues. When employees voice their concerns but then feel like they are not listened to and have little control over their jobs and others in the workplace, they can become apathetic, depressed, and disengaged with the people they work with. However, when colleagues communicate social support and compassion, employees are possibly less likely to engage in presenteeism behavior because they feel as if their contributions are valued by others in the organization.

Workplace Bullying

Workplace bullying is defined as "verbal or nonverbal acts, such as name calling, teasing, etc., that are persistent over time, intense, and include a power disparity between the worker involved" (Vorell et al., 2014, p. 307). Workplace bullying is a communicative phenomenon that is created and sustained through discourses and everyday talk between bullies and targets. Bullies feed off discourses that support employee abuse (Lutgen-Sandvik & McDermott, 2008), and bullying occurs as a cyclical process that often keeps bystanders silent due to a fear of retaliation (Lutgen-Sandvik, 2006). Indeed, workplace bullying is talked into existence by employees, and it usually involves many organizational members working collectively to bully one target (Namie & Lutgen-Sandvik, 2010).

Workplace bullying is relatively common within organizations, with about 10% of employees experiencing abuse within a year and 35% of employees experiencing bullying at some point during their careers (Lutgen-Sandvik & Tracy, 2012). Bullying is a traumatic experience that can constrain an employee's QWL, which can cause negative impacts on employee health. For example, workplace bullying can increase problems with employee mental health (such as depression), physical health (such as heart problems), and prevalence of substance abuse (Gruber & Fineran, 2008).

Research using metaphor analysis of experiences of people targeted by bullies found that they described bullying like a battle, water torture, nightmare, and a noxious substance; they named bullies as narcissistic dictators, two-faced actors, and devil workers; and they labeled themselves as vulnerable children, slaves, prisoners, animals, and heartbroken lovers (Tracy, Lutgen-Sandvik, & Alberts, 2006, p. 148). These metaphors paint a vivid picture of the trauma and dis-ease bullying can create for targets on a daily basis and also reveal that people often feel powerless and out of control in bullying situations at work—leading to stress at work and in some cases even burnout.

Even though many targets feel a lack of control, they sometimes attempt to reclaim their QWL through resistance to bullying. Indeed, most targeted workers fight back, but the effectiveness of their resistance strategies varies greatly (Cowan, 2009; Lutgen-Sandvik, 2006). One strategy that seems to help targets is receiving social support from others. Social support makes targeted individuals feel better about their experience and helps to reduce stress. And while social support from family and friends is important, individuals name social support from positive coworkers as most beneficial for improving their QWL (Lutgen-Sandvik & Tracy, 2012). Take a moment to consider Theorizing Practice 7.2, asking yourself questions about how you would survive workplace bullying.

Theorizing Practice 7.2
How to Survive Workplace Bullying

Workplace bullying is a traumatic experience for targets and also witnesses in the workplace. One of the biggest challenges of workplace bullying for targets is deciding how to handle the situation and when to come forward (Lutgen-Sandvik & Tracy, 2012). Research suggests that targets should keep detailed logs of events and also work to tell credible and clear stories about their bullying experiences at work (Tracy, Alberts, & Rivera, 2007).

Credible stories include several key components (see Tracy et al., 2007, p. 14 for a complete list). First, the story must have a clear beginning, middle, and end—making it easier for the manager or human resources (HR) employee to follow the time line of events. Second, the story should have a clearly identified bully and focus on the bully's destructive behavior (Tracy et al., 2007, p. 14). Third, the story should include specific details and anticipate objections from individuals outside of the experience. Fourth, the story is vivid, but it is presented in such a way that the target does not appear overly emotional. Fifth, the story is consistent and includes detailed quotes and times of events. Sixth, and finally, the story should mention the negative effects of bullying on the target's workplace productivity and overall wellness. Indeed, if a manager recognizes that workplace bullying is decreasing employee morale and the productivity of not only the target but other employees as well, they are more likely to try to stop the bad behavior (Tracy et al., 2007). If you experience workplace bullying, be sure to keep these tips in mind for telling a credible story to your managers or HR coworkers.

While this is excellent advice, often it is difficult for victims of bullying to follow these steps to create a believable story they are ready to report to someone in authority, and as a result, all aspects of their health suffers.

(continued)

Imagine you have experienced bullying at work and consider how you might answer the following questions:

1. What impacts do you think bullying would have on your health? Your work?

2. What would keep you from writing down the specifics of your experiences of being bullied?

3. What steps could you take to address those constraints and begin keeping a list?

Now imagine that someone has accused you of being a bully, and consider the following questions:

1. What steps do you take to find out why you are perceived that way?

2. What strategies of self-reflection might you engage in to consider the truth/falsity of the statement?

3. Do you have someone you can talk with whom you believe is willing to be open with you in assessing the accusation?

Sexual Harassment

Sexual harassment is another form of emotional, physical, and/or psychological abuse that can constrain quality of work as we have seen through Allyson's narrative. Sexual harassment is defined as "unwelcome sexual advances, requests for sexual favors, and other verbal or physical harassment of a sexual nature" (EEOC, n.d.). There are two types of sexual harassment—quid pro quo and hostile work environment. Quid pro quo, or literally this for that, is the exchange of sexual favors for workplace rewards. Allyson experienced quid pro quo sexual harassment as she fended off her professor's inappropriate behavioral patterns of hugging, kissing her neck, and following her to her hotel room at a conference. The second form of sexual harassment, hostile work environment, is any behavior that involves unwelcome sexual advances and creates an uncomfortable, intimidating, or aggressive environment at work. For example, in Allyson's story her professor's attempts to get a hug after every meeting had created a hostile work environment.

In Allyson's case, it is clear that she is being harassed not only in these two ways, but in other ways as well. The harassment escalated to forms of sexual abuse that led her to seek out a lawyer and begin a process of suing the university. In her final semester, she had to take a seminar with this professor that was required for her master's program, but was only offered every two years.

So I thought, I'm in a class, it's just a seminar, no big deal. Of course, it was terrible. I would walk to my car with my friends and he would be waiting at my car, and these are other people that are in the class so they would leave because he's the professor. So they would leave and every single class I was begging somebody to walk with me, begging my friends not to leave. . . . And he'd proceed to go and get drunk during class. . . . We sat at a table and he'd take his shoes off and put his foot between my legs at the table, and I'd scoot back from the table and push his foot down. I would move to another end of the table during break, and he'd move and ask the student to move so that he could sit by me. As I said, he would follow me to my car. He'd put notes on my car if I parked in a different parking lot. One time he was drunk and didn't let me shut the

*door to my car, and he grabbed me behind the back of my head and started French kissing me. I
was shoving him away, and I started crying, and I said, "Leave me alone." [And he said] "If I
told somebody that there was some threat, I could kiss my career goodbye," or something like
that, and I thought, "Oh my God."*

The saga of Allyson's sexual harassment, in terms of a hostile working environment and the quid pro quo encounters, prompted her to seek help, through the department chair, the assistant dean, the dean, and the ombudsperson. In every case, she
was not supported. It wasn't until she told the whole story to another professor in the
department that she found the support and strength she needed to move forward to
make a formal complaint. The harassment continued, and she kept notes about every
instance. In the end, she faced intimidation from individuals at high levels of the university and settled out of court. One of her demands in the settlement was for the sexual harassment policy to be rewritten and that sexual harassment complaints be
handled through a central office. This was for Allyson a victory, but at the time of the
interview, she had not gotten into any PhD programs, causing her to question her own
capability of continuing in the profession.

While this narrative shows a common type of sexual harassment—male harasser
and female victim—sexual harassment happens to both men and women, and it can
be same-sex or opposite-sex harassment. Male victims are less likely to come forward
with charges because they are often embarrassed and feel as if they should be able to
handle the situations themselves (Scarduzio & Geist-Martin, 2008, 2010). Race also
impacts sexual harassment because many women of color experience sexual and
racial harassment at the same time (Richardson & Taylor, 2009). One study found
that "at least one participant quit her job rather than fulfill the stereotype of angry
black woman" (Richardson & Taylor, 2009, p. 266). Lastly, sexual harassment is more
common in certain (traditionally female) occupations such as nursing—where
patients may actually sexually harass their nurse (Dougherty, Baiocchi-Wagner, &
McGuire, 2011).

Communication plays a role in sexual harassment because the act of harassing
someone occurs through distinct verbal and nonverbal behavior. Sexual harassment
encompasses verbal comments, touching, gestures, and many more communicative
behaviors. Sexual harassment is also perpetuated in the ways that people discuss it at
work. In other words, if people at work downplay the severity of harassment, it will
likely make the victim feel as if nothing will be accomplished if she/he comes forward
with charges. On the other hand, if victims feel socially supported and specific policies
are in place to give them a step-by-step guide of how to press charges, they may feel
more comfortable coming forward with accounts of their experiences.

Sexual harassment creates various health consequences for employees, too. For
instance, it can lead to increased physical and psychological problems. One study
found that women who have been sexually harassed are more likely to report psychological distress than men who have been sexually harassed (Nielsen & Einarsen,
2012). Yet, despite this difference, it seems that both men and women who have experienced sexual harassment can experience problems with their mental health due to
the trauma of the experience and also increased substance abuse, which leads to a
variety of health consequences (Gruber & Fineran, 2008).

Violence

Workplace violence is a serious problem for organizations and employees that impacts QWL. Yet many workplaces do not have formal organizational policies to help deal with and prevent incidences of violence. Workplace violence is defined as "any behavior initiated by employees that is intended to harm another individual in their organization or the organization itself" (Dillon, 2012, p. 15). Violence can encompass both psychological and physical acts, and it is more often perpetuated by lower status employees than higher status employees (Howard & Wech, 2012). Lower status employees often feel as if they have been wronged by the company in some way and therefore are more likely to react with violence (Howard & Wech, 2012).

There are four primary types of workplace violence (Dillon, 2012). The first type, called criminal violence, occurs when crime happens at work, such as a robbery at gun- or knifepoint or a shooting (Dillon, 2012). The second type, domestic violence, happens when an employee's partner or coworker comes to the workplace to cause harm to the worker, and other workers not involved in the relationship get caught in the crossfire. The third type is customer or client violence, and it manifests when someone from outside the company comes inside and causes the violence—usually a client or customer. The fourth type is also the most common—it involves violence between coworkers.

Workplace violence has a negative impact on the health and QWL for employees. Workplace violence creates physical health problems such as headaches, stomachaches, and pain (Lanctot & Guay, 2014). In terms of psychological consequences on employee health, workplace violence most commonly leads to posttraumatic stress disorder, or PTSD. Additionally, a violent experience at work can create negative changes in mood, recurring memories and flashbacks, hypervigilance or the tendency to be overcautious and anxious, fatigue and sleep disturbances, depression, burnout, and higher levels of stress in some cases (Lanctot & Guay, 2014). In sum, employees who experience workplace violence have a higher chance of "physical and mental health issues including insomnia, high blood pressure, gastrointestinal symptoms, insecurity, crying spells, weight loss, depression, increased use of alcohol, and in severe cases suicide" (Dillon, 2012, p. 16). Employees also demonstrate lower levels of effort at work when they are targets of violence and engage in behaviors that impact their social wellness, such as being more concerned about violence in the community and constantly worrying about their personal safety, behaviors that impact their ability to foster relationships with others (Lanctot & Guay, 2014).

■ Dimensions of Communicating Wellness at Work

Quality of life as a health outcome demands a focus on people's physical, emotional, and social well-being. In fact, quality of life as a health outcome has been extensively studied through the health-related, quality of life (HRQOL) measure, which is a multidimensional, patient-reported outcome that measures the "extent to which a patient's physical, emotional, and social well-being and function are impacted by a condition, disease, or treatment" (Passalacqua, 2014, p. 1149). In fact, the U.S. Centers for Disease Control promote quality of life through the objectives of Healthy People 2020, explicitly acknowledging HRQOL as a "pragmatic and humanistic imperative" (Passalacqua, 2014, p. 1151). While organizations have a history of placing emphasis on employees' physical health, increasingly, organizations today are recognizing the need to focus more on employees' emotional/psychological and social well-being as well. In our view, these three dimensions of well-being (physical, psychological, and social) are essential. So, too, are the less emphasized but essential forms of well-being—spiritual and ecowellness. Life quality is flourishing as work demands consideration and encouragement of all five dimensions of communicating health.

As Chapter 1 of this text indicates, communicating health is a process that demands our attention to all dimensions of health. We must reconsider worksite health promotion in ways that recognize the significant role that communication plays in creating and sustaining a healthy workplace (Geist-Martin & Scarduzio, 2014). The following subsections of this chapter offer a more complete description of each of these five dimensions in communicating workplace wellness and quality of life at work.

Communicating Physical Wellness

Communicating about physical wellness in organizations, one of the most prominent ways that organizations consider the quality of life for employees, places emphasis on employees' biological and bodily health and fitness. Inevitably, people get physically sick and cannot perform their work well; they either take days off or come to work, performing less efficiently and, in the process of communicating with others, exposing them to their illnesses. At the same time, organizations employ individuals who may suffer from a wide range of chronic diseases and illnesses such as obesity, diabetes, heart conditions, arthritis, and other often invisible forms of physical illness. Chronic diseases are responsible for more than 60% of deaths around the world (Malouf, 2011). Some of these chronic diseases are caused or exacerbated by employees' levels of stress, and often individuals do not possess knowledge about effective coping mechanisms (Farrell & Geist-Martin, 2005; Geist-Martin, Horsley, & Farrell, 2003). In some cases, employees turn to chemicals, such as alcohol or cigarettes, to cope with occupational stress (Ray & Miller, 1994). These chronic conditions can also be worsened by environmental stressors such as improper equipment, lighting problems, temperature, and noise levels that may negatively impact employees' physical wellness ("Overcoming Ergonomics Risks," 2012).

Organizations across the nation are offering a wide range of programs to help address these illnesses or conditions that negatively impact their employees' physical health. Wellness programs could include exercise meetings, stress management programs, on-site fitness centers, health screenings (e.g., diabetes, heart disease, cholesterol), and cessation programs for smoking, drugs, alcohol, and other addictive behaviors. Employee Assistance Programs (EAPs) are workplace initiatives that focus on evaluating employees' workplace wellness, designing initiatives to promote healthy behaviors, and offering bonuses for healthy behavior, such as losing weight, lowering cholesterol, and quitting smoking (Geist-Martin & Scarduzio, 2014). While this focus on improving physical health may in turn enhance the other dimensions of workplace well-being, it is essential to realize that only focusing on the naming of illnesses and directing our attention to those illnesses, conditions, and aspects of people's physical functioning becomes a focus on biology and not biography (Zook, 1994). Rather than medicalize individuals at work, we consider wellness at work "in terms of employees' biographies, including ruptures at work and at home, such as an injury, a death, a family crisis, caring for elderly parents, a new assignment, or a new supervisor" (Geist-Martin & Scarduzio, 2014, p. 1479).

Communicating psychological, social, spiritual, and ecowellness at work offers opportunities to engage people in their work as a form of preventive medicine. Even though we offer a definition of each of these dimensions, in reality for employees, these dimensions overlap. For example, in communicating any one of the dimensions of workplace wellness, the other dimensions of wellness may be accomplished as well.

Communicating Psychological Wellness

The fact that employees are working more hours than ever before can lead to higher levels of stress, burnout, and ultimately deteriorating psychological wellness (Scarduzio & Geist-Martin, 2016). Psychological health at work is the "absence of distress or a disability otherwise caused by a behavioral, psychological, or biological dysfunction in an individual" (Farrell & Geist-Martin, 2005, pp. 547–548). Symptoms of psychological illness can include anxiety, lower self-esteem, depression, and boredom, among others. In a recent autoethnography, Jago (2015) discusses her own personal experience with mental illness and anxiety, and how that can lead to extreme levels of medication. Indeed, problems with psychological health can impact employees' relationships both inside and outside of work.

More prevalent today is the home–work conflict that results as individuals attempt to balance the competing roles and demands in their personal and professional lives. The finite resources of time, energy, and attention lead to an "inherent tension between work and home [which] often culminates in stress and psychological burnout" (Omilion-Hodges, 2014, p. 1341). Rather than overemphasizing the objective features of work, the physical health of workers, and the bottom-line aspects of workplace communication (Thornton & Novak, 2010), more organizations are recognizing the need to communicate with employees in ways that recognize and appreciate their lived experiences at work and the issues they face related to work–life balance (Cowan & Hoffman, 2007; Edley, 2001, 2003; Golden, Kirby, & Jorgenson, 2006; Hoffman & Cowan, 2008; Medved & Kirby, 2005). Another way to offer employees ways to manage stress is to focus on what they consider to be meaningful work and thus their subjective well-being. According to Cheney, Zorn, Planalp, and Lair (2008), "The attainment of meaningful work goals contributes to subjective well being" (p. 141). Organizations may offer services (e.g., counseling services, bereavement services, mental health services), programs (e.g., book reading groups, travel excursions, or special interest clubs), or weekly classes (e.g., meditation, yoga, and dance) that contribute to psychological wellness. Not surprisingly, any one of these services, programs, or classes could also contribute to communicating social or spiritual wellness.

Communicating Social Wellness

The relationships among people in the organization and the organizational culture are included in social health. Social wellness is defined as the "quality of an individual's network of professional and personal relationships" (Farrell & Geist-Martin,

2005, p. 549). One way that coworkers can enhance each other's social wellness is through the communication of social support. However, as recent research shows, the burden to provide too much social support can also be difficult for employees (see Wittenberg-Lyles, Washington, Demeris, Oliver, & Shaunfield, 2014). In addition, while communicating compassion may contribute to individuals' social wellness, the phenomenon of *compassion fatigue,* characterized as physical and psychological exhaustion resulting from professional demands (Leon, Altholz, & Dziegielewski, 1999), is prevalent in certain helping professions such as social work, hospice, child care, the clergy, or working with the elderly. Tompkins's (2009) work as a volunteer in a Denver homeless shelter captures well the compassion fatigue experienced by volunteers at the shelter; at the same time, he offers understandings of the evolution of community and hopefulness. In this case, as well as in many others, we see that when this support or compassion is provided in the context of friendship, it may be a way of creating a supportive, caring, and compassionate workplace.

In his book, *The Best Place to Work,* psychologist Ron Friedman (2014) emphasizes the value of friendships at work and what it takes for employees to flourish. Following his advice, organizations could communicate social wellness through holiday parties, spring picnics, monthly social gatherings (during work time), rewards for productivity that include social aspects such as lunches, break rooms that encourage socialization, and interior design elements that encourage open communication.

Once again, it would not be surprising if, through communicating social wellness, an organization's employees might experience spiritual wellness as well.

Communicating Spiritual Wellness

Spiritual health is not necessarily connected to religion. Rather, organizational spirituality is "an ongoing process of growth and nourishment; its quintessence is wisdom, connectedness, integration, independence and a holistic apprehending of organizational life" (Geist & Freiberg, 1992, p. 2). For many, flourishing in the organization is about connecting what they do to what they love. For some that means their work is play; for others that means that they feel passionate about the work they do, no matter what the pay, no matter what the hours. Their spiritual wellness is that their work is something that feeds their soul—they believe in what they are able to accomplish at work. In fact, research reveals that our identification with our place of work has a spiritual dimension when we feel a sense of oneness or a connectedness with our work (Tompkins, 2015). Theorizing Practice 7.3 on the following page asks you to track your passion. Take a moment to check it out.

In their film project, *The Next US,* David Mackenzie and Susan Perkins traveled throughout the country to gain stories of people doing what they love at work (Mackenzie & Perkins, 2009). *The Next US* is a journey into the heart of America to find those who are thriving while supporting high standards of community, sustainability, ecology, and cultural evolution. In Mackenzie's perspective, "Greatness is not about the size of a company, it's about the spirit of innovation in action, a modern version of the 'can do' legacy that built this country and is still alive in creative individuals who refuse to quit" (quoted in Willkinson, 2009). *The Next US* website (http://thenext-us.com/) offers short films of individuals who search for and discover what they are "meant to do," what they are "passionate about," and what they create in their "canvas for artistic

---

Theorizing Practice 7.3
Track Your Passion

Martha Beck (2012a), the author of the book *Finding Your Way in a Wild New World,* offers advice to anyone who is seeking to find his/her source of passion. She believes that finding your passion is a methodological practice involving at least four steps:

1. Notice if you're on a cold, or joyless trail. If so, use step two to go back in your memory.

2. Recall a hot track. Try to remember experiences where you lost track of time—signs that you are connected with your passion.

3. Spot the patterns. Think back to memories that had a similar kind of energy. You remember them well, you enjoy reliving what you were doing in those moments.

4. Warm up your life. When you examine your schedule you will find activities that range from cool to warm. She suggests that each week you cancel one cool thing and do something warm instead. In this way you can explore your passions without leaving the position you are in.

In Beck's view, small steps might lead you to big changes down the road, changes that help you find ways to a good life at work and at home (Beck, 2012b).

Take a moment to write about a recent moment when you lost track of time because you were so passionately engaged in the activity or project, then answer the questions below:

1. What were you doing?

2. What emotions did you feel at that moment?

3. Brainstorm a list of what you believe are "warm" activities in your life.

4. What "cool" activities do you want to replace with "warm" activities?

5. What impact do you believe these replacements will have on your overall health?

---

expression," whether they are driving a truck, building a pizza, or designing automobiles. Jeff Kelley, founder of the Sanuk shoe company, advises people to "follow your passion and don't let anyone tell you it won't work. It's better to try and fail than always wonder if" (quoted in Stanger, 2011, C1). Kelley also suggests that when he hires employees, he will "take passion over education 100 percent of the time" (quoted in Stanger, 2011, C1). He chose the name Sanuk, because it means "fun" in Thai.

Wellness programs that focus on communicating spiritual wellness could offer employees autonomy; spaces for creativity; time to engage in yoga, meditation, or riding a bike during work time; and a library of books and materials that promote wisdom, creativity, and learning. Employers could work to create healthcare plans that offer employees the opportunity to participate in integrative medicine practices such as chiropractic, acupuncture, yoga, meditation, and nutrition. Innovative companies like Google offer free, healthy food options for all of its employees and has created well-stocked microkitchens where employees have access to these healthy options and the capability of creating their own selected food creations. Google has taken spiritual wellness one step further by creating the nonprofit organization, Search Inside Yourself (SIY) Leadership Institute, which uses "practices of mindfulness to train Emotional Intelligence skills, leading to resilience, positive mind-set, and centered leadership" (https://siyli.org). The SIY Leadership Institute's methods have been offered in more than a dozen countries to organizations, teachers, and the general public.

In the same way that the organization is a palate for creativity and promoting spiritual wellness, the organization can be structured and constructed in ways that create an ecological environment that sustains physical, psychological, social, and spiritual wellness.

Communicating Ecowellness

Ecowellness is becoming what many are referring to as the missing factor in holistic wellness models (Reese & Myers, 2012). Ecowellness has been defined as "a way of life oriented toward optimal health and well-being, in which body, mind, and spirit are integrated by the individual to live life more fully within the human and natural community" (Myers, Sweeney, & Witmer, 2000, p. 252). Research from a number of different disciplines is finding that there are health benefits from working and spending part of our day in natural environments or from creating natural environments (Brymer, Cuddihy, & Sharma-Brymer, 2010; Buzzell & Chalquist, 2009; Faber Taylor & Kuo, 2011; Grahn & Stigsdotter, 2003; Guite, Clark, & Ackrill, 2006; Leather, Pyrgas, Beale, & Lawrence, 1998; Reese, Lewis, Myers, Wahesh, & Iversen, 2014; Wilson, Ross, Lafferty, & Jones 2008). This emphasis on ecowellness can be as simple as having access to natural light—for patients, a quicker recovery from surgery (Ulrich, 1984) and for employees, greater alertness and less stress (Friedman, 2014; Leather et al., 1998). Ecowellness may even go as far as encouraging employees to take more time off from work by giving them a "paid, paid" vacation; that is, giving them a stipend of $1,000 or more in addition to their paid vacation (Harvey, 2014).

Ecowellness may also be created through an enticing and comfortable physical environment for employees. One of the most common ways that companies and wellness programs can address ecological health is through a consideration of ergonomics. Ergonomics helps employees maximize the relationship between the tools, the equipment, and the environment they work in and their overall health. In order to prevent workplace injury and stress, employers need to consider the physical layout of the space in which employees work (Galea, 2011). For example, if you work at a desk all day, there are specific behaviors you can engage in to increase your workplace wellness such as providing lumbar support, using the rule of 90 degrees, and ensuring a proper line of sight (Meghji, 2007). The rule of 90 degrees suggests that "while typing, ensure your elbows are supported at 90 degrees, your feet are flat on the floor with your knees at 90-degree angles, and your hips are at right angles to your body" (Meghji, 2007, p. 151). Employers have a responsibility to be cognizant of the temperature, lighting, noise, and equipment that could impair an employee's ability to function effectively at work.

An uncomfortable workplace station could create negative feelings and moods. In contrast, a well-organized and ecologically healthy environment could help employees feel invigorated and decrease stress levels (Galea, 2011). One suggestion is to use some simple practices of feng shui—the Chinese system for harmonizing your surroundings (Galea, 2011). Suggestions as simple as removing clutter from your desk, organizing your work at the end of the day for the next day, and putting plants near your desk could create an entirely more peaceful work environment (Galea, 2011). Advice offered by

Friedman (2014) about the best workplaces suggests that employees need exposure to natural daylight. As a psychologist, his research reveals that "exposure to daylight puts us in a better mood, fights stress by lowering our blood pressure, and reduces the production of melatonin—the hormone that makes us drowsy" (quoted in Harvey, 2015).

The individual health benefits of ecowellness are mounting, and organizations are beginning to make changes to facilitate these benefits. The epitome, and in most cases unattainable, exemplar of ecowellenss is Google, Inc., which strives to create work environments that are playful, open, and interactive, very much like the environment of start-up companies. Environments are created in ways that fit with interests/needs of employees, including "bring the outdoors in," "you can be serious without a suit," and "you don't need to be at your desk to get an answer." Google builds places to think, play, and interact, including terraces that house chickens and herbs, a pub-style lounge, a mother's room, a bowling alley, a music room, meeting pods for small group meetings, and the opportunity and freedom to personalize their workspaces. Google's gold standard of ecowellness is being shared with others through a foundation they have established to offer training and education to other companies that want to follow their lead. But other companies, like Google, that have been on *Fortune* magazine's list of the best companies to work at for multiple years, such as Wegmans, an 84-store grocery chain established in 1916, tend to operate on the same principle of leading with the heart, empowering employees to give their best, let no customer leave unhappy, and to do the right thing regardless of cost (Bock, 2015).

Of course, it is important to recognize that not all companies have the same financial resources as Google and cannot provide their employees with as many wellness opportunities. However, there are still many companies finding ways to address ecowellness. In terms of larger companies, Kaiser Permanente, a nationally known healthcare system, provides healthy recipes and allows users to track personal wellness goals and join group fitness challenges; Microsoft offers flexible work hours, paid membership to full-service gyms, a full health package that includes physician house calls, and free on-campus health screenings and flu shots; and Genetech, a biotechnology pharmaceutical firm, hosts a farmer's market where employees can purchase local produce (Thorpe, 2015). In terms of small companies, Sparks, an exhibit and event planning company based out of Philadelphia, makes sure its employees get to experience summer BBQs, chili cook-offs, and holiday parties, among other festivities that keep the work environment lively; the software company, SolidFire, located in Boulder, Colorado, provides unlimited paid-time-off and weekly on-site massages; minitrampolines, scooters, and flash fitness workouts for a minute or less allow Limeade's employees to participate in a "fun zone" experience (Thorpe, 2015).

In today's workforce, individuals desire a more positive and enriching experience at work. Organizations across the nation are constructing goals and practices that enhance employees' wellness at work. As well, consultants are offering services to help organizations build happy, joyful, and enriching experiences for their employees (see, for example, Schenk Consulting Group, http://www.schenkconsulting.com/about.html).

The popularity and prevalence of this emphasis on flourishing at work is represented well in recently published books. Rich Sheridan, CEO of Menlo Innovations, a small software company in Ann Arbor, Michigan, published a book, *Joy, Inc.: How We Built a Workplace People Love* (Sheridan, 2013), which describes his explicit goal of replacing fear and ambiguity with joy in his organization. In fact, every year thousands of visitors travel to Ann Arbor to tour the organization and learn of its success with a radically different approach to company culture, as well as to attend the class, Deep Dive into Joy. Other recently published books offer insight into designing new, enriching organizational cultures that tap into one or more of the dimensions of wellness, including *Love 2.0* (Fredrickson, 2013), *The Happiness Advantage* (Anchor, 2010), and *The Desire Map* (LaPorte, 2014). Psychologist, Barbara Fredrickson (2013) suggests that love, even more than happiness and optimism, is instrumental to improving our health and lengthening our lives. Psychologist Shawn Anchor (2010) indicates that happiness fuels success; in his view, our brains become more engaged, creative, motivated, energetic, resilient, and productive when we are positive. Danielle LaPorte (2014), an inspirational speaker, poet, former think tank executive, and business strategist, tells us that mapping our personal and professional desires allows us to engage in empowered choices that take into consideration our minds, bodies, and souls.

While the five dimensions of wellness—physical, psychological, social, spiritual, and eco—offer health benefits to individuals at work, constraints on these dimensions can negatively impact the health and quality of life for anyone. Communication is key to creating workplace wellness and flourishing at work. As well, communication plays an important role in addressing the constraints that may minimize the sense of well-being that has been created.

■ Epilogue

While there was no real satisfying solution for Allyson, she did report that at one point, she realized she had the power to do something:

I realized that this was extensive history [of this professor's sexual harassment]. It wasn't just all hearsay. So then I started thinking something major is going to have to happen in order for it to really stop. But you know when I really thought I've got something here and I've got power, it was one of those flashbulb kind of things, Oh, I get it. . . . On the day that I went to the dean's office, I brought everything.

Allyson gave the dean the list of everything she had documented and told him that she hired a lawyer and would be filing a suit against the university. She had communicated with the chair, the ombudsperson, the assistant dean, and the dean. In the end, she was convinced by upper level administration not to file suit because of the impact of the whole ordeal on herself and her family. But in that settlement, the sexual harassment policy was changed and centralized, and the professor's file now had clear documentation of this case. While not a complete victory in Allyson's view, she was relieved to put this experience behind her. We have no idea where she is today. We can only hope that she did go on for her PhD and the career she had always hoped for.

■ Conclusion

Quality of work life (QWL) is essential if organizations are committed to the holistic well-being of their employees. In the past, communicating workplace wellness focused predominantly on the physical well-being of employees, compartmentalizing individuals in terms of the health conditions that organizations assumed these individuals wanted to address. Not surprisingly, employees have resisted the medicalization of their lives and in some cases have resented or resisted the assumptions and incentives offered for them to change their physical health.

Communication is essential to constructing QWL, not only in terms of creating appropriate messages communicated to employees, but also in terms of creating mechanisms for employees to communicate their perceptions of what they need to work toward creating QWL. Employees need to feel empowerment to change organizations, especially in the face of constraints upon QWL such as in the case of Allyson's experience. It is essential that instead of one-shot, short-term programs, the mission, vision, values, and goal statements of any organization integrate and communicate a working-well philosophy. In addition to gaining support from upper management, there needs to be a system in place, clearly communicated to employees, that allows for continuous evaluation and improvement of each of the five dimensions of communicating wellness. If individuals at all levels of the organization recognize that everyone benefits when a focus is placed on all components of health identity (the physical, psychological, social, spiritual, and eco), then flourishing will follow.

Discussion Questions

1. When you think of your best moments at work, moments when you are flourishing, what are you doing?

2. Which dimension of health (physical, psychological, social, spiritual, or ecological) is the most important to your own personal experience of wellness at work?

3. What are some ways that you feel this dimension could be better integrated into your current place of work?

4. How can companies integrate a consideration of work/life issues into wellness programs?

5. What types of incentives do you think are ethical to provide for participation in wellness programs? Which incentives are unethical? What are some other potential incentive ideas for wellness program participation besides the ones currently provided in this chapter?

NOTE

[1] We use the term "we" to refer to both authors, and first names are used to designate a specific author.

REFERENCES

Ahmad, S. (2013). Paradigms of quality of work life. *Journal of Human Values, 19,* 73–82.

Anchor, S. (2010). *The happiness advantage: The seven principles of positive psychology that fuel success and performance at work.* New York, NY: Crown.

Aristotle. (1566/1999). *Nicomachean ethics* (T. H. Irwin, trans.). Introduction. Indianapolis: Hackett.

Beck, M. (2012a). *Finding your way in a wild new world: Reclaim your true nature to create the life you want.* New York, NY: Free Press.

Beck, M. (2012b, January 1). This is the year to track your passion. *Parade.* Retrieved from http://parade.com/121507/marthabeck/track-your-passion/

Belita, A., Mbindyo, P., & English, M. (2013). Absenteeism amongst health workers: Developing a typology to support empiric work in low-income countries and characterizing reported associations. *Human Resources for Health, 11,* 34–44.

Bock, L. (2015). *Work rules: Insights from inside Google that will transform how you live and lead.* London, UK: John Murray.

Brymer, E., Cuddihy, T. F., & Sharma-Brymer, V. (2010). The role of nature-based experiences in the development and maintenance of wellness. *Asia-Pacific Journal of Health, Sport and Physical Education, 1,* 21–28.

Buzzell, L., & Chalquist, C. (2009). Psyche and nature in a circle of healing. In L. Buzzell & C. Chalquist (Eds.), *Ecotherapy: Healing with nature in mind* (pp. 17–21). San Francisco, CA: Sierra Club Books.

Candrian, C. (2014). *Communicating care at the end of life.* New York, NY: Peter Lang.

Cheney, G., Zorn, E. E., Planalp, S., & Lair, D. L. (2008). Meaningful work and person/social well-being: Organizational communication engages the meanings of work. In C. Beck (Ed.), *Communication yearbook 32* (pp. 137–186). New York, NY: Routledge.

Cherns, A. B., & Davis, L. E. (Eds.). (1975). *The quality of working life* (2 vols). New York, NY: Free Press.

Cowan, R. L. (2009). "Rocking the boat" and "continuing to fight": Un/productive justice episodes and the problem of workplace bullying. *Human Communication, 12,* 283–302.

Cowan, R., & Hoffman, M. F. (2007). The flexible organization: How contemporary organizations construct the work/life border. *Qualitative Research Reports in Communication, 8,* 37–44.

Davis, L. E. & Taylor, J. C. (Eds.). (1972). *Design of jobs: Selected readings.* Harmondsworth, UK: Penguin Books.

Dillon, B. L. (2012). Workplace violence: Impact, causes, and prevention. *Work, 42,* 15–20.

Dougherty, D. S., Baiocchi-Wagner, E. A., & McGuire, T. (2011). Managing sexual harassment through enacted stereotypes: An intergroup perspective. *Western Journal of Communication, 75,* 259-281.

Dunn, D. S., & Dougherty, S. B. (2008). *Flourishing:* Mental health as living life well. *Journal of Social and Clinical Psychology, 27,* 314–316.

Edley, P. (2001). Technology, employed mothers, and corporate colonization of the lifeworld: A gendered paradox of work and family balance. *Women and Language, 24,* 28-35.

Edley, P. (2003). Entrepreneurial mothers' balance of work and family: Discursive constructions of time, mother, and identity. In P. M Buzzanell, H. L. Sterk, & L. H. Turner (Eds.), *Gender in applied communication contexts* (pp. 255–273). Thousand Oaks, CA: Sage.

EEOC. (n.d.). Sexual harassment. Retrieved from: http://www.eeoc.gov/laws/types/sexual_harassment.cfm

Faber Taylor, A., & Kuo, F. E. (2011). Could exposure to everyday green spaces help treat ADHD? Evidence from children's play settings. *Applied Psychology: Health and Well-Being, 3,* 281–303.

Farrell, A., & Geist-Martin, P. (2005). Communicating social health: Perceptions of wellness at work. *Management Communication Quarterly, 18,* 543–592.

Fisher, C. D. (2010). Happiness at work. *International Journal of Management Reviews, 12,* 384–412.

Ford, J. L., & Scheinfeld, E. (2016). Exploring the effects of workplace health promotions: A critical examination of a familiar organizational practice. In E. L. Cohen (Ed.), *Communication yearbook 40.* New York, NY: Routledge.

Foster, E. (2007). *Communicating at the end of life: Finding magic in the mundane.* Mahwah, NJ: Erlbaum.

Fredrickson, B. L. (2013). *Love 2.0: Creating happiness and health in moments of connection.* New York, NY: Hudson Street Press.

Fredrickson, B. L., & Losada, M. F. (2005). Positive affect and complex dynamics of human flourishing. *American Psychologist, 60,* 678–686.

Friedman, R. (2014). *The best place to work: The art and science of creating an extraordinary workplace.* New York, NY: Perigee.

Galea, M. (2011, February). Workplace wellness: Putting your health on the agenda. *Alive: Canada's Natural Health and Wellness Magazine, 340,* 55–59.

Geist, P., & Freiberg, K. L. (1992, October). *The saving grace of organizational communication.* Paper presented at the annual convention of the Speech Communication Association, Chicago, IL.

Geist-Martin, P., Horsley, K., & Farrell, A. (2003). Working well: Communicating individual and collective wellness initiatives. In T. L. Thompson, A. M. Dorsey, K. I. Miller, & R. Parrott (Eds.), *Handbook of health communication* (pp. 423–443). Mahwah, NJ: Erlbaum.

Geist-Martin, P., & Scarduzio, J. A. (2014). Working well. In T. Thompson (Ed.), *Encyclopedia of health communication, Volume III* (pp. 1478–1479). Los Angeles, CA: Sage.

Geist-Martin, P., & Scarduzio, J. A. (2011). Working well: Reconsidering health communication at work. In T. L. Thompson, R. Parrott, & J. F. Nussbaum (Eds.), *Handbook of health communication* (2nd ed., pp. 117–131). Mahwah, NJ: Erlbaum.

Golden, A. G., Kirby, E. L., & Jorgenson, J. (2006). Work–life research from both sides now: An integrative perspective for organizational and family communication. In C. S. Beck (Ed.), *Communication yearbook 30* (pp. 143–195). Mahwah, NJ: Erlbaum.

Grahn, P., & Stigsdotter, U. A. (2003). Landscape planning and stress. *Urban Forestry and Urban Greening, 2,* 1–18.

Gruber, J. E, & Fineran, S. (2008). Comparing the impact of bullying and sexual harassment victimization on the mental and physical health of adolescents. *Sex Roles, 59,* 1–13.

Guite, H. E, Clark, C, & Ackrill, G. (2006). The impact of physical and urban environment on mental well-being. *Public Health, 120,* 1117–1126.

Hall, J., Giovannini, E., Morrone, A., & Ranuzzi, G. (2010). A framework to measure the progress of societies. *OECD Statistics Working Papers, 5.* Retrieved from http://www.oecd.org/officialdocuments/publicdisplaydocumentpdf/?cote=std/doc(2010)5&docLanguage=En

Harvey, K. P. (2014, October 27). Unlimited vacation not a fantasy at some jobs. *The San Diego Union Tribune,* pp. A1, A8.

Harvey, K. P. (2015, January 5). Creating the best place to work in 2015. *The San Diego Union Tribune.* Retrieved from http://www.sandiegouniontribune.com/news/2015/jan/05/how-to-create-the-best-workplace/

Hashemi, S. M., Schuler, S. R., & Riley, A. P. (1996). Rural credit programs and women's empowerment in Bangladesh. *World Development, 24,* 635–653.

Healthier Worksite Initiative. (2015). The Center for Disease Control and Prevention healthier worksite initiative. Retrieved from: http://www.cdc.gov/nccdphp/dnpao/hwi/

Hoffman, M. F., & Cowan, R. (2008). The meaning of work/life: A corporate ideology of work/life balance. *Communication Quarterly, 56,* 227–246.

Howard, J. L., & Wech, B. A. (2012). A model of organizational and job environment influences on workplace violence. *Employee Responsibilities and Rights Journal, 24,* 111–127.

Hughes, E. (1971). *The sociological eye.* Chicago, IL: Aldine Atherton.

Hursthouse, R. (1999). *On virtue ethics.* Oxford, UK: Oxford University Press.

Jago, B. (2015). My sleep fest: An autoethnographic short story. *Health Communication, 30,* 96–99.

Lanctot, N., & Guay, S. (2014). The aftermath of workplace violence among healthcare workers: A systematic literature review of the consequences. *Aggression and Violent Behavior, 19,* 492–501.

LaPorte, D. (2014). The desire map: A guide to creating goals with soul. Boulder, CO: Sounds True.

Lawler, E. E. (1982). Strategies for improving the quality of work life. *American Psychologist, 37,* 486–693.

Leather, P., Pyrgas, M., Beal, D., & Lawrence, C. (1998). Windows in the workplace. *Environment and Behavior, 30,* 739–763.

Leon, A. M., Altholz, J. A. S., & Dziegielewski, S. F. (1999). Compassion fatigue: Considerations for working with the elderly. *Journal of Gerontological Social Work, 32,* 43–62.

Loch Lomond Villa. (2013). Accomplishments. Retrieved from: http://www.lochlomondvilla.com/accomplishments.html

Lutgen-Sandvik, P. (2006). Take this job and . . . . Quitting and other forms of resistance to workplace bullying. *Communication Monographs, 73,* 406–433.

Lutgen-Sandvik, P., & McDermott, V. (2008). The constitution of employee-abusive organizations: A communication flows theory. *Communication Theory, 18,* 304–333.

Lutgen-Sandvik, P., Riforgiate, S., & Fletcher, C. (2011). Work as a source of positive emotional experiences and the discourses informing positive assessment. *Western Journal of Communication, 75,* 2–27.

Lutgen-Sandvik, P., & Tracy, S. J. (2012). Answering five key questions about workplace bullying: How communication scholarship provides thought leadership for transforming abuse at work. *Management Communication Quarterly, 26,* 3–47.

Mackenzie, D., & Perkins, S. (Directors). (2009). *The next US.* Ashland, OR: Every Day Wonder Productions. www.thenextus.com

Malouf, M. (2011). Implementing a strategic approach to employee wellness—Globally and locally. *Benefits Quarterly, 27,* 13–16.

May, S. (1998). Health care and the medicalization of work: Policy implications. *Marriner S. Eccles biennial policy yearbook* (pp. 5–36). Salt Lake City, UT: University of Utah.

May, S. K. (Ed.). (2012). *Case studies in organizational communication: Ethical perspectives and practices* (2nd ed.). Thousand Oaks, CA: Sage.

May, S. (2015). Corporate social responsibility and employee health. In T. R. Harrison & E. Williams (Eds.), *Organizations, health, and communication* (in press). New York, NY: Routledge.

Medved, C. E., & Kirby, E. L. (2005). Family CEOs: A feminist analysis of corporate mothering discourses. *Management Communication Quarterly, 18,* 435–478.

Meghji, R. K. (2007, April). Wellness inc., healing companies: Smart companies make health a priority. *Alive: Canada's Natural Health and Wellness Magazine, 294,* 150–151.

Mirivel, J. (2014). *The art of positive communication: Theory and practice.* New York, NY: Peter Lang.

Myers, J. E., Sweeney, T. J., & Witmer, J. M. (2000). The Wheel of Wellness counseling for wellness: A holistic model for treatment planning. *Journal of Counseling & Development, 78,* 251–266.

Namie, G., & Lutgen-Sandvik, P. (2010). Active and passive accomplices: The communal character of workplace bullying. *International Journal of Communication, 4,* 343–373.

Nielsen, M. B., & Einarsen, S. (2012). Prospective relationships between workplace sexual harassment and psychological distress. *Occupational Medicine, 62,* 226–228.

Noguchi, Y. (2015, May 29). When are employee wellness incentives no longer voluntary? *All Things Considered.* National Public Radio. Retrieved from http://www.npr.org/sections/health-shots/2015/05/29/410334545/when-are-employee-wellness-incentives-no-longer-voluntary

Nussbaum, J. F. (2007). Life span communication and quality of life. *Journal of Communication, 57,* 1–7.

Nussbaum, J. F., Robinson, J. D., & Grew, D. J. (1985). Communication behavior of the long-term health care employee; Implications for the elderly resident. *Communication Research Reports, 2,* 16–22.

Omilion-Hodges, L. M. (2014). Stress and burnout: Home-work conflict. In T. Thompson (Ed.), *Encyclopedia of health communication, Volume III* (pp. 1341–1343). Los Angeles, CA: Sage.

Overcoming ergonomics risks improves workplace safety. (2012). *Professional Safety, 57*(9), 16.

Parse, R. R. (2013). Living quality: A humanbecoming phenomenon. *Nursing Science Quarterly, 26,* 111–115.

Passalacqua, S. S. (2014). Quality of life as a health outcome. In T. Thompson (Ed.), *Encyclopedia of health communication, Volume III* (pp. 1149–1151). Los Angeles, CA: Sage.

PetersonLund, R. R. (2014). Living on the edge: A Parse method study. *Nursing Science Quarterly, 27,* 42–50.

Ray, E. B., & Miller, K. I. (1994). Social support, home/work stress, and burnout: Who can help? *Journal of Applied Behavioral Science, 30,* 357–373.

Reese, R. F., Lewis, T. F., Myers, J. E., Wahesh, E., & Iversen, R. (2014). Relationship between nature relatedness and holistic wellness: An exploratory study. *Journal of Humanistic Counseling, 53,* 63–79.

Reese, R. F., & Myers, J. E. (2012). Ecowellness: The missing factor in holistic wellness models. *Journal of Counseling and Development, 90,* 400–406.

Richardson, B. K., & Taylor, J. (2009). Sexual harassment at the intersection of race and gender: A theoretical model of the sexual harassment experiences of women of color. *Western Journal of Communication, 73,* 248–272.

Robinson, D. N. (1989). *Aristotle's psychology.* New York, NY: Columbia University Press.

Scarduzio, J. A., & Geist-Martin, P. (2008). Making sense of fractured identities: Male professors' narratives of sexual harassment. *Communication Monographs, 75,* 353–379.

Scarduzio, J. A., & Geist-Martin, P. (2010). Accounting for victimization: Male professors' ideological positioning in stories of sexual harassment. *Management Communication Quarterly, 24,* 419-445.

Scarduzio, J. A., & Geist-Martin, P. (2016). Workplace wellness campaigns: The four dimensions of a whole person approach. In T. Harrison & E. Williams (Eds.), *Organizations, health, and communication* (pp. 172–186). New York, NY: Routledge.

School Employee Wellness Awards Program. (n.d.). The director of health promotion and education (DHPE): School health and employee wellness. Retrieved from: http://www.dhpe.org/?Programs_SEWAward

Schultz, A. B., Chen, C.-Y., & Edington, D. W. (2009). The cost and impact of health conditions on presenteeism to employers: A review of the literature. *Pharmacoeconomics, 27,* 365–378.

Seligman, M. E. P. (2011). *Flourish: A visionary new understanding of happiness and well-being.* New York, NY: Free Press.

Sheridan, R. (2013). *Joy, Inc.: How we built a workplace people love.* New York, NY: Penguin.

Simpson, A. V., Clegg, S., & Pitsis, T. (2014). "I used to care but things have changed": A genealogy of compassion in organizational theory. *Journal of Management Inquiry, 23,* 347–359.

Stanger, S. (2011, September 13). Innovator put best foot forward: Founder of shoe company blended equal parts function and fun. *San Diego Union-Tribune,* pp. C1, C3.

Suttle, J. L. (1977). Improving life at work: Problem and prospects. In H. R. Hackman & J. L. Suttle (Eds.), *Improving life at work: Behavioural science approaches to organizational change* (pp. 1–29). Santa Barbara, CA: Goodyear.

The causes and costs of absenteeism in the workplace. (2013, July 10). *Forbes.* Retrieved from http://www.forbes.com/sites/investopedia/2013/07/10/the-causes-and-costs-of-absenteeism-in-the-workplace/#223568ef3bd3

The Transformation Project. (n.d.). Retrieved from: https://humancommunication.clas.asu.edu/research-initiatives/transformation-project

Thornton, L. A., & Novak, D. R. (2010). Storying the temporal nature of emotion work among volunteers: Bearing witness to the lived traumas of others. *Health Communication, 25,* 437–448.

Thorpe, A. (2015, October 27). *The 44 healthiest companies to work for in America.* Retrieved from: http://greatist.com/health/healthiest-companies

Tompkins, P. K. (2009). *Who is my neighbor? Communicating and organizing to end homelessness.* Boulder, CO: Paradigm.

Tompkins, P. K. (2015). *Managing risk and complexity through open communication and teamwork.* West Lafayette, IN: Purdue University Press.

Tracy, S. J., Alberts, J. A., & Rivera, K. D. (2007). *How to bust the office bully: Eight tactics for explaining workplace abuse to decision-makers.* Distributed to workplace bullying websites and media outlets internationally. Retrieved from: http://humancommunication.clas.asu.edu/aboutus/wellnesspublications.shmtl

Tracy, S. J., Lutgen-Sandvik, P., & Alberts, J. K. (2006). Nightmares, demons, and slaves: Exploring the painful metaphors of workplace bullying. *Management Communication Quarterly, 20,* 148–185.

Ulrich, R. S. (1984). View from a window may influence recovery from surgery. *Science, 224,* 420–421.

U.S. Bureau of Labor Statistics. (2014, June 18). *American time use survey—2013 results.* Washington, DC: U.S. Department of Labor.

Vorell, M., Carmack, H., & Scarduzio, J. A. (2014). *Surviving work: Toxic workplace communication.* Dubuque, IA: Kendall Hunt.

Way, D., & Tracy, S. J. (2012). Conceptualizing compassion as recognizing, relating and (re)acting: An ethnographic study of compassionate communication at hospice. *Communication Monographs, 79,* 292–315.

Wellness Council. (n.d.). Well workplace awards. Retrieved from: https://www.wellnesscouncilwi.org/Pages/13/Well_Workplace_Awards.aspx

Wellness at heart. (2015). Wellness at heart awards. Retrieved from: http://www.heartandstroke.nb.ca/site/c.kpIPKZOyFkG/b.4183795/k.73A5/Workplace_Wellness_NB.htm

Wild, R. (1975). *Work organization: A study of manual work and mass production.* New York, NY: Wiley.

Willkinson, W. (2009, July 13). Ashlanders look for "everyday genius." *Ashland Daily Tidings.* http://www.dailytidings.com/apps/pbcs.dll/article?AID=/20090713/LIFE/907130304/-1/LIFE

Wilson, N. M., Ross, M. K., Lafferty, K., & Jones, R. (2008). A review of ecotherapy as an adjunct form of treatment for those who use mental health services. *Journal of Public Mental Health, 7,* 23–35.

Wittenberg-Lyles, E., Washington, K., Demeris, G., Oliver, D. P., & Shaunfield, S. (2014). Understanding social support burden among family caregivers. *Health Communication, 29,* 901–910.

Wood, A. M., Froh, J. J., & Geraghty, A. W. (2010). Gratitude and well-being: A review and theoretical integration. *Clinical Psychology Review, 30,* 890–905.

Zook, E. G. (1994). Embodied health and constitutive communication: Toward an authentic conceptualization of health communication. In S. A. Deetz (Ed.), *Communication yearbook 17* (pp. 244–377). Thousand Oaks, CA: Sage.

8

Communicating Stigma and Acceptance

Christine S. Davis & Margaret M. Quinlan

I give Maggie a quick hug as she gets in my Miata. "Sorry I'm late," I say with a grimace. I'm always late.

"It's not a problem at all," she says cheerfully. Maggie is always cheerful. I pull out of her driveway as she adjusts her seat belt over her growing belly.

"Look at you!" I exclaim. "You're finally starting to show! How far along are you?"

"Five months," she says.

We chat as I drive out of her neighborhood. I motion toward the lake peeking behind the houses. "I am so jealous! If I lived here, I'd be on the water every single day!" I say.

She laughs. "It's great! I saw your kayaking picture on Facebook last week. It looked like you were having a great time."

I grimace. "I was tagged. I wouldn't have posted that picture of me. I loved kayaking but I swear I looked eight months pregnant in that picture! Where did that stomach come from? I must have been slouching down in the kayak. See? I'm not that fat!" I point to my stomach as I suck it in.

She nods her head. "You looked great in that picture!! Strong!"

I smile at her. I don't believe her, but I'm not in the mood to prolong the fat talk right now. I change the subject. "You look great. Any morning sickness?"

"No, I feel really good," she says. "But, speaking of fat and pregnancy, it's really interesting that people have been asking me how much weight I've gained. I'm really afraid about gaining too much weight. I saw an article in The New York Times *this morning that talked about the dangers of being overweight and pregnant* [Brody, 2014]. *And I've read other research that says that there's a relationship between obesity and birth defects"* [Oddy, DeKlerk, Miller, Payne, & Bower, 2009].

I sigh. "First of all, you are nowhere, not at all, in danger of being overweight. Listen to us and our fat talk! Secondly, I read that article also and saw that it admitted that most mothers who are overweight have healthy babies. Even with an increased risk from excess weight to the mother and the baby, the rhetoric about it is overblown. For example, I've read that the increased risk for neural tube defects in babies of pregnant women who are fat is about 1%. That means 99% of pregnant women with excess weight won't have babies with that defect [Vireday, 2011]. *Pregnant women of all sizes need support and information, not rhetorical scare tactics. This is really part of the stigma the medical profession has against obesity and fat. Articles like that are dangerous because weight-loss diets during pregnancy are harmful for the fetus."*

"This is a timely conversation, isn't it?" Maggie asks. "Since we're on our way to meet your sister and talk about her experience with weight."

"It really is," I agree. "Maybe that's why we brought it up, but conversations about extra pounds are ones women have all the time."

"Fat talk often leads to us assuring each other that we aren't fat," Maggie mentions.

I laugh. "Just like we did!"

■ Fat Talk

Fat talk—negative remarks about our body shapes—is a pervasive social norm that both contributes to and results from body dissatisfaction and lower self-esteem. Fat talk also reinforces the thin body ideal, and the resulting dissatisfaction with our bodies can lead to disordered eating (Salk & Engeln-Maddox, 2011). We engage in fat talk interpersonally, intrapersonally (self-talk), and socially.

I (Cris) can personally relate to body dissatisfaction. I've struggled with weight issues my whole life. I've been smaller than I am now, and I've been heavier. I've been on one diet or another most of my life. When I was growing up, my mom told me constantly I was fat, which I wasn't. She had body issues herself. She had me on diet pills when I was eight years old. I was a size 6 when I was in my 20s, but when I was in my mid-30s, I was heavy enough to be categorized as obese. In recent years, I've maintained a mostly normal size and even got in good enough shape to run a half marathon a few years ago. But in order to keep my size close to normal, I have to exercise extensively and be obsessive about my eating. Sometimes I think I have eating control issues. Sometimes I wonder why, at my age, I bother. I frankly struggle with being a feminist and a scholar who is supportive of the field of fat studies and still being preoccupied about my body size.

The cultural rhetoric surrounding body size, fat, and obesity exacerbates that struggle. On the one hand, excess weight is related to all sorts of health problems. Obesity or excess weight is statistically associated with heart disease (Ghandehari, Le, Kamal-Bahl, Bassin, & Wong, 2009), cancer (Heron et al., 2009; Leitzmann et al., 2009), type II diabetes (Nguyen, Magno, Lane, Hinojosa, & Lane, 2008), esophageal reflux (Chung et al., 2008), diverticulitis and diverticular bleeding (Strate, Liu, Aldoori, Syngal, & Giovannucci, 2009), hypertension (Nguyen, Magno, Lane, Hinojosa, & Lane, 2008), kidney stones (Asplin, 2009), poor wound healing (Wilson & Clark, 2003), periodontal disease (Ylostalo, Suominen-Taipale, Reunanen, & Knuuttila, 2008), and other chronic diseases (Field et al., 2001). However, research does not confirm that people's obesity is the *cause* of these disorders.

One explanation for the connection between weight and poor health is that, unrelated to any health implications of excess weight, people who are fat avoid or delay going to the doctor when they need healthcare or even routine screenings because of their past bad experiences and expectations of discrimination by healthcare providers, and that may result in worse health outcomes (Creel, 2010; Fontaine, Heo, & Allison, 2001). People who are fat frequently report having difficulty finding doctors who will provide good healthcare without imparting value judgments on their size (Lupton, 2013), and this can prevent a patient who is fat from receiving decent healthcare (Puhl & Brownell, 2006). Researchers argue that doctors blame the patient for his/her excess weight and admit perceiving that patients who are fat are dishonest, hostile, unhygienic, indulgent, lacking in willpower, lazy, possessing emotional problems and unresolved anger, unsuccessful, worthless, bad, ugly, and awkward (Brownell, 2005; Epstein & Ogden, 2005; Fabricatore, Wadden, & Foster, 2005). Frequently, physicians ignore other physical symptoms and only focus on pushing patients who are fat to lose weight, as if all a patient's problems are related to his/her weight. Healthcare providers also blame people who are fat, if they are unable to lose weight, as if the inability to lose weight represents the patient doing something wrong (Thomas & Wilkerson, 2005).

HCIA 8.1

Loose-ing Weight

Bonnie Creel

One year, early in my teaching career, I got a student evaluation that has stuck with me. There was a question on the form that asked, "What could this instructor do to improve his or her teaching?" And this student wrote: "Loose weight." Of course, it was a misspelling. But really, isn't that the problem? "Loose" weight?

Out of my own personal experience as well as revelations over many years from other women affected by overweight and obesity, I became concerned that the healthcare needs of women who struggle with weight issues are not being adequately met. I wondered if avoidance or postponement of medical care might well contribute to the poor health outcomes often reported for overweight patients. The central research questions of my dissertation were: How is an overweight/obese (OW/O) woman's weight implicated in her self-identity? How does she make sense of the experience of being overweight? What role does her identity and her understanding of her weight play in her health-seeking behaviors and interactions with physicians and other health professionals?

I employed multiple methods of analysis and multiple genres of representation of the data I collected, an approach described by Laura Ellingson as "crystallization." I used autoethnography, in-depth interviews, narrative analysis, and grounded theory. I learned that the pernicious effects of social bias against OW/O people do, indeed, play a role in personal identity and in health-seeking behaviors of affected patients and that the attitudes communicated by many medical practitioners contribute to a vicious cycle of reinforcing negative identity and avoidance/postponement of healthcare.

As a final chapter to my dissertation, I developed a performance script capturing the voices of several of my informants. The excerpt below is an example of stories that were represented in the script.

So I went to the appointment and, of course, first the nurse comes in and takes your history and does your blood pressure and all of that sort of preliminary thing. And when

(continued)

she was taking my blood pressure she came up with a higher reading than was typical for me. And I was kind of surprised by that, so she took it another time or two, and then the whole time she was acting very frustrated, kind of "hhhh," making little sounds that made me think that she was really kind of distressed. And she left the room for a few minutes, and then she came back and she said, "Well, we're just going to have to go with the reading that we've got because I can't find the blood pressure cuff that we have—we don't use it very often so I'm not sure where it is, but it's especially designed for large women. So I think maybe the reading is because this blood pressure cuff that we're using for you is really too small, and maybe it's because you're nervous since you haven't seen a doctor in some time."

And I remember thinking that I felt like a freak. I was heavy, there's no question about that. But I had never felt freakishly heavy. But I did at that moment. I was so big that a normal blood pressure cuff would not fit around my arm!

So then the doctor came into the room and she was performing the exam. And the whole time she was performing it she was kind of—I don't know how to describe it. She wasn't rude. But there came a point during the exam where I had the sense from the kind of sounds she was making—the kind of sounds that people make when they're doing something physical that requires a lot of effort, so they have these little kind of "unhhh, unhhh," little exhaled breath that you do when you're exerting a lot of effort on something? And then she said, "I'm afraid I'm not going to be able to do a very good exam on you because it's very difficult to palpate fat."

And I remember, when she said that, that I felt so terribly sorry that I was putting her through that. I realized that touching me was disgusting to her. I felt like I was an unpleasant object that she had to deal with. And that she was doing her best to be nice about it, but really, deep down, she was just terribly disgusted to have to be touching me. And I don't really know that it was anything that she did. I couldn't even say that I think now that she necessarily was. But that's how I felt at the time. I felt like she was disgusted with me. Or not disgusted with me, but disgusted with having to touch me.

So, the next time I had a well-woman check was five years later in the summer of 2000. My general practitioner's nurse practitioner did my well-woman check, and she was very good. But it came back with a suspicious result on my Pap smear. So I had to take some medication for several months and then go back for a follow-up Pap smear, and this time I had to have another doctor because of insurance carrier issues. And I really couldn't stand him. And I had a very definite impression when I left his office that he was very worried. There were things that he said and things that he didn't say that made it sound like he was very deeply concerned.

So for several weeks while I waited for the results of that Pap smear—that follow-up Pap smear—I remember thinking, "It's my own fault. I didn't get a well-woman check for so many years, and if this Pap smear comes back bad it's my own fault, because I didn't go to the doctor." But then I thought, "It's so hard to go to the doctor. Because you feel like you're so disgusting."

But the Pap smear came back OK.

QUESTIONS TO PONDER

1. What do you think is the basis of the narrator's perception of her doctor's response to her? Is it because of the way the doctor communicated with her? Or is it more related to her self-identity as an overweight/obese woman? Based on your answer, discuss what you might advise clinicians to consider when interacting with patients affected by overweight or obesity.

2. Do you think that men affected by overweight/obesity have similar stories to tell about their interactions with healthcare providers?

3. All other factors being equal (e.g., access to healthcare, financial ability to pay for healthcare, etc.), do you think that avoiding or postponing medical screenings and other preventive care is more likely to be a problem for people affected by overweight/obesity than it is for people of normal weight? What other physical conditions do you think might create the same sort of health-seeking or health-avoiding behaviors?

Source: Creel, B. (2010). *Suffering, hoping, resisting and accepting: Perceptions of overweight women about personal identity and medical care.* Unpublished dissertation: Texas A & M University, College Station, TX.

We're not disputing that obesity is a pervasive phenomenon; almost seven out of ten adults in the U.S. over age 20 weigh more than the medical guidelines suggest they should, and almost half of them would be termed obese ("Prevalence of Overweight," 2006). However, research suggests that obesity is not increasing to the extent many people claim. Body Mass Index (BMI), determined by the Centers for Disease Control and Prevention (2009), is calculated based on a person's weight and height and indicates whether someone is overweight, obese, or morbidly obese. When authorities generate claims around obesity rates increasing, they do not acknowledge the fact that a great deal of this increase is due to the BMI categories arbitrarily changing, resulting in many more people being labeled as overweight, obese, or morbidly obese, without any changes at all to their body weight (Lupton, 2013).

Further, in perpetuating the claims that fatness places people at risk for various health and medical conditions, medical researchers are ignoring, misrepresenting, and misinterpreting the myriad of research that *disputes* that the weight is the cause of the medical problems and suggests that, instead, the medical problems might be the *cause* of the weight gain, or other phenomena may contribute to both excess weight and related health problems. They are confusing association with causality.

In this chapter, we discuss issues of fat talk, hegemony and medicalization of fat, social construction of body size, stigma, and the biomedical model, related to obesity primarily, but also to the body generally. We introduce you to the concept of fat studies and suggest a new way to view and interact with people who have more body fat than the "norm" or who live with other stigmatizing conditions.

■ Hegemony and Medicalization

I take the upcoming exit off the interstate. "Well, my sister certainly lives the fat body experience, so it will be interesting to see what she has to say about it."

"So, fill me in with a little background information," Maggie says.

"Kelli is my younger sister. She's in her early 50s. She's been overweight her entire life, ever since she was a very small child. I can remember her being two years old and being picked on by other kids about her weight. When she was in her 20s and 30s, she was large but very strong. If you wanted something heavy lifted or moved, you'd ask Kelli. In the past 20 years she's had quite a few serious and chronic health problems that have made her pretty much obese. And now she's battling breast cancer too."

"I can't wait to meet her," says Maggie as I pull my Miata into the parking space at the Village Tavern.

I'm relieved that Kelli smiles as we walk in. She's already at the table and I know from her text messages she got there early and has been waiting for us for almost an hour.

"There you are!" Kelli says as we walk up and take our seats. I introduce her to Maggie.

"I ordered some food," Kelli says. "I hope you don't mind. My blood sugar was getting low. Diabetes," she explains to Maggie. "Help yourself." She passes a bowl of homemade potato chips to our side of the table.

Maggie helps herself to a chip as I set up the tape recorder and open my menu.

The waitress stops by our table.

"Water, no lemon," I order. "And an order of sweet potato fries as well," I add.

We turn to Kelli to begin our questions.

"How are you doing?" I ask.

Kelli shakes her head. "Fair." I'm going in for my pre-op on Wednesday." She turns to Maggie to explain. "I'm having a port put in to start chemotherapy."

"I'm so sorry to hear you're going through all that," Maggie says.

"Tell her about all your health issues," I prod.

Kelli frowns. "Let's see if I can remember them all." She recites. "Type 2 diabetes, osteoarthritis in both hips, degenerative disc disease, patellofemoral arthritis in both my knee caps, chronic venous insufficiency in both my legs, stasis dermatitis, pyoderma gangrenosum."

"An autoimmune skin disorder," I interrupt to explain to Maggie.

Kelli nods and continues. "Obstructive sleep apnea, psoriasis, rosacea, and a couple other skin disorders, whose names I can't remember and are a mile long. I also have a history of a rare reoccurring viral meningitis, which came back several times over the years, resulting in a total of nine spinal taps."

"And now breast cancer," I add.

"Wow." says Maggie. "Do you think of your weight as a health issue as well?"

"From my experience," says Kelli, "it is all related. My weight is related to my health conditions—going back as far as I can remember." She pauses. "Being overweight is a result of other issues, not a cause of them."

"Are you open to talking more about that?" I ask. "Give us the history?"

Kelli nods. "When I was in my early, mid-twenties, about 25 years ago, doctors discovered I have very severe obstructive sleep apnea. I was born with it and it was a birth defect. They told me then that my weight was probably a result of that. All of my health issues since have been a result of all those years of lack of sleep—causing all kinds of issues. When they did the sleep study, I stopped breathing over 500 times in six hours. As far back as I can remember, I had a long history of having severe out-of-body experiences during the night—probably from dying in my sleep over and over again. When the sleep apnea was discovered, I stopped having these experiences."

Kelli's numerous health issues are not uncommon. There is a plethora of research about the relationship between excess weight and sleep issues (e.g., sleep apnea) (Carter & Watenpaugh, 2008; Hirshkowitz, 2008). However, while some medical researchers claim that obesity causes sleep apnea, others argue that studies like these conflate findings of association with causation. In Kelli's case, they may be related, but it is possible the sleep problems are causing the obesity rather than the other way around, as Kelli said was true for her. We also note that Maggie has sleep apnea as well, and she is at the low end of the BMI standards for her height and age.

"Let's talk about your weight," I say to Kelli. "When you think of your weight, what do you think?"

Kelli frowns. "I think I don't like it. I am not happy with it. And I need to keep trying harder to fix it."

"What do you mean by fix it?" Maggie asks.

"Lose it, get healthy," Kelli says.

"Do you think of yourself as overweight or fat?" I ask, searching for the terminology she uses to describe herself.

"Yes," Kelli says. "I think of myself as very overweight. Obese."

"Is that a term you use?" I ask.

"It's a term other people use," she answers. "It's a term I really do not like." She sits for a minute. "It is what it is. I don't like it because it is close to the truth."

"Is there a word you would prefer?" Maggie asks.

"No, not really." Kelli says. "I would prefer to not talk about it." She pauses. "It's not something you dive in and generally advertise."

There is an area of academic scholarship called "fat studies," similar to cultural studies and gender studies in that they all are populated by critical scholars who examine *hegemonic* (i.e., influence or authority exerted by a dominant group) language and discourse within these areas of study (Rothblum & Solovay, 2009). Fat studies scholars analyze how society, supported by the biomedical model of medicine, communicates in hegemonic ways to marginalize people with differently sized bodies. Critical fat studies scholars have a lot in common with activists and critical scholars in LGBTQ (lesbian, gay, bisexual, transgender, questioning, queer), cultural, disability, aging, and gender studies in that they all are concerned with the way hegemonic (hidden) norms constrain, control, and marginalize bodies that are different from the dominant view.

The story of difference, stigma, discrimination, and marginalization is one we can relate to, as it touches all of us (Green, Davis, Karshmer, Marsh, & Straight, 2005). As we and our loved ones age, our bodies are less under our control, and we are all a few short steps from being older, larger, or less-abled than we would like to be. Other than fat bodies, many disabling conditions have their own specific social difficulties. Speech and hearing difficulties make interpersonal communication challenging, piling an additional awkwardness onto an already stigmatizing situation. Hearing impairments are socially isolating. Wheelchair users have the danger of being embarrassed by committing social transgressions such as tipping over, bumping into people, or knocking things over (Green et al., 2005). Many people with different appearing bodies (and behaviors)—people with mental illness or mental disorders, people with physical disabilities, people who are older, as well as people with larger bodies—often find themselves in social situations in which they are treated as being not quite human. This results in "nonperson" treatment, with people frequently either completely ignoring the person with a disability or larger body, mistreating him/her, or treating the person with civil inattention (a glance followed by the immediate withdrawal of visual attention) (Cahill & Eggleston, 1995; Goffman, 1963; Marks, 1999; Susman, 1994). Barnes (1996) suggests that the ideals of our Western society worship the perfect body, and a body that is less than perfect—older, larger, impaired in some way—tends to be stigmatized.

In addition, there is a relationship between thin bodies and gender, ethnicity, and socioeconomic status. Fat studies scholars claim that an insistence that all bodies must be thin ignores genetic differences and therefore marginalizes minorities such as females, nonwhites, and individuals with lower socioeconomic status who are more likely to be larger (Donaghue, 2014; Farrell, 2011).

Critical fat scholars pay a significant attention to language usage and tend to avoid using the terms *overweight* or *obese,* because these terms have diagnostic and medicalizing implications. Labeling people with larger bodies "obese" has connotations that a larger body size is always a medical issue, and that's simply not true. These scholars often prefer to use the term *fat,* because that is more of a descriptive term. Although labeling someone else as "fat" has other cultural meanings, fat studies scholars reclaim that word and change the denotation to one that is less negative (LeBesco, 2004; Lupton, 2013). To *medicalize* means to turn something natural into a medical condition to be treated and fixed, like the way pregnancy, menopause, and aging are now medical conditions rather than just normal parts of the life span. The terms *overweight* and *underweight* imply there is a normal weight to be desired, and *obesity* implies abnormality, pathology, or a medical problem. Ironically, the term *obesity* comes from a Latin word that implies that larger people always consume more than thinner people, and that's not necessarily true either. The words we use to describe others and ourselves have real implications (Lupton, 2013; Wann, 2009), as we further discuss in the next section.

■ Social Construction of Body Size

"Do you ever talk about your weight to people?" Maggie asks Kelli.

Kelli frowns. "Yes, I do have private conversations about my weight, with close friends. I don't discuss it with people I'm not close to."

"What do you talk about, when you talk about your weight?" I ask.

"I generally talk to people who have lost weight or can give me advice. Pointers or tips to lose weight," Kelli says.

"Oh, it's always about losing it?" I ask.

"Oh, yes," Kelli says. "For instance, I've talked to people who have had gastric bypass surgery, about their adventures with that. And my best friend CJ is a professional bodybuilder and a fitness fanatic. I've talked to him about what to do in terms of exercising, fitness."

"Do you have friends who are fat?" I ask.

Kelli nods.

"It's interesting," Maggie says. "Women like to sit around and talk about weight. It becomes a bonding thing, to one up each other, to ask each other 'do I look fat in this,' in dressing rooms."

"I have not experienced that," Kelli says. "Maybe I don't because I am obese and it isn't a conversation that comes up with me. Maybe that's something that thin women discuss."

Some health communication scholars suggest that obesity is a social construction (Campo & Mastin, 2007; Kim & Willis, 2007). When we interact socially with each other, through communication, we share our experiences and knowledge (Laing, Phillipson, & Lee, 1966). Our identities—how we see ourselves and how we think others see us—are constructed through those interactions with others. Cultural communication, especially via media outlets—TV shows, movies, books, magazines, the Internet, and so on—also affects our identity. All of us live within our socially constructed meanings (Davis, 2013). We all communicate with others to construct our meanings of health, illness, ability, obesity, and normal weight. Your body might be a certain size. That is a fixed reality. What that size *means* is a product of communication. The fact that people look down on others because of the size of their bodies is a social construction. For example, the BMI cutoffs that are used to classify people by the labels of overweight, obese, or morbidly obese were arbitrarily determined and based on population parameters rather than on any health conditions related to weight. In addition, BMI is an inaccurate guide for health, as it does not distinguish between fat and muscle, body frame, age, gender, good health, or ill health (Lupton, 2013). Several medical researchers (Campos, 2011; Gaesser, 2002; Oliver, 2006) claim that obesity is *not* increasing to the extent many people contend; that there is *no* evidence that obesity or fat shortens life spans or increases health risks; that there is some evidence that excess weight has some protective health benefits (doctors call this the "obesity paradox"); that research shows that attempts to lose weight, which result in weight cycling, are themselves detrimental to health and, ironically, frequently result in ultimately higher weight; and that fatness is often a *symptom* of health problems rather than their cause (Lupton, 2013).

The social construction of fat does not take into account how people's weight is affecting their health; it is the *meaning* attached to the body size that creates a problematic situation, often through social stigma. The meaning is socially constructed, but it still has effects on people, both physically and socially (Freedman & Combs, 1996). An example of the physical effects of stigma is that while women in all cultures go through a period in their lives that we call menopause, women in cultures other than ours do not experience distress from the phenomenon. And American women today experience less menopausal distress than did our mothers and grandmothers, because the ability to bear children is not the identity-ending experience it was to them (Kleinman, 1988). In an example of the social effects of stigma, people with mental illness and disabilities, for example, are frequently perceived to have characteristics that others look down on and are treated differently as a result—often devalued, disrespected, or treated as if they are less than fully human (Green et al., 2005).

When we label and classify each other, we marginalize and create cultural narratives that depict certain groups of people as unwanted or undesirable, separate from their actual physical properties. Sometimes, for medical conditions or mental disorders, labeling is perceived as positive, because without the label (diagnosis), the person cannot be treated and possibly relieved of her/his symptoms. But, concurrently, labeling categorizes people into social hierarchies. As Foucault (1995) pointed out, labeling people as somehow "deviant" led to the long-term confinement of people with mental illness (labeled "the insane") in mental hospitals, of people who were ill in hospitals, of people who were older-aged in nursing homes. Szasz (1987) noted that "the primary function of the public mental hospital has always been, and still is, to provide room and board for society's misérables—the homeless, the unskilled, the unemployed, those unable or unwilling to care for themselves and for whom no one else is willing to care" (p. 358). Separating out the deviant other makes us feel more "normal" (Szasz, 1970).

Space for deviant others is not only created by physical location, however. It is also created in language, by referring to people with illness or disability by their illness or disability, or by pointing out their difference through language, rendering people "less human, more a collection of body parts" (Marks, 1999, p. 57). Theorizing Practice 8.1 invites you to consider people-first language as a way of challenging dehumanizing references.

Theorizing Practice 8.1
People First Language

"Sticks and stones will break my bones, but words will never hurt me." Chances are you've heard this childhood chant, and chances are you know it's not true. Words *do* hurt. They can also stigmatize, stereotype, and dehumanize, whether as purposeful insults or as thoughtless labels. "People First Language" is one way to avoid prejudicial and hurtful terms, particularly when communicating about disabilities. While many champion this terminology, believing it eliminates generalizations and assumptions by focusing on the person rather than the disability, some critics reject it (e.g., autism activists who argue that "person with autism" suggests that autism can be separated from the person). Regardless, thoughtful word usage communicated with sensitivity and respect should always be the rule. Some suggestions include:

- Refer to the person before the disability (e.g., girl with Down syndrome or boy with epilepsy).
- Avoid terms and phrases that equate the person with the disability (e.g., the disabled or autistic) or that carry negative connotations (e.g., she *suffers* from mental illness or he's *confined* to a wheelchair).
- Emphasize abilities rather than limitations (e.g., he walks with crutches).
- Consider whether the disability is relevant and necessary to mention when referring to or describing individuals.

Conduct a search of stories about individuals with disabilities in a variety of media formats. Note the use of appropriate and inappropriate terminology. Did anything in your findings surprise you? Why or why not?

Labels reinforce the traditional medical hierarchy because the process of diagnosing privileges medical terminology and creates dependence on professionals. Labels are products of social practice and discourse. While there are advantages to medical labeling, as we've stated, all of these medical labels still construct the person as deviant (Davis, 2013). While impairment can be seen as a "real" physical fact, disability due to that impairment is believed by social constructionists to be a negative label used to enforce social marginalization (Barnes, 1996). As Cris observed in her research on children with mental illness, we blame people for their problems (poor people for their poverty, people with physical or mental impairments for their disabilities), rather than acknowledging the social issues that contribute to their situation (Davis, 2013).

Lupton (2013) also reminds us that in other times and places, additional weight has been considered a sign of health and beauty. She reminds us that "in and of itself, fat has no meaning" (p. 3), and she asserts that the significance of differently sized bodies is culturally constructed. Not all people with excess weight are gluttons, or are unhealthy. Scholars such as Lupton (2013) and Wann (2009) argue that society needs to accept *biodiversity*—a diversity of sizes and shapes. For example, many of the difficulties that people who carry more weight have are not due to conditions inherent in their bodies but rather are the result of architectural and spatial decisions that render spaces too small, tight, and unmanageable for people of many body sizes (Lupton, 2013). Think of airplane seats and turnstiles. Being larger-sized would not matter if design engineers made spaces generously large. Fat studies researchers suggest the stigma against obesity has a lot to do with space issues. Fat bodies take up more space (Lupton, 2013), and as the population gets larger, people get increasingly concerned about who's taking more than their share—of space, resources, or healthcare. Also, when a person is fat, his/her body size is a master status (Hiller, 1982), overpowering all other characteristics she/he may have and affecting his/her whole life (Macionis, 1995). People with fat bodies are constructed as being out of control, lazy, ugly, monstrous, and emotionally unstable (Lupton, 2013). We are in what Lupton (2013) terms a "fat-phobic society" (p. 3) in which if you are not fat, you are afraid of becoming fat.

■ Stigma

Kelli frowns. "I can see a size-12 woman in a dressing room whose weight is up from a size 10 being concerned about it. But at my size I would never ask anyone if this makes me fat because the answer will be, 'Well, duh.'"

"What do you think are some people's misconceptions about obesity?" Maggie asks.

Kelli nods her head. "The biggest one is that it's my fault; it's something I've deliberately done to myself. And people think it's very easy to fix and I'm this size simply because I eat too much. None of that is true."

Stigma, a social construct, is defined as an undesirable differentness, an adverse reaction to the perception of a negatively evaluated difference (Goffman, 1963). Of course, the experience of stigma is not only experienced by people with larger bodies. All sorts of differently appearing bodies, including older, larger, and injured bodies, and differently acting behaviors (as people with mental illness or cognitive disorders), are potentially implicated in socially constructed and stigmatizing meanings. It is not about the attribute of the person who is stigmatized but rather about the way other people evaluate whatever is different about her/him in negative terms (Goffman, 1963). In a society in which health, youth, and beauty are highly valued, people with bodies that look different in a variety of ways—various sizes, shapes, impairments, or imperfections—are seen as having negatively valued traits (Barnes, 1996). The stigma itself can have a negative effect on a person's well-being and sense of self. In the conversation among Kelli, Cris, and Maggie, examples of stigma are pervasive.

Link and Phelan (2001) identify five components of stigma: labeling, stereotyping, separation, status loss and discrimination, and power differential. Stigma occurs when people with these differences believe that they are labeled, stereotyped, and separated from others. They feel a loss of status when the labeling, stereotyping, and separation interfere with their ability to participate fully in the social and economic life of their community. In qualitative research on people with disabilities, Green et al. (2005) heard distressing examples of Link and Phelan's (2001) five components: social awkwardness resulting from labeling; pity resulting from stereotyping; violence, hostility, mistreatment, and shunning resulting from separation ("othering"); deterred social and economic participation related to status loss and discrimination; inequitable power relationships that marginalize people with disabilities; and subsequent lower self-worth, depression, and social isolation. Green et al. (2005) quoted one participant with a disability describing the experience of separation: "People have a preconception of [the individual] not being a whole person when they see somebody on crutches or in a wheelchair so you have to kind of overcome that. Show them that you are a person and not an object to be pitied" (p. 205). Stigma can have long lasting negative consequences on employment, quality of life, and self-esteem. Being stigmatized results in negative outcomes including shame, depression, and social isolation, as well as mistreatment and discrimination (Puhl & Heuer, 2009).

HCIA 8.2

Experiencing Transgender Microaggressions

Lucy J. Miller

As a graduate student, I once visited the campus health clinic for treatment of a sinus infection. The doctor began the examination and then paused, looked up at me, and asked, "You do know your body is male, right?" I froze and mumbled a quiet "yes." The rest of the examination proceeded normally, but I still left the clinic in shock at the doctor's inappropriate and irrelevant question. While one would hope for more sensitivity from a healthcare provider, such microaggressions are unfortunately not uncommon for me as a transgender woman.

Microaggressions are brief, interpersonal expressions of disgust, distrust, or dislike of the identity of another person, usually along the lines of race, gender, class, sexual orientation, religion, or other individual characteristics. While interpersonal in nature, microaggressions are part of societal systems whose master narratives force the individual to conform to commonly held norms. These experiences often place a great deal of physical stress and psychological discomfort on people. I have an abundance of personal experience with microaggressions as a transgender woman, and they have certainly affected my health—I feel self-conscious, disembodied, and stigmatized every day.

The microaggressions directed at me are intended to force me to conform to the expectations of the gender binary in order to fit with societal expectations of what it means to be male or female. Microaggressions are often intended to make me feel self-conscious about my gender performance. For example, I stopped once at a fast-food restaurant in a small Texas town in the early stages of my transition. The cashier, noticing my short hair, commented that I would look better with long hair; her microaggression was performed for an audience of her coworkers who chuckled behind her the entire time. While the comment was not overtly aggressive, its intention was to make me feel nervous and self-conscious about my appearance and, along with other comments, make me second-guess my perceived "choice" to violate social gender norms.

Microaggressions are also directed at transgender people by treating them as exotic. Doing so attaches a stigma to the individual's identity by bringing attention to the way she or he differs from the norm. When I am in public spaces, people often do double takes as they pass by, stopping to look over their shoulder to verify what they have seen. Some people are not discreet and openly gawk at me as I walk through a store or across a college campus. In all of these situations, I am treated as if I am a novelty, almost as if I were on display in a zoo or museum and must be stared at in order to be understood. People frequently take my picture without my consent in public. I have been followed through stores by people attempting to get a clear shot, and even had a man get verbally upset with me when I denied his request to take my picture in a supermarket. These actions clearly communicate that others see transgender people are bizarre, like mythical creatures whose presence must be documented. This kind of attention can be devastating for someone just trying to go about her or his daily routine. After experiences like these, I am often anxious in public spaces, looking over my shoulder constantly for any sign of unwanted attention.

Disapproval and discomfort represent the most common types of microaggressions experienced by transgender people. While shopping in a discount store, a mother said, "That's just wrong!" under her breath as I walked by, and a cashier at a fast-food drive-thru laughed and exclaimed, "Ah, hell no!" when I pulled up to get my food. Expressions like these make it clear that some people are not comfortable with my presence in public spaces and cannot constrain themselves as they communicate their aggression. Even something as simple as calling me by my correct name can be a clear indicator of whether or not someone approves of or is comfortable with my identity as a transgender woman. I have had to accept food orders for "Lucian" or "Lucius" many times because cashiers were unwilling to call me by my (rather uncomplicated) name.

What can be done about microaggressions? Personally, I often just avoid people who engage in this behavior, and I try to exit the situation as quickly as possible. I wish I could address these issues more directly, but the anxiety I feel in those situations is already high enough without confronting the perpetrator directly. I think sometimes people have just never encountered a transgender person before and would regret their actions if they were made aware of my perception of them. I know I would feel better if I witnessed people sincerely trying to understand me, but I am not yet able to take that risk, fearing increased mental stress or even physical violence. Victims often experience microaggressions similarly to abuse and require active coping strategies to deal with the negative psychological effects. What I believe is really needed is a way for people to understand that gender identities exist outside of the male/female binary. This could help reduce the negative reactions to transgender people because everyone wouldn't be expected to express their gender identities in the same way.

QUESTIONS TO PONDER

1. Do you know any transgender people personally? How have these personal relationships helped you reconsider any assumptions held about these individuals?

2. How would treating microaggressions as a health crisis instead of an interpersonal conflict open up new possibilities for addressing the issue?

3. Focusing on the serious health effects of microaggressions, how might you design a media campaign intended to raise public awareness of these negative impacts?

Source: Miller, L. J. (2015). Disciplining the transgender body: Transgender microaggressions in a transitional era. In A. R. Martinez & L. J. Miller (Eds.), *Gender in a transitional era: Changes and challenges* (pp. 133–149). Lanham, MD: Lexington Books.

Fat stigma is prevalent across media. Even children's television depicts people with larger bodies as evil, lazy, weak, unattractive, unfriendly, cruel, unimportant, stupid, uneducated, unsophisticated, and unlikeable (Fouts & Burggraf, 2000; Fouts & Vaughan, 2002; Robinson, Callister, & Jankoski, 2008; Spinetta, 2013; Veverka, 2014). Scholars criticize the reality television show *The Biggest Loser* because it treats people like children and humiliates and punishes them as motivational techniques. It teaches us that people with excess weight are not "normal," that it is justifiable to mistreat people who are large because it is for their own good, and that certain people, because of size, are not worthy of being loved, which perpetuates fat shaming and anti-fat attitudes (Domoff et al., 2012; Lupton, 2013). Also, shows like *The Biggest Loser* sustain the misconception that excess weight is a direct result of simply eating more calories than you burn, despite the fact that much research shows that body size is much more complex. In fact, many people mistakenly attribute obesity to lack of willpower (Veverka, 2014).

Another example is Michelle Obama's "Let's Move" campaign, which targets children. It has been criticized for its emphasis on weight loss rather than healthy eating and exercise, resulting in potential stigma against children who are larger sized and propagating eating disorders in youth. In addition, the "Let's Move" campaign also communicates, again, that fat is always negative and people who are fat are inevitably less healthy and they are to blame for their overeating and lack of exercise. It constructs a war on fat and, by association, on people who are fat (Jette, Bhagat, & Andrews, 2014). Unfortunately, this kind of discrimination and stigma has been shown to result in the bullying of children (Doty, 2014). Many individuals who are fat experience depression, lower self-esteem, body dissatisfaction, eating disorders, negative social relationships, reduced physical activity, higher blood pressure, and suicidal behaviors (Matthews, Salomon, Kenyon, & Zhou, 2005; Puhl & Latner, 2007).

The concept of "deviance" is related to our social emphasis on productivity. Part of the reason for the stigmatization of people who have bodies that are ill, impaired, or different is the value placed on productivity in our society. If individuals' bodies (or minds, or emotions) do not allow them to be productive, such as when they have mental illness, impairments, or disabilities (especially hidden disabilities, as Theorizing Practice 8.2 demonstrates), they are often blamed for their bodies. Of course, this is paradoxical because by stigmatizing them, these individuals are held back from jobs and earning money, which in turn makes them less productive, and frequently even more sick and differently abled. The medical model of care reinforces this dilemma through its emphasis on loss and inability rather than on ability (Barton, 1996; Foucault, 1973).

People cope with being stigmatized in many different ways. They may attempt to hide their differentness (Goffman, 1963), educate or manage the emotions of others in public encounters (Cahill & Eggleston, 1995), withdraw from others (Link, Struening, Cullen, & Shrout, 1989), or mostly associate with people they know understand what they're going through (Goffman, 1963). Ironically, stigma against individuals who are fat makes them much more likely to become and remain fat (Smith, 2011), which is why the public health messages against being fat and public discrimination against fat people often backfire.

Theorizing Practice 8.2
"People Think I Look Fine, So I Am Not Sick"

Consider the following Facebook post by Julie McGovern, who hopes to raise compassion and awareness for people like herself with hidden disabilities. After reading Julie's story, formulate your response to the following questions:

- Have you ever questioned someone's abilities based solely on their appearance?
- Do you think people with hidden disabilities or illnesses have a responsibility to announce their condition? Would you want your hidden disability or illness known to strangers or casual acquaintances?
- Julie says, "It is up to us to share our story and to raise awareness." What stories of discrimination could you tell? What do you take away from hers?

My name is Julie. My entire life I have been an athlete. I have excelled in all things athletic. I was on the track team in high school and college, as well as a cheerleader in high school and college. In the summer of 2005 I was diagnosed with mononucleosis. Until then, I was unaware of this and continued to train hard in my collegiate sports. I thought my excessive fatigue, sore throat, headache, and overall sickness was due to being a freshman living in the dorms. It is not uncommon to get sick in that environment. However, my symptoms progressed and I went to the doctor. As soon as I learned about the mono, I immediately stopped these activities.

Six months later I began fainting, my heart would race, I was nauseous, had migraines, along with other debilitating symptoms. I knew something was wrong when I could no longer walk to my mailbox without being short of breath and having to sit down for several minutes before I made my way back to my house. I went to the doctor and they told me it was nothing. They said if I had anything, it was anxiety. I knew they were wrong. I knew my body and I knew something was very wrong. After many months searching for answers, I finally found a doctor who changed my life with a few simple words, "I believe you." Together he and I began the journey to find out why my quality of life had decreased in such drastic ways. After many tests, I was diagnosed with Postural Orthostatic Tachycardia Syndrome (POTS). My physician believed because of the mono and my continued activity, the mono destroyed my autonomic system, which controls all things in the body that are automatic. This illness affects literally every organ in the body.

It causes my blood pressure to be dangerously low and my heart rate critically high. I have GI issues and my body cannot withstand the pull of gravity, so the blood drops to my feet, which can cause a loss of consciousness. Due to this, I am unable to stand for long periods of time or walk long distances. Being a young person with an invisible chronic illness is one of the hardest things I've ever dealt with. People think I look fine, so I am not sick. It isn't that I'm looking for sympathy, but respect and compassion. It has been an incredible odyssey going from a vibrantly healthy person to someone living with a chronic illness. My life before I was sick is much different now that I am.

I am unable to keep up with my friends and my pride often keeps me from asking for help. Sadly, the disbelief of others around me has caused me to remain silent about my illness. It is like I am being punished for being sick. They think if I just eat better or sleep more, I would be cured, but that couldn't be further from the truth. POTS symptoms are always changing, they come and go, and appear in many different combinations. No one POTS patient is treated medically the same. The symptoms I have today, I may not have tomorrow. I can be fine one minute and on the floor the next. It is very hard to make plans due to the unpredictably of this horrible syndrome.

(continued)

My doctor issued me a handicap parking tag. I have always been afraid of what others would say and I often sit in my car until I feel no one is around so that they won't judge me or accuse me of using the system. I am sick. I didn't choose this and it isn't my fault. I would give anything to be healthy again. I would give anything to have one day of freedom. Just because a person looks fine does not mean they are. There are many illnesses that go unnoticed to the untrained eye. Being handicapped isn't always a wheelchair or crutches. Some illnesses manifest themselves internally and destroy the body from within. I have one of those illnesses.

Today my fear came true. So many emotions flooded my mind. I was hurt, I was angry, I wanted my voice to be heard, but this person is a coward and could not tell me what he/she thought to my face. This person incorrectly perceived my situation, because it is impossible for someone my age to have an illness. This person doesn't know me or my struggles. They don't know what this illness has taken from me. They don't see the countless nights I cry myself to sleep, soaking my pillow with tears, pleading—praying for God to heal me. They don't see the weakness, the pain, the symptoms that are very real, but only I can feel. They don't understand, and until it happens to them they never will.

However, it is up to us to tell our story and to raise awareness. As I said, not all things are visible. The person who wrote me such a hateful note is also handicapped. This person has a mental handicap disguised as ignorance. And even though I am sick, I don't always park in the handicapped parking. I only do so on my bad days. And sometimes even on my bad days I won't park there because someone else might be having a worse day. And other times, I am just too afraid to be attacked, ridiculed, and judged like I was today.

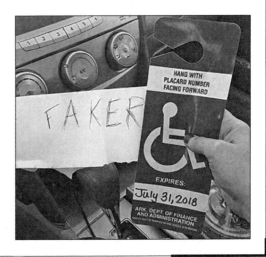

To the person who wrote me that note. Shame on you! I pray you are never faced with the struggles I am every minute of every day. I pray that someone you love who is ill is never treated the way you have treated me. I pray you open your eyes and your heart to the people around you and exercise compassion, as you abandon your need to hurt others. You are obviously a very angry and unhappy soul. I pray you find peace and love in your life. And finally, I hope you are never a victim to a life-altering illness and experience the cruelty I experienced today because of you.

"In many ways, I'm strong and tough on the outside, but on the inside, of course, it does hurt when people say cruel things about me. I am an emotional eater and I swallow my depression and that is a problem. That has contributed a lot to this," Kelli says.

"Do you know where your depression started?" Maggie asks.

"It's a domino effect," Kelli says. "I'm depressed because I'm fat, so I eat more because I'm depressed. Go figure. I'm depressed because I don't like myself so I'm going to self-sabotage it."

I nod sympathetically. "That's very, very common, when people try to get other people to lose weight; it just makes them eat more."

Maggie adds, "3–5 are my eating hours."

"This is what strikes me," I say. "All three of us do the same things. We sometimes eat what we shouldn't, when we shouldn't. We probably all do emotional eating sometimes. And we probably all beat ourselves up for it when we do it. But because Kelli's behaviors manifest visually, she gets social blame and Maggie and I don't."

"Well, I know I have been the recipient of a great deal of hatred, discrimination, and bullying because of my weight," says Kelli.

"Do you think there are other misconceptions people have about people with excess weight?" Maggie asks Kelli.

Kelli nods. "There are misconceptions about overweight people in general—there is a prejudice about overweight people. There are people who think they are superior to us."

"How do you know that?" Maggie asks.

"It's their attitude," Kelli says. "I have a very early childhood memory of being in nursery school and having this little girl actually whip me with her jump rope. Beat me up against a tree. That was when I was six years old. I still remember that. That memory has stayed with me all these years. Now that I'm older, I want to beat her up."

I laugh, feeling very big-sisterly protective. "Tell us her name and we'll do it."

"Bullying against larger sized children is a real problem," Maggie says. "There's been a lot of recent cases of kids being bullied over their weight, and some even committing suicide because of it" [Doty, 2014; Puhl, Luedicke, & Heuer, 2011].

"Unfortunately, it's not just children who are bullies," Kelli says. "I still get bullied today, as an adult. People look at me as an easy target. The prejudice against my body size has made me tougher growing up. I never dated a lot. The men I always wanted never wanted me," Kelli adds.

"I have a lot of friends, "Kelli says. "I have been very blessed. In some ways, my weight and health issues have helped me be a little luckier. The friends I have are true friends. You find out who your friends are when you go through tough times. I have a handful of very close, very dear friends, and then I have a world of so-so friends. I have learned over the years to be more aware, more discriminating of people, as far as choosing my friends. I am not needy. I don't need to have a lot of friends. I think being overweight has strengthened me. You get a thick skin. I try not to think about things. I try not to let it get to me."

"Are there times when it does get to you?" Maggie asks.

"I'm sure there have been." Kelli pauses to think. "People can be cruel or ignorant. Recently, I went to a convention in New Orleans right after my initial cancer surgery and I was not well while I was there. I had just had the lumpectomy the week before."

"You got on a plane a week after the surgery?" Maggie interrupts to ask.

Kelli nods. "I barely survived it. It was very rough. I had a couple friends at the convention sit me down and let me have it about coming to the convention and being so far gone."

"What do you mean, far gone?" I ask.

"Being so sick. They told me it was my fault that I let myself go this far to get cancer. I didn't know what to say to that."

"Wow," Maggie and I both say.

"I was sitting there minding my own business and this person came walking up. The day before, a couple friends and I had gone sightseeing and I was pretty well wiped out. I just couldn't walk and I got a wheelchair, although it didn't work on the cobblestone streets, so we ended up walking. But this woman came up to me and said 'I heard you were in a wheelchair yesterday,' and she just dove in. She said, 'What do you think you're doing? I don't want to ever hear anything like that again. How can you do this to yourself?'" Kelli pauses. "She meant well."

I grimace. "If that is someone meaning well, I'd hate to see someone who didn't mean well. Why did she have to say anything at all?"

"Couldn't she have said, 'I'm sorry to hear you're in a wheelchair; are you OK?'" Maggie says.

I frown. "What is it with people who think it's OK to say things like that? Here's how you want to respond: 'Thank you for telling me I've put on some weight. Thank you for telling me my health is bad. I have been waiting and waiting for someone to tell me.'"

"Do strangers ever say anything to you about your weight?" I ask.

"Well," says Kelli. "There are things I won't do because of I'm afraid of reactions to my weight. Not that people usually say anything out loud, but I may get looks. I don't go to public swimming pools or the beach."

"That's a shame," I say. "Swimming would help your arthritis and would be great gentle exercise for you."

"Yes, but I'm not going to a pool," Kelli says.

"That's such an example of weight stigma making it harder for people of size to get healthier," I protest. "I remember when I was heavier, trying to exercise to lose weight; it was impossible to find workout clothes in my size."

"But I do other stuff," Kelli says.

"Like what?" Maggie and I ask.

"Well, at our convention, there was a party with a live band, and CJ and I got up on the dance floor and danced."

I smile at the picture. "Flying itself, how was that?"

Kelli continues. "I have learned this last year, Southwest Airlines will give me a second seat for free. That is something special they do. I can be first on the plane and choose the seat I want. No one says a word. I have to ask for it, but I've never had a problem. On other airlines, I haven't been able to have two seats without paying for both of them."

"Do you have other space issues with your size?" I ask.

"When I go out to eat, I can't sit at a booth so I always ask for a table. Sometimes, the table is fixed and I can't move it to make more room for me." She pauses thoughtfully. "Sometimes when I'm riding with someone, people try to let me sit in the front seat but I can't use their seat belt. In my car, I have a seat belt extension. If I sit in the back seat, I can get away without a seat belt"

I nod, thinking about how that situation puts her at risk for injury in case of an accident.

"What about at work?" Maggie asks.

Kelli nods her head. "I have had suspicions that I have been turned down for jobs or promotions. When it goes to the younger, cuter looking girl with no experience, when I have years of experience, it makes you wonder. Things like that."

Theorizing Practice 8.3 invites you to consider how the Americans with Disabilities Act of 1990 (ADA) has afforded protection from discrimination in a variety of ways. Still, as Kelli demonstrates, weight stigma is one of the most pervasive types of stigma in our culture (Seacat, Dougal, & Roy, 2014). Puhl and Brownell (2006) report that if people think another's excess weight is due to a medical issue out of her/his control, then they have fewer negative opinions of the fat person, similar to reactions to breast versus lung cancer, for example, or differentiating causes of HIV, STIs, and so on. In interpersonal relationships, people who are fat are the recipients of discriminating behavior from family members and so-called friends (Puhl, Moss-Racusin, & Schwartz, 2007). Individuals who are fat have difficulty dating and are believed to be

---

Theorizing Practice 8.3
Equal Opportunity for Persons with Disabilities

The Americans with Disabilities Act of 1990 (ADA) prohibits discrimination and ensures equal opportunity for persons with disabilities in employment, state and local government services, public accommodations, commercial facilities, and transportation. Spend a day committed to noticing ADA provisions in your usual environment and regular routine. What taken-for-granted accommodations exist? What resources are available? What, if anything, surprised you?

---

less warm and sexually attractive (Puhl et al., 2011). The discrimination individuals who are fat experience results in their being less likely to be hired, paid lower wages, given lower performance evaluations, less likely to be promoted, and more likely to be fired (Puhl & Heuer, 2009).

In addition, if individuals who are fat also have health problems, often society takes a moralistic standpoint, blaming their ill health on excess weight, when the health problem may be due to stress induced by the stigma against their weight. In fact, medical research has produced evidence that acute and chronic stress contributes to conditions such as cardiovascular disease, depression; lowered immune response; digestive, endocrine, circulatory, respiratory, gastrointestinal, genitourinary, and musculoskeletal disorders; and impaired brain structure and functioning (D'Andrea, Sharma, Zelechoski, & Spinazzola, 2011; Lupton, 2013; Schnurr & Green, 2004; Wann, 2009). In addition, research has shown that chronic stress from stigma and discrimination contributes to overeating as well as to lower metabolism, thus contributing to weight gain (Torres & Nowson, 2007).

Biomedical Model of Weight Loss

Maggie asks, "Do you think if obesity were talked about more as a disease that would change the way people think about it?"

Kelli shakes her head. "I actually read an article online where they were talking about that idea. The general consensus was that people with excess weight didn't want to think of it as a disease. I don't think of obesity as a disease. I think of it as an outcome, a result, a side effect of lots of other issues. I do think some people are fat because they do not take care of themselves; they don't eat right. But not all fat people."

Maggie and I nod as Kelli continues.

"People have different metabolisms. Food affects different people differently."

I nod as I think of friends I have who eat what we would call "fattening" foods regularly but don't gain weight as a result.

"But does that make obesity itself a disease?" Kelli asks. "For me, I think of it as a birth defect. Everyone is different. Some people can eat whatever they want and be as thin as a rail. Other people can eat lettuce and gain five pounds."

I nod. I'm one of those people.

Kelli continues. "The medical community doesn't really know why people are obese. And if it takes calling it a disease to find out, maybe that's OK. But I don't think it's a disease. I think it is a result of something else, maybe different metabolisms or whatever. I don't think it's just because I eat too much. That is a very unfair generalization. It's especially unfair for someone with a size 2 body to sit with a bag of donuts in front of them and call me fat because they say I eat too much. I wish people would have more compassion in general."

"It's biodiversity," I say. "Whatever size we are is OK; we don't all have to be the same size. Get over it. My body is not anyone else's business."

"I am not healthy," Kelli says after a pause.

"Do you think your health problems are weight-related?" Maggie asks.

"I think to a certain extent they are," Kelli says. "They have proven some are weight- related. Like diabetes." She pauses. "But then there are thin people with diabetes as well."

I sit thoughtfully. "Lots of people in our family struggle with weight, but Dad was not obese. He had type 2 diabetes and he ate pretty healthy. Blood sugar issues run in our family. I don't think you can say excess weight always causes diabetes. And I don't think you can say eating unhealthy foods always causes excess weight. As I said, lots of thin people eat unhealthy also."

"What do you think your life would have been like if you had been thin?" Maggie asks.

"Would I still be working, not out on disability?" Kelli asks rhetorically. "Would I still have these health issues? I don't know how much my weight affects these health issues. Would I still have arthritis? Yes. Degenerative disk disease? Yes. Circulation problems? Yes."

"Moving forward," I ask, "if you were able to miraculously lose the weight, what would life look like for you?"

"I'm hoping it would make enough of a difference that I could get back to work, be less dependent, not so needy. I could make more money, support myself better, get back to my regular wages and achieve other goals like get a job I like. Get my own place, get a dog. Date." Kelli pauses. "I don't know. Be out of pain hopefully."

"There is a perception that people who receive disability benefits would choose that rather than a job," Maggie notes. "Talk to us about being on disability."

"Many days, I'm in a lot of pain. I have to keep my legs up, which means I sleep a lot. I can go days without even getting out of the house. When I'm feeling better, I can go to the gym and try to exercise. I can go maybe 15 minutes on a treadmill and play around with the equipment. But if I do too much then I am laid up for days. It is a vicious cycle. It is not really living. When I went on that trip to New Orleans I was so ill I didn't know if I could make it home. This is not living." Kelli thinks for a minute. "My income was cut by 40% when I went on disability. I am living on 60% of my pay and I don't know how much longer I'll be approved for that. I put in for an extension of my disability income. They may say OK or not. If I don't get approved for permanent disability, I'll have to find a job whether I can physically work or not. Or I'll be out on the street. I might be in big trouble. This is no way to live. If I lose my disability, I'll lose my health insurance and I'll really be in big trouble."

"But there's the Affordable Care Act, right?" I say.

Kelli nods. "As of right now, I don't qualify for it because I make too much money on disability. If I lose it all, I'll have to go on welfare and hope I qualify for Medicaid."

"North Carolina politicians chose not to expand Medicaid," I say. "That's the reason you don't qualify for the ACA now. The original intent of ACA was to care for people in your situation. Politicians playing with people's lives."

"You have a lot of health issues," Maggie notes. "Where does your weight fall in the list?"

"I think about it 24/7," Kelli says. "It's the number one thing in my subconscious that I'm always thinking about. It's the one thing about myself that I hate the most."

"Why?" I ask.

"I know that if I can lose the weight it would help some of these other problems," Kelli says. "And, it is an image thing. It is the elusive goal that I want to achieve the most. Of everything. I think about it more than other health issues. I'd like to lose weight; I can't."

"You haven't been able to?" Maggie asks.

"I haven't yet," Kelli says.

"What attempts have you made?" Maggie asks.

Kelli shrugs. "Not a lot."

"So you haven't done yo-yo dieting," Maggie clarifies.

Kelli shakes her head. "I consider myself a moral failure. I see myself doing it in my mind. But then the day goes by and I haven't done enough."

"I feel like a failure," Kelli says, grimacing. "I know what I'm supposed to eat and what I'm not supposed to eat. I know how much exercise I'm supposed to do. I know I'm supposed to get off my butt and go to the gym every day. I do it for a while and I'm doing great and wonderful, and then something happens. Lately it's been health-related. I threw my back out at the gym. Then something else happened. Now I have cancer."

I interrupt her. "You consider yourself a moral failure because health issues stopped your exercise? You have cancer, for goodness' sake!"

"You sound like you're struggling with being self-disciplined," Maggie says. "Nobody has 100% self-discipline 100% of the time!"

Kelli shakes her head. "My friend CJ is very disciplined. He doesn't care about food. He will have a little grilled chicken and a salad. He could eat that seven days a week. If he were here, that is what he would eat. He doesn't care about taste and flavor. And I am a foodie."

Maggie laughs. "I get up in the morning and the first thing I think about is what I am going to eat." Kelli and I laugh with her. "That actually sounds like CJ is the one with food issues."

"Yeah, well, maybe," Kelli says. "He has his moments, but for the most part he is not consumed with it. His food issues aren't hurting anyone."

"Yours aren't hurting anyone else, either," I say with a grimace. "What is it about our society that—for some people with certain body sizes only—it is considered a moral failing to like food?" I shake my head.

Maggie changes the subject. "So, you bring it up to friends? To doctors?"

Kelli nods. "My doctor and I talk about it a lot. A couple months ago I started the process to do gastric bypass surgery. As part of the prep with that I have to talk with my doctor once a month about my weight, because we have to document that I'm trying to lose weight. I was moving forward with that until I got the breast cancer diagnosis."

I turn to Maggie. "Now they won't talk to her until her cancer treatments are over with."

"I'm not sure I want to do it," Kelli says. "I keep changing my mind. Something inside me is telling me not to. I think it is too dangerous. I'm concerned with all my other health issues that it could be a serious problem doing surgery that drastic. I'm afraid it would do more harm than good." Kelli adds, "And there's no guarantee it's going to work. A lot of people have the surgery and it comes right back. You can still have problems."

Kelli is not alone in her efforts to lose weight. Fewer than 5% of the people losing weight through dieting have been able to maintain their weight loss (Bacon, 2012). Further, research suggests that gastric bypass surgery leads to health problems later, such as regained weight, nutritional deficiencies, alcoholism, and substance abuse, even in people who never had those problems before the surgery (Hagedorn, Encarnacion, Brat, & Morton, 2007). Also, many people require additional surgeries to remove excess skin, which usually is not covered by insurance (Bishop, 2005).

The desire to medically fix weight is part of the biomedical model of illness. Excess weight is labeled as "unhealthy," as a medical problem. Weight is discussed as a temporary biological condition that can be cured by medical intervention. This model stresses cure; a dominant, paternalistic physician role; and a passive patient role, rather than prevention (Mischler, 1984). Foucault (1995) said that, in this model, the body serves as an object and target of power in which professionals disempower and marginalize the patients. This creates a distance between people who are healthy and people who are ill, who are considered to be "deviant" in some way—in this case, in their body size.

We pause our conversation as the waitress brings our salads and refills our unsweetened iced tea.

Kelli takes a sip of her tea. "One thing I wanted to add about the surgery," she says, as Maggie and I take a bite. "I don't think I've tried hard enough on my own and I would feel like I was giving up. A cop-out. It goes back to I know what to do. I just seem to have a mental block. I try to eat better. Like bread; I should cut out bread. I have food sensitivities and allergies to wheat. I think I'm addicted to it."

I nod. I know I feel much better all the way around when I am not eating wheat.

Kelli continues talking between bites of her salad. "When I first became a diabetic, giving up sugar was very easy. I'm fine with fake sweeteners. Giving up pasta, not a problem, I don't like it anyway. I never eat rice or potatoes. I don't bake potatoes. All of that was easy to give up. But it's all those other carbs and sugars. Any form of bread, I cannot stop, and that is my biggest issue."

"What's the longest you've been successful in healthier eating?" I ask, purposefully avoiding the term "diet."

"Four months," Kelli says.

"What triggers you to stop eating healthier?" I ask.

"I eat one thing I shouldn't, and it's hard to stop," Kelli says.

I make a mental note of her continued use of moralistic language (e.g., "shouldn't"). I wonder if it would be easier to have a healthy lifestyle if stigmatizing, moralizing judgments were removed from the equation.

"What could doctors do to help patients?" Maggie asks.

"It would be nice if they could try harder to actually help. Just sitting and talking to the doctor isn't doing anything. The local hospital does have a medical diet center, but my health insurance won't pay for it. It costs $2,500 out of pocket. If something like that was covered, I would be the first one in line."

"Yet your insurance covers gastric bypass," I say.

Maggie nods. "They want the quick fix."

"They will pay $25,000 for the surgery," Kelli says. "But they won't pay $2,500 for the non-surgical route. To me that is crazy."

"But we're still talking about trying to fix fat," I say in protest. "It's still the medical model. Whether it's The Biggest Loser, *or gastric bypass surgery, or medical weight loss clinics, we're using language that identifies excess body weight as a medical problem that needs medical intervention to fix."*

"And that language stigmatizes people," says Maggie.

■ Addressing and Reducing Stigma

Just as language stigmatizes, it can also connect and heal. Sharing personal experiences through story—in various forms—is a great way to minimize stigma and encourage inclusivity and biodiversity. Providing space for people with stigmatizing conditions to be seen as fully human lessens their experiences of separation, othering, marginalization, discrimination, and negative stereotypes (Davis, 2013; Green et al., 2005). Hearing others' stories, such as in this chapter, is an effective way to get to know someone as a person beyond his/her body size, shape, age, or ability. Cris's work with poetry, drama, and fiction (see, for example, Davis, Delynko, & Cook 2010; Davis & Warren-Findlow, 2011, 2012) has shown the importance of providing opportunities for people who are not frequently afforded a voice to tell their story. Storytelling lets us reframe our versions of reality—either our own or someone else's, and it helps us better understand someone else's experience. Storytelling acts as resistance discourse because it lets us substitute our personal narratives for the canonical (official) narratives (Davis & Warren-Findlow, 2011, 2012).

Maggie is interested in the ways in which numerous forms of aesthetic storytelling, including dance, can do the work of social movements (Quinlan, 2010a, 2010b; Quinlan & Harter, 2010). For example, she conducted an in-depth case study of Dancing Wheels—the first modern dance company to integrate professional stand-up (able-bodied) and sit-down (wheelchair) dancers, based in Cleveland, Ohio. She is interested in the ways in which the performing arts, particularly dance, have a history of engaging only the "physically elite" (i.e., able-bodied) as performers. She has explored how Dancing Wheels positions performance as artistic vocation, individual expression, and social change. Dance offers employment but also allows individuals to creatively express themselves, connect with others, and challenge stereotypes and enlarge possibilities for individuals marked as disabled (Quinlan, 2010a, 2010b; Quinlan & Bates, 2015; Quinlan & Harter, 2010).

HCIA 8.3

Communicating Disability and Health through Wheelchair Rugby

Kurt Lindemann

I grew up communicating with physically and mentally disabled people. My father was paralyzed from the waist down in a motorcycle accident when I was seven. While he still had to go through physical therapy during his time at the spinal cord rehabilitation center, an equal part of his recovery had to do with the mental adjustments he had to make. His doctors recommended sports and hobbies as ways he might learn that he could, indeed, live what could be considered by most accounts a "normal" life. So, while growing up in a culture of disability, I also came of age in a world of sport participation: first wheelchair basketball, then wheelchair road racing competing in marathons. I eventually realized that, while all these activities were just a way of life for me, most able-bodied people were shocked that people in wheelchairs could accomplish such demanding physical feats.

(continued)

Years later, I came across an article in a Phoenix-area newspaper about wheelchair rugby and read the words of the athletes interviewed. I knew this was a subject I wanted to research. The sport, sometimes called Murderball (as popularized in the 2005 Oscar-nominated documentary of the same name), is played on a basketball court and consists of players strapped into tank-like wheelchairs smashing into each other and knocking each other over as they try to get the ball past a goal line. Using my in-group status as someone who had grown up around athletes in wheelchairs, I was granted access by the athletes on several teams to observe and interview them. I also talked to referees, coaches, and physical trainers who work with the athletes. In total, I spent about two-and-a-half years traveling the country to tournaments, attending practices, and hanging out with the athletes.

Being so immersed in the culture, I became privy to a lot of communication interaction: on the sidelines, during practices, at parties, in hotels, in bars, and waiting to board planes. It occurred to me that athletes' communication was as much about health practices as it was about playing the game. Players took pride in the rough, aggressive, and dangerous aspects of the game; they appeared to relish shattering people's perceptions about what those in wheelchairs are capable of. The ways the players talked about their play on the court seemed to frame their bodies as invulnerable. I heard players say, over and over, "What's the worst that can happen? I break my neck again?" This phrase illustrates what my coauthor and I call a "daredevil masculinity," which pushes some players to downplay the potential injuries that may arise from playing the sport. Considering many of the players I interviewed told me that their doctors recommended the sport as a form of physical therapy and rehabilitation, the way players talked about the potential for injury is ironic. Nonetheless, such talk illustrates the power of communication to frame health experiences.

One of the most interesting insights into health communication we found is the ways new players are taught to live the quad rugby "lifestyle." Veteran players on the teams also have experienced living life in a wheelchair with quadriplegia, or impairment in all four limbs of the body. As such, the experienced players not only teach new players the ins and outs of the game, they also teach the newly disabled players how to live life with a disability. This may include transferring themselves from their wheelchairs to the bathtub and back, getting into bed, and other everyday activities most people take for granted. These shortcuts taught by veteran players often contradict the "safe" way doctors recommend to do such things. These shortcuts aren't potentially hazardous to players' health like the attitude of "daredevil masculinity." But it still seemed ironic to us that a sport recommended by doctors to help quadriplegic persons regain some of the strength, mobility, and self-confidence they might have lost due to their disability would be at odds with what was communicated in that very same sport.

Sex and communication about sex is an important part of understanding health. The athletes in the sport, who are mostly male (there is a small percentage of females playing the sport), definitely talked about sex; most of us probably know the term "locker room talk" as a phrase that refers to sometimes graphic, crude, humorous, and often sexist language. These players told stories that sometimes involved tales of sexual conquests. The difference in Murderball athletes' talk is that these athletes more or less admitted in their storytelling that they weren't able to "perform" like a "normal" able-bodied man. However, they made sure to emphasize other sexual abilities. For example, when I was waiting to board a plane after one tournament, some players and I were passing around a bag of Starburst candy. While I could unwrap one easily with my fully functioning hands and fingers, the same task was considerably more difficult for some players with hardly any dexterity. They explained that they had to do the same task with their mouths, and that this skill translated into the ability to please a woman with a good oral sex technique.

We concluded that quad rugby athletes' off-court talk and on-court displays communicate to the able-bodied world that they can not only do the same things "normal" men can do but in some cases can do them better. In the process, however, they sometimes reaffirm somewhat narrow versions of what it means to be "healthy," including an emphasis on the aggressive athletic prowess of the male athlete whose body is invulnerable to pain, and the sexual prowess of the heterosexual male. In both cases, society is likely to imagine an able-bodied male at the center, making the wheelchair athletes' communication doubly ironic.

QUESTIONS TO PONDER

1. Do a Google search for a video clip of the film *Murderball*. What are your first reactions? Where do those reactions come from? Stereotypes? Personal experience? Can you think of any other portrayals in television and film of people in wheelchairs? How would you describe them?

2. What are your perceptions about the health of people in wheelchairs? Do you imagine them to be any less healthy than able-bodied people? In what ways? How might the concept of "health" be fluid and dependent on a person's situation?

3. There have been a lot of news stories about NFL athletes dying young from complications related to head trauma, including concussions. Many of us would imagine most professional athletes to be the epitome of health in terms of physical fitness. In what ways might sport participation lead to unhealthy personal choices?

Source: Lindemann, K., & Cherney, J. L. (2008). Communicating in and through "Murderball": Masculinity and disability in wheelchair rugby. *Western Journal of Communication, 72*, 107–125.

Taking an active role in our own care can also reduce stigma (Davis, 2013). Puhl (2015) suggests that people with stigmatizing conditions can address bias by educating others, challenging negative attitudes, obtaining social support, participating more fully in enjoyable activities even when it is challenging to do so, practicing self-talk and self-acceptance, being vocal and assertive about needs, responding assertively to people who make unkind or hurtful remarks, participating in advocacy groups, and getting professional help from a therapist.

Puhl (2015) has several suggestions for healthcare providers to address the bias that comes with stigmatizing conditions. Healthcare providers should: (1) directly address stigma with their patients by encouraging them to share their experiences, offering social support, and helping them identify ways they can cope; (2) address stigma within themselves by identifying their own biases; (3) better support patients by improving their own environments and making sure they are accessible to and appropriate for people of all sizes and abilities; and (4) improve their interpersonal skills to better communicate with patients in a nonjudgmental supportive manner. Given that communication research demonstrates the prevalence of stigma and the harm it creates (Smith, 2011), it is ultimately the responsibility of all of us to recognize and eliminate stigmatizing attitudes, messages, and behaviors.

■ Epilogue

"Bottom line—what do you want us to know?" Maggie asks Kelli.

"Get the insurance companies to pay for better treatment—preventative treatment. Know that we are all different and there are many factors that enter into it." Kelli pauses thoughtfully for a minute, "We need to quit playing naming and blaming games and be compassionate to each other." Kelli takes a deep breath. "I need to stay hopeful that all my health problems will be OK."

■ Conclusion

Although attempts to encourage others to lose weight may be well intentioned, they are based on questionable science and are ill-advised in many ways. The medicalization of fat—the assumption that people's fat is an inherent medical problem that is entirely under their control to fix—results in stigma, hate, prejudice, and in treating fat people like they are not human and do not have rights (Cooper, 1998). As Wann (2009) reminds us, "It is not possible to hate a group of people for their own good" (p. xiv). Interpersonal and mediated communicative attempts to persuade people to lose weight result directly in stigma and marginalization of people who are fat, and indirectly in stress-related medical problems, and ironically, related weight gain. One exception to this is a relatively new social movement called Health at Every Size, which focuses attention on healthy eating and physical fitness for everyone rather than reducing body size for people who are larger sized or assuming that thin automatically equates with health. Health at Every Size also supports biodiversity and acceptance of people of many different body sizes and shapes (Thomas & Wilkerson, 2005).

Discussion Questions

1. This chapter focuses on the stigma associated with body size. Why do you think this stigma, perhaps more than others, is so prevalent in our society?

2. How can stigma affect our health in negative ways? What communicative strategies can help to resist the stigma?

3. Have you experienced a stigmatizing condition? How were your experiences similar to Kelli's? How were they different?

4. Think of a natural process (e.g., aging, childbirth, or weight gain) that has been medicalized in our society. What are the consequences? How have people taken back control? How might we develop strategies for taking back control?

REFERENCES

Asplin, J. R. (2009). Obesity and urolithiasis. *Advances in Chronic Kidney Disease, 16,* 11–20.
Bacon, L. (2012). The contrarian: Health at any size: Why diets are harmful and counterproductive. *Discover Magazine.* Retrieved from http://discovermagazine.com/2012/dec/25-health-at-any-size-why-diets-are-harmful-and-counterproductive#.UyChHeddUt0
Barnes, C. (1996). Theories of disability and the origins of the oppression of disabled people in western society. In L. Barton (Ed.), *Disability and society: Emerging issues and insights* (pp. 19–43). New York, NY: Longman.

Barton, L. (1996). Sociology and disability: Some emerging issues. In L. Barton (Ed.), *Disability and society: Emerging issues and insights* (pp. 3–17). New York, NY: Longman.

Bishop, R. (2005). A philosophy of exhibitionism: Exploring media coverage of Al Roker's and Carnie Wilson's gastric bypass surgeries. *Journal of Communication Inquiry, 29,* 119–140.

Brody, J. E. (2014, July 8). The perils of being obese and pregnant. *The New York Times,* p. D5. Retrieved from http://well.blogs.nytimes.com/2014/07/07/overweight-and-pregnant/?_php=true&_type=blogs&_r=0

Brownell, K. D. (2005). The chronicling of obesity: Growing awareness of its social, economic, and political contexts. *Journal of Health Politics, Policy and Law, 30,* 955.

Cahill, S. E., & Eggleston, R. (1995). Reconsidering the stigma of physical disability: Wheel-chair use and public kindness. *Sociological Quarterly, 36,* 681–698.

Campos, P. (2011). Does fat kill? A critique of the epidemiological evidence. In E. Rich, L. Monaghan, & L. Aphramor (Eds.), *Debating obesity: Critical perspectives* (pp. 36–59). London, UK: Palgrave Macmillan.

Campo, S., & Mastin, T. (2007). Placing the burden on the individual: Overweight and obesity in African American and mainstream women's magazines. *Health Communication, 22,* 229–240.

Carter, R., & Watenpaugh, D. E. (2008). Obesity and obstructive sleep apnea: Or is it OSA and obesity? *Pathophysiology, 15,* 71–77.

Centers for Disease Control and Prevention. (2009). *Defining overweight and obesity.* Retrieved from http://www.cdc.gov/obesity/defining.html

Chung, S. J., Kim, D., Park, M. J., Kim, Y. S., Jung, H. C., & Song, I. S. (2008). Metabolic syndrome and visceral obesity as risk factors for reflux oesophagitis: A cross-sectional case-control study of 7078 Koreans undergoing health check-ups. *Gut: An International Journal of Gastroenterology and Hepatology, 54,* 1360–1365.

Cooper, C. (1998). *Fat and proud: The politics of size.* London, UK: The Women's Press.

Creel, B. R. (2010). *Suffering, hoping, resisting and accepting: Perceptions of overweight women about personal identity and medical care.* Unpublished doctoral dissertation, Texas A&M University.

D'Andrea, W., Sharma, R., Zelechoski, A. D., & Spinazzola, J. (2011). Physical health problems after single trauma exposure: When stress takes root in the body. *Journal of the American Psychiatric Nurses Association, 17,* 378–392.

Davis, C. S. (2013). *Communicating hope: An ethnography of a children's mental health care team.* Walnut Creek, CA: Left Coast Press.

Davis, C. S., Delynko, K. M., & Cook, J. (2010). Oral history of McCreesh Place, apartment building for (formerly) homeless men: Advancing the warp and balancing the weave. *Cultural Studies-Critical Methodologies, 10,* 508–519.

Davis, C. S., & Warren-Findlow, J. (2011). Coping with trauma through fictional narrative ethnography: A primer. *Journal of Loss and Trauma, 16,* 563–572.

Davis, C. S., & Warren-Findlow, J. (2012). The mystery of the troubled breast: Examining cancer and social support through fictional narrative ethnography. *Qualitative Communication Research, 1,* 291–314.

Domoff, S. E., Hinman, N. G., Koball, A. M., Storfer-Isser, A., Carhart, V. L., Baik, K. D., & Carels, R. A. (2012). The effects of reality television on weight bias: An examination of *The Biggest Loser. Obesity, 20,* 993–998.

Donaghue, N. (2014). The moderating effects of socioeconomic status on relationships between obesity framing and stigmatization of fat people. *Fat Studies, 3,* 6–16.

Doty, L. (2014). *Addressing the elephant in the room: A descriptive analysis of weight-based harassment on college campuses.* Unpublished doctoral dissertation, West Virginia University.

Epstein, L., & Ogden, J. (2005). A qualitative study of GPs' views of treating obesity. *The British Journal of General Practice: The Journal of the Royal College of General Practitioners, 55,* 750–754.

Fabricatore, A. N., Wadden, D. A., & Foster, G. D. (2005). Bias in healthcare settings. In K. D. Brownell, R. M. Puhl, M. A. Schwartz, & L. Rudd (Eds.), *Weight bias: Nature, consequences, and remedies* (pp. 29–41). New York, NY: The Guilford Press.

Farrell, A. E. (2011). *Fat shame: Stigma and the fat body in American culture.* New York: NYU Press.

Field, A., Coakley, E., Must, A., Spadano, J., Laird, N., Dietz, W., . . . Colditz, G. A. (2001). Impact of overweight on the risk of developing common chronic diseases during a 10-year period. *Archives of Internal Medicine, 161,* 1581–1586.

Fontaine, K. R., Heo, M., & Allison, D. B. (2001). Body weight and cancer screening among women. *Journal of Women's Health and Gender-Based Medicine, 10,* 463–470.

Foucault, M. (1973). *The birth of the clinic: An archaeology of medical perception* (A. M. S. Smith, Trans.). New York, NY: Pantheon Books.

Foucault, M. (1995). *Discipline and punish: The birth of the prison* (A. Sheridan, Trans.). New York, NY: Random House.

Fouts, G., & Burggraf, K. (2000). Television situation comedies: Female weight, male negative comments, and audience reactions. *Sex Roles, 42,* 925–932.

Fouts, G., & Vaughan, K. (2002). Television situation comedies: Male weight, negative references, and audience reactions. *Sex Roles, 46,* 439–442.

Freedman, J., & Combs, G. (1996). *Narrative therapy: The social construction of preferred realities.* New York, NY: Norton.

Gaesser, G. A. (2002). *Big fat lies: The truth about your weight and your health.* Carlsbad, CA: Grüze Books.

Ghandehari, H., Le, V., Kamal-Bahl, S., Bassin, S. L., & Wong, N. D. (2009). Abdominal obesity and the spectrum of global cardiometabolic risks in US adults. *International Journal of Obesity, 33,* 239–248.

Goffman, E. (1963). *Stigma: Notes on the management of spoiled identity.* Englewood Cliffs, NJ: Prentice-Hall.

Green, S., Davis, C. S., Karshmer, E., Marsh, P., & Straight, B. (2005). Living stigma: The impact of labeling, stereotyping, separation, status loss and discrimination in the lives of individuals with disabilities and their families. *Sociological Inquiry, 75,* 197–215.

Hagedorn, J. C., Encarnacion, B., Brat, G. A., & Morton, J. M. (2007). Does gastric bypass alter alcohol metabolism? *Surgery for Obesity and Related Diseases, 3,* 543–548.

Heron, M. P., Hoyert, D. L., Murphy, S. L., Xu, J. Q., Kochanek, K. D., Tejada-Vera, B. (2009). Deaths: Final data for 2006. *National Vital Statistics Reports, 57*(14). Retrieved from http://www.cdc.gov/nchs/data/nvsr/nvsr57/nvsr57_14.pdf

Hiller, D. V. (1982). Overweight as master status: A replication. *The Journal of Psychology, 110,* 107–113.

Hirshkowitz, M. (2008). The clinical consequences of obstructive sleep apnea and associated excessive sleepiness. *Journal of Family Practice, 57* (Aug Supplement), S9–S16.

Jette, S., Bhagat, K., & Andrews, D. L. (2014). Governing the child-citizen: "Let's Move!" as national biopedagogy. *Sport, Education and Society, 19,* 1–18.

Kim, S. H., & Willis, L. A. (2007). Talking about obesity: News framing of who is responsible for causing and fixing the problem. *Journal of Health Communication, 12,* 359–376.

Kleinman, A. (1988). *The illness narratives: Suffering, healing, and the human condition.* New York, NY: Basic Books.

Laing, R. D., Phillipson, H., & Lee, A. R. (1966). *Interpersonal perception: A theory and a method of research.* London, UK: Springer.

LeBesco, K. (2004). *Revolting bodies? The struggle to redefine fat identity.* Amherst: University of Massachusetts Press.

Leitzmann, M. F., Koebnick, C., Danforth, K. N., Brinton, L. A., Moore, S. C., Hollenbeck, A. R., . . . Lacy, J. L., Jr. (2009). Body mass index and risk of ovarian cancer. *Cancer, 115,* 812–822.

Link, B. G., & Phelan, J. C. (2001). Conceptualizing stigma. *Annual Review of Sociology, 27,* 363–385.

Link, B. G., Struening, E., Cullen, F. T., & Shrout, P. E. (1989). A modified labeling theory approach to mental disorders: An empirical assessment. *American Sociological Review, 54,* 400–423.

Lupton, D. (2013). *Fat.* New York, NY: Routledge.

Macionis, J. J. (1995). *Sociology.* Englewood Cliffs, NJ: Prentice-Hall.

Marks, D. (1999). *Disability: Controversial debates and psychosocial perspectives.* London, UK: Routledge.

Matthews, K. A., Salomon, K., Kenyon, K., & Zhou, F. (2005). Unfair treatment, discrimination, and ambulatory blood pressure in black and white adolescents. *Health Psychology, 24,* 258–265.

Mischler, E. (1984). *The discourse of medicine: Dialectics of medical interviews.* Norwood, NJ: Ablex.

Nguyen, N. T., Magno, C. P., Lane, K. T., Hinojosa, M. W., & Lane, J. S. (2008). Association of hypertension, diabetes, dyslipidemia, and metabolic syndrome with obesity: Findings from the National Health and Nutrition Examination Survey, 1996–2004. *Journal of the American College of Surgeons, 207,* 928–934.

Oddy, W. H., DeKlerk, N. H., Miller, M., Payne, J., & Bower, C. (2009). Association of maternal pre-pregnancy weight with birth defects: Evidence from a case-control study in Western Australia. *Australian and New Zealand Journal of Obstetrics and Gynaecology, 49,* 11–15.

Oliver, J. E. (2006). *Fat politics: The real story behind America's obesity epidemic.* New York, NY: Oxford University Press.

Prevalence of overweight and obesity among adults: United States, 2003–2004 (2006). Centers for Disease Control and Prevention/National Center for Health Statistics. Retrieved from http://www.cdc.gov/nchs/products/pubs/pubd/hestats/overweight /overwght_adult_03.htm

Puhl, R. (2015). *Understanding the negative stigma of obesity and its consequences.* Tampa, FL: Obesity Action Coalition. Retrieved from: http://www.obesityaction.org/educational-resources/resource-articles-2/weight-bias/understanding-the-negative-stigma-of-obesity-and-its-consequences

Puhl, R. M., & Brownell, K. D. (2006). Confronting and coping with weight stigma: An investigation of overweight and obese adults. *Obesity, 14,* 1802–1815.

Puhl, R. M., & Heuer, C. A. (2009). The stigma of obesity: A review and update. *Obesity, 17,* 941–964.

Puhl, R. M., & Latner, J. D. (2007). Stigma, obesity, and the health of the nation's children. *Psychological Bulletin, 133,* 557–580.

Puhl, R. M., Luedicke, J., & Heuer, C. (2011). Weight-based victimization toward overweight adolescents: Observations and reactions of peers. *Journal of School Health, 81,* 696–703.

Puhl, R. M., Moss-Racusin, C. A., & Schwartz, M. D. (2007). Internalization of weight-bias: Implications for binge eating and emotional well-being. *Obesity, 15,* 19–23.

Quinlan, M. M. (2010a). Dancing Wheels: Integration and diversity. In L. Black (Ed.), *Group communication: Cases for analysis, appreciation, and application* (pp. 43–48). Dubuque, IA: Kendall/Hunt.

Quinlan, M. M. (2010b). Fostering connections among diverse individuals through multi-sensorial storytelling. *Health Communication, 25,* 91–93.

Quinlan, M. M., & Bates, B. R. (2015). Unsmoothing the cyborg: Technology and the body in integrated dance. *Disability Studies Quarterly.* http://dsq-sds.org/article/view/3783/3792

Quinlan, M. M., & Harter, L. M. (2010). Meaning in motion: The embodied poetics and politics of Dancing Wheels. *Text & Performance Quarterly, 30,* 374–395.

Robinson, T., Callister, M., & Jankoski, T. (2008). Portrayal of body weight on children's television sitcoms: A content analysis. *Body Image, 5,* 141–151.

Rothblum, E., & Solovay, S. (Eds.). (2009). *The fat studies reader.* New York: NYU Press.

Salk, R. H., & Engeln-Maddox, R. (2011). "If you're fat, then I'm humongous": Frequency, content, and impact of fat talk among college women. *Psychology of Women Quarterly, 35,* 18–28.

Schnurr, P. P., & Green, B. L. (2004). *Trauma and health: Physical health consequences of exposure to extreme stress.* Washington, DC: American Psychological Association.

Seacat, J. D., Dougal, S. D. & Roy, D. (2014, online ahead of print). A daily diary assessment of female weight stigmatization. *Journal of Health Psychology.* Retrieved from http://hpq.sagepub.com.librarylink.uncc.edu/content/early/2014/03/17/1359105314525067.full.pdf+html

Smith, R. A. (2011). Stigma, communication, and health. In T. Thompson, R. Parrott, & J. Nussbaum (Eds.), *The Routledge handbook of health communication* (2nd ed., pp. 455–468). New York, NY: Routledge.

Spinetta, C. M. (2013). *Fat and fit: A culture-centered approach toward a new paradigm of health and the body.* Unpublished doctoral dissertation, Purdue University.

Strate, L. L., Liu, Y. L., Aldoori, W. H., Syngal, S., & Giovannucci, E. L. (2009). Obesity increases the risk of diverticulitis and diverticular bleeding. *Gastroenterology, 36,* 115–122.

Susman, J. (1994). Disability, stigma and deviance. *Social Science and Medicine, 38,* 15–22.

Szasz, T. (1970). *The manufacture of madness.* New York, NY: Harper & Row.

Szasz, T. (1987). *Insanity: The idea and its consequences.* New York, NY: John Wiley.

Thomas, P., & Wilkerson, C. (2005). *Taking up space: How eating well and exercising regularly changed my life.* Nashville, TN: Pearlsong Press.

Torres, S. J., & Nowson, C. A. (2007). Relationship between stress, eating behavior, and obesity. *Nutrition, 23,* 887–894.

Veverka, A. (2014, August 25). Here's the truth on obesity research. *The Charlotte Observer,* p. 2C.

Vireday, P. (2011, June 10). Maternal obesity: A view from all sides. Retrieved from http://www.scienceandsensibility.org/?p=3030

Wann, M. (2009). Foreword. Fat studies: An invitation to revolution. In E. Rothblum & S. Solovay (Eds.), *The fat studies reader* (pp. ix–xxv). New York: NYU Press.

Wilson, J. A., & Clark, J. J. (2003). Obesity: Impediment to wound healing. *Critical Care Nursing Quarterly, 26,* 119–132.

Ylostalo, P., Suominen-Taipale, L., Reunanen, A., & Knuuttila, M. (2008). Association between body weight and periodontal infection. *Journal of Clinical Periodontology, 35,* 297–304.

9

Communicating through Health Challenges

Elissa Foster

■ My Eyes Cry without Me[1]

The First Ultrasound: August 2008

Holding hands with [my partner] Jay in a darkened exam room; staring at a large flat screen monitor high on the opposite wall; lying prone beside an enormous piece of computer equipment. The technician[2] gently folds down my trousers and folds up my shirt.

"This may be a bit cold," she says, and squirts gel onto my lower abdomen. "You're only eight weeks along, so we may not be able to find the baby from the outside."

I shoot a look at Jay. I didn't know there was an alternative. The "inside" version of the ultrasound is never shown in the movies or on TV.

She pushes the transducer impossibly low and I can see why they ask women to empty their bladders. In seconds, she is clicking the computer to show us our baby. After three years of "trying"—the moment feels both unreal and intensely real.

"There's the Cheerio!" Jay exclaims. Although the baby is now the size of a bay shrimp, the size analogy in our pregnancy book for week seven—when the baby was "the size and shape of a Cheerio cut in half" [Shanahan, 2000, p. 48]—was so surprising that the name stuck. Jay grins and squeezes my hand. Our eyes focus on the center of the "body," where a butterfly appears to flutter its wings in happy agitation.

"Ready to hear the heartbeat?" she asks, and, before we can respond, half the screen fills with pulsating lines as the room beats with an instant, rapid rhythm.

"Chill out dude!" Jay urges.

"Actually, 170 beats per minute—that's perfect," she says.

I don't say anything. I just try to absorb the "other-ness" of this little being—that heartbeat, coming from me but not of me. I think, "You go little Cheerio! You go."

The Second Ultrasound: September 2008

Three weeks after the initial ultrasound I walk a short block to the clinic, grateful to have a doctor who is also a friend. Holly is not seeing patients today, but after four days of slight bleeding and "watchful waiting" she asks me to come for an exam.

"It doesn't sound like there's anything to worry about, but let's just have a look and see what might be going on."

This week, I searched my pregnancy books to find information about spotting. I turned from one book's index to the indicated page to find myself in a chapter called "Dashed Hopes" [Shanahan, 2000, p. 55], which indicates that 80 percent of miscarriages occur before the eighth week, but that 20 percent will occur later. I skillfully compartmentalize my reaction to this text and wait for information that is not based on statistics but is specifically about me.

Holly is in charge of the family medicine maternity care curriculum, so I expect that I will experience the definitive gyn exam—feet in the footrests ("Not stirrups," she explains, "No one's riding a horse here"), announcements of every step, slow and reassuring. My cervix is "closed," she tells me, so it's not clear what the bleeding portends.

"Let's have a listen," Holly suggests, picking up the handheld Doppler ultrasound that she used during last month's exam. She listens intently and for a long time as she moves the transducer across my belly. Last month it was too early to hear the heartbeat [with the Doppler handheld ultrasound in Holly's office] and I remember this as she continues the exam. "Come on little Cheerio!" Holly says quietly, and something in the tone of her voice ignites the tinder of anxiety that I had not yet acknowledged.

Holly turns off the Doppler saying, "Why don't you get dressed and I'll be back in a moment?" I hear her speaking to someone outside but only one phrase distinguishes itself from the others—"if the pregnancy is still viable."

Re-entering the room she asks, "What else do you have going on today?"

I quickly dismiss my next meeting. She explains that not finding the heartbeat is "a bit concerning," so she has arranged for us to go to the women's center at the hospital across the street for a more complete ultrasound, just to be sure.

"But what do you have going on today?" I ask.

"This is what I have going on today," Holly smiles and dissolves any protest.

* * *

After a short wait, a dark-haired technician escorts us back to an exam room, larger but quite similar to the one that Jay and I visited only a few weeks ago.

The technician asks, "How are you feeling?"

"A little nervous," I admit. "I am an 'elderly primigravida,'"[3] I note, only semi-seriously. She smiles kindly.

I lie back and feel the gel, followed by the transducer moving fairly quickly across my abdomen. My eyes are focused on the wall monitor, so I'm surprised when the technician stops and says, "I'd feel better if we do this transvaginally."

"Have you had one of these before?" she asks. I shake my head; she holds up the clearly phallic transducer and declares seriously, "As you can see, it's nothing too different from what you would have already experienced."

I laugh; grateful for some levity. The technician raises an eyebrow.

I go to the adjacent change room and disrobe from the waist down. I return and quickly position myself on the exam table. Holly stands beside me—ready.

The exam proceeds and I am, again, transfixed by the screen, strangely oblivious to the presence of the transducer between my legs. Holly takes my hand. I watch as this technician, like the first, identifies the baby and clicks the computer to record measurements. No one speaks. I stare at the screen and wonder why it looks like the baby has turned its back on us and, at the same moment, I realize that the butterfly is gone. Tears escape across my temples as I turn my face to the ceiling. An intense internal struggle begins as I tell myself that "no one has said anything yet; I don't really know anything," and yet, somehow, my eyes continue to cry.

Like before, the technician flips a switch, but, this time there is no insistent rhythm and the lines on the screen are flat.

"You can get dressed now," the technician says quietly. I go into the change room and dress in a fog, refusing to allow any thoughts to form in my mind. My body, in contrast, is internally frenzied as my pulse roars and my hands shake.

Holly turns as I emerge from the change room. "It's not good news," she says.

Holly holds me. The technician leaves the room. I wail with abandon as I feel the stories, plans, and hopes we have constructed for our family dismantled and discarded by waves of realization—"It's over. It's over. It's over."

I regain enough composure to ask Holly, "What happens now?"

Holly explains that she can schedule a D and C [dilation and curettage] or that I can wait for the miscarriage to happen on its own.

"When will it happen?" my voice is small, like a child's.

"There's no way to know exactly," she tells me gently, "But if it doesn't happen in the next five days, we'll need to schedule the D and C anyway." As she continues to explain the details, I note that Holly uses the term "products of conception" to describe what will be "passed" during the miscarriage or D and C. So quickly, we have moved on from referring to "the baby." The Cheerio has disappeared.

When we leave the exam room, the technician is right outside the door. "I'm so sorry." She reaches out to hug me and whispers in my ear, "Please don't despair."

Becoming a parent and growing a family is a life transition that is celebrated, promoted, and, for most people, taken for granted as an essential part of maturing and participating in society. Beyond this dominant narrative of reproductive success are the *personal complexities* of those who face unplanned pregnancy, difficulty conceiving or sustaining a pregnancy, or the loss of a baby through premature labor or stillbirth. As illustrated in this opening narrative—in which I was an older mother (an "elderly primigravida" at 38 years old), who had been trying to conceive for three years—individuals transitioning to parenthood have unique stories and experiences. In turn, these experiences are negotiated through communication with a myriad of healthcare professionals, and navigated through a range of *cultural and political complexities*. When individuals and families face healthcare challenges or transitions, including pregnancy and childbirth, the quality of their communication with others contributes greatly to their capacity to create meaning and attain health-affirming outcomes.

In this chapter, I address communication surrounding challenging healthcare events, including receiving "bad news" such as a negative test outcome or terminal diagnosis, working through a stressful life transition, or facing the end of life. In many cases, I focus on the communication between healthcare practitioners[4] and patient; however, members of a patient's family and social support network are also an important part of the communication system and are addressed throughout the chapter. Across all topics, I emphasize the importance of maintaining a balance between attending to the content of a message as well as its implications for the relationship (Watzlawick, Beavin, & Jackson, 1967)—a perspective that aligns with relational communication theory (Bochner, 1978, 1984; Millar & Rogers, 1976; Rogers & Escudero, 2004).

Although the content and relationship dimensions of a message are inseparable, the relationship dimension of the message is more implicit, less observable, and more difficult to control. As a result, many efforts at assisting people to improve communication, including aspects of the models present in this chapter, tend to focus on content and process. Although scripts and checklists can help people know *what* to say when navigating a health crisis, it is also extremely important that communicators attend to *how* they are communicating—the implicit messages that let others know that an individual is present, listening, and honoring another's unfolding story.

■ Breaking Bad News: Practitioner–Patient Communication

In the days and weeks following the second ultrasound procedure described in the opening narrative, my mind returned to the moment of seeing the ultrasound image and the struggle I experienced between the grief in my body (my eyes crying without me) and my mind's refusal to accept the evidence that our baby was lost. Performance theory draws attention to the body as a site of meaning in relation to mothering and grief (e.g., Holman Jones, 2005; Pineau, 2000; Pollock, 1999; Spry, 2000). Furthermore, the performative power of communication is identified in speech act theory (Austin, 1983), which explains that certain realities come to exist through the speaking of the words that declare them to be (e.g., "I declare you husband and wife"; "The defendant is guilty"). The construct of "breaking bad news" centers on the speech act of diagnosis, prognosis, or sharing life-altering information, recognizing that a new reality for the patient is created through the speaking of the words. Although the reality of my miscarriage preceded the diagnosis by many days, my physician's declaration created the reality for me. Holly's words marked the end of the pregnancy even more profoundly than viewing the ultrasound image or the physical loss of the pregnancy that came later. This same power to create reality through words is the purview of any healthcare practitioner delivering a diagnosis, any member of a support network offering comfort or advice, or any stranger responding to an evident crisis.

The medical sonographer in the second scene of the opening narrative stuck very close to her professional script as she conducted my examination. Although sonographers must be able to correctly identify the conditions that they are seeking to image, because of the *political complexities* related to their position within the medical hierarchy, they are not permitted to "diagnose," nor are they permitted to communicate to the patient any information pertaining to the images (Foster & McGivern, 2014). Typically, a patient in my situation would be sent for her ultrasound examination, then left to wait in uncertainty for minutes or hours until the results could be communicated back—from the radiographer, to the nurse or primary care provider, to the patient. Although this professional boundary is established in some ways to protect the patient from potential misdiagnosis or receiving only partial information, in other ways it can profoundly isolate the patient as well as silence the sonographer at a time when compassion is desperately needed. The emotional labor (Hochschild, 2003) associated with this silencing of sonographers increases the stress of an already difficult clinical situation. I was extremely fortunate to have a physician who was willing to walk beside me—literally and figuratively—as I faced the loss of a much-wanted pregnancy. Not all patients are so lucky, and some will argue that the current limitations and *political complexities* of the healthcare system mean that not all physicians are empowered to go the extra mile that Holly did with me. And as for the sonographer, she could easily have left that exam room and gone to see her next patient having completed a professional and proficient examination—but she stayed, and communicated her compassion and support of me in a manner that I will always remember.

Breaking bad news (Buckman, 1984) to patients and family members is one of the inevitable and unenviable aspects of providing healthcare. Perhaps for this reason, a number of models have been developed to assist healthcare practitioners, particularly physicians to whom this responsibility mostly falls (Narayanan, Bista, & Koshy, 2010; VandeKieft, 2001). In the following sections, I present the protocol most widely taught in the medical context (SPIKES), and then introduce the COMFORT approach, which has been developed, tested, and disseminated by health communication scholars and takes a comprehensive approach to the task of navigating difficult communication. I also discuss the role of empathy in the delivery of bad news, and offer an additional model—BATHE—as a structured method of framing and delivering an empathic response, whether you are a practitioner, a family member, or a member of a support network.

The SPIKES Protocol

The SPIKES protocol for delivering bad news (Baile et al., 2000; Kaplan, 2010; Shetty & Shapiro, 2012) is widely taught in the medical education context as an approach to breaking bad news. The six letters of the acronym stand for: S—Setting up the interview; P—assessing the patient's Perception (what the patient already knows about her condition); I—obtaining the patient's Invitation (making sure that the patient is ready to receive the news); K—giving Knowledge and information to the patient; E—addressing the patient's emotions with Empathic responses; S—Strategy and Summary (if the patient is ready, moving the conversation toward a plan of treatment or next steps). The SPIKES protocol encompasses *process* elements (specifically, making sure that the physical and emotional context of the conversation is appropriate and supportive), *content* elements (specific scripting), and *relational* elements (attending and responding to the emotional cues of the patient). However, the protocol has been critiqued because it tends to fulfill its function of reducing physician anxiety while delivering bad news, while not sufficiently facilitating the development and delivery of emotionally supportive messages (Goldsmith, Wittenberg-Lyles, Villagran, & Sanchez-Reilly, 2008).

The COMFORT Approach

In response to limitations of existing protocols intended to guide clinicians (physicians, nurses, and others) in the breaking of bad news, Villagran, Goldsmith, Wittenberg-Lyles, and Baldwin (2010) developed COMFORT—a set of competencies grounded in interaction adaptation theory (Burgoon, Stern, & Dillman, 1995) and centered on principles of relational communication (Rogers & Escudero, 2004; see also, Goldsmith, Ferrell, Wittenberg-Lyles, & Ragan, 2013; Wittenberg-Lyles, Goldsmith, Richardson, Hallett, & Clark, 2013). The emphasis of the COMFORT competencies is on the practitioner's ongoing adaptation to the communication of the patient. "COMFORT is not a linear guide for BBN [breaking bad news] performance by clinicians, but rather a set of competencies that should occur reflexively and concurrently by patients, family members, and providers" (Villagran et al., 2010, p. 225). This approach is designed to facilitate a co-constructed series of encounters that meets the essential requirements of the BBN conversation but avoids a routinized or clinician-driven orientation. Although the COMFORT model was developed primarily for guiding communication education related to palliative care, in most of the descriptions that follow I link each of the COMFORT competencies back to the example of acute care and delivering bad news in the narrative that began this chapter.

In the COMFORT approach, C—Communication—refers to core skills of communicating clear verbal (content) messages in concert with nonverbal (relational) messages that maintain a sense of immediacy and connection among the communicators. One of the least successful aspects of breaking bad news efforts by medical students (Goldsmith et al., 2008; Villagran et al., 2010) is in presenting bad news clearly and unambiguously (particularly when it comes to disclosing a terminal diagnosis) and also in communicating supportive emotional messages. An important emphasis within the COMFORT approach is understanding that content and relational messages are always being communicated simultaneously and therefore must be attended to with equal care.

In the opening narrative of this chapter, Holly (my physician) remained physically present throughout the examination and knew from my nonverbal cues that I must have suspected the worst. Although the words of her diagnosis—"It's not good news"—were ambiguous, they were enough to convey clearly and without delay that the pregnancy was over and, at the same time, communicate the information with sufficient gentleness and empathy to let me know that she understood what I had been hoping to hear and that she was about to shatter my hopes.

O—Orientation and Opportunity—encompasses the orientation of the patient and practitioner with respect to culture and health literacy. The emphasis in this step is on adapting to the situation by recognizing that the patient/family member and practitioner may not (almost certainly do not) share the same orientation to the patient's condition, nor do they share the same understanding of health and illness. Nothing should be assumed at this point; rather, the conversation should include a dialogue through which practitioner and patient explore opportunities to reach a shared understanding of the situation and available options.

Although from a cultural and political perspective, I was a well-educated patient and somewhat higher on the health literacy scale than many, when it came to facing my personal story of miscarriage, I felt overwhelmed and in need of guidance. Patients and family members may react in ways that run counter to their expressed values when faced with the actuality of a life-changing diagnosis or terminal prognosis, and so, according to the model, all options should be offered and engaged through dialogue. Holly was able to understand and respond to each of my questions as they arose. Because she was my friend as well as my practitioner, she already suspected that I would be resistant to undergoing a D and C; nevertheless, she presented me with both options for responding to the loss of my pregnancy.

M—Mindfulness—in this case refers to the capacity to be "in the moment" with a patient and represents a key difference between the articulation of the COMFORT model and other protocols described here. Although the various BBN protocols emphasize that they *are not* scripts and that practitioners will need to improvise and respond spontaneously to the patient and family members, they reinforce the expectation with step-by-step phases that the "bad news conversation" should at the very least proceed in an orderly sequence. Given the highly emotional nature of conversations around life-changing health events, it can be extremely difficult for practitioners and patients alike to remain "in the moment" with one another. Mindfulness requires attending to both the cues of the patient and the practitioner's own internal cues in order to respond with authenticity, even if it means "abandoning the script" (Wittenberg-Lyles, Goldsmith, & Ragan, 2010, p. 287).

In the opening narrative, the medical sonographer abandoned her professional script by waiting for the opportunity to acknowledge my loss and offer words of comfort. Although other sonographers later critiqued this act when I shared my story with them on the grounds that it was "unprofessional" (Foster & McGivern, 2014), her witnessing and honoring of my grief in that moment was essential to my capacity to cope both then and going forward. Note that the words exchanged are far less significant to this aspect of communication than the person's capacity to demonstrate that she/he is willing to "be there" with the other (Goldsmith et al., 2013, p. 167).

F—Family—encapsulates a set of competencies that relate to communicating with the patient and family as part of what is known in hospice and palliative medicine as the unit of care. In most challenging health situations, and particularly in cases of chronic or terminal illness or disability, family members are implicated because of their essential role in offering social support and hands-on caregiving. The key components of conducting a family meeting are described later in this chapter; however, an additional perspective on family communication offered by the COMFORT model is worth elaborating here. Family communication patterns can be identified according to two characteristics: conversation and conformity (Goldsmith et al., 2013; Wittenberg-Lyles, Goldsmith, Parker Oliver, Demeris, & Rankin, 2012). The conversation characteristic describes how much or how little a family shares with one another and what they choose to discuss. The conformity characteristic describes the extent to which the family desires to be in agreement with one another as a group. Understanding how the family enacts each of these two characteristics can aid considerably in helping clinicians navigate the complexity of sharing bad news and facilitate subsequent decision-making.

Although family members were not a key feature of the interaction during the opening narrative, my partner Jay was a profound presence-in-absence at the moment of receiving the diagnosis. I was fortunate that he was working nearby and, rather than finding him and having to break the news to him alone, that Holly stayed with me, walked with me, and was present to answer Jay's questions when we were able to meet together. Sadly, we then undertook the necessary task of contacting the friends and family members who knew about the pregnancy to break the news to them. At one point, I recall that we asked a member of Jay's family to contact others because, as

Jay put it, we "could not face uttering the words one more time." As with other instances of "bad news," the repercussions of a challenging health event can ripple out beyond immediate family members and those who might be involved in a family meeting. Helping family members to identify and call on support can be a significant step in establishing an emotional and practical safety net.

The second O in COMFORT has been variously labeled as Ongoing (Villagran et al., 2010), Openings (Goldsmith et al., 2013), and Oversight (Wittenberg-Lyles et al., 2010). Despite the various terms, however, this competency relates to the important work of communicating to ensure support beyond the exigencies of the immediate diagnosis or health transition. Sometimes, this involves the practitioner's assurances of support, and it also includes dialogue with the patient and family around the coordination of care and social support needs related to the challenging health situation. The commitment to ongoing care of the patient has become particularly important in the current U.S. healthcare system where increased specialization of roles may lead to significant gaps in care (Wittenberg-Lyles et al., 2010). The mindful communication that transitions a patient from direct care of health practitioners to her/his home environment is also referred to as "safety-netting" (Miller, 2004).

R refers to Reiterative communication (Villagran et al., 2010), Reiteration and Radically Adaptive messages (Wittenberg-Lyles, et al., 2010), and Relating (Goldsmith et al., 2013). In this competency, practitioners are encouraged to view "bad news" communication with patients and family members as an ongoing process rather than as a one-time event. Not only are patients and family members unlikely to be able to take in the full implications of their health challenge in a single sitting, but their needs for information and support will change over time. Even in a single meeting, practitioners may need to repeat information in several different ways in order to have the best chance that patients and family members will fully understand the content and its implications. A significant emphasis of this competency is *nonlinearity*—meaning that a simple sequence of communication is unlikely to result in successful coordination of meaning between the practitioner/healthcare team and the patient. As with the principle of mindfulness, the concept of radically adaptive messages makes the COMFORT approach different from the other models for breaking bad news.

T—Team structure and processes of care—is an aspect of the COMFORT approach that speaks particularly to the context of communication in hospice and palliative care (see section later in this chapter), but as more patients face complex and chronic illness, it is an increasingly important aspect of primary care as well. An important feature of the shift to a team-based approach to communication and care is a shift in the physician role from the top of a chain of command to a more collaborative and facilitative role. Depending on the circumstances, a nurse practitioner, nurse, social worker, chaplain, physical therapist, or other health professional may be called on to advise and lead a team responding to the needs of a patient and family.

In sum, the COMFORT approach—although it is presented as a method for breaking bad news—is a set of guiding principles that can assist individual practitioners and teams in communicating effectively in the context of patients' health challenges. The principles are grounded in a relational approach to communication that perceives meaning as emerging between practitioners and patients in a nonlinear, mutually influencing, and highly individualized process.

The BATHE Model: Responding with Empathy

An essential capacity or competency of practitioners who are called to respond to patients' health challenges is *empathy* for others. At its core, empathy encompasses skills of attending to the emotions of another person (relational), understanding those emotions (cognitive), and responding to those emotions (communicative) (Buckman, Tulsky, & Rodin, 2011; Suchman, Merkakis, Beckman, & Frankel, 1997). As with skills of breaking bad news, however, physicians are often not skilled at responding to the emotional cues of patients and will tend to focus on responding to clinical questions and providing information rather than addressing expressions of feeling (Buckman et al., 2011). Friends and family members may also find themselves struggling when confronted by the many difficult emotions that can accompany a challenging health situation—be it a miscarriage or infertility, diagnosis of a chronic or life-limiting condition, or the impact of mental illness. This section introduces a set of guidelines to help communicators both perceive and respond empathically to expressions of emotion.

One approach (Suchman et al., 1997) begins with the capacity to attend to the communication of patients or family members in order to identify and respond to *empathic opportunities* (explicit expressions of emotion) or *potential empathic opportunities* (implied expression of emotion). Once these opportunities are identified, practitioners and others may respond with an *empathic response,* a *potential empathic opportunity continuer,* or an *empathic opportunity terminator.* For example, if a patient is silent immediately after receiving a diagnosis, this would constitute a potential empathic opportunity to which family members or practitioners could respond by inviting an explicit expression of emotion with a potential empathic opportunity continuer (e.g., "I can tell that this is a lot for you to take in; how are you feeling about what I've just told you?"). If the patient bursts into tears after the diagnosis, this constitutes an empathic opportunity, because it is clear that the patient is feeling a strong emotion, although family members or practitioners should not assume to know what it is. An empathic response would be, "I am so sorry to have brought you such distressing news," or possibly "I can understand why this is so difficult for you," or even simply reaching out a hand and a box of tissues to offer comfort. The empathic opportunity terminator is any response that ignores the emotions in the room (of both the patient and the practitioner) and steamrolls ahead with a task-oriented agenda.

Another technique that has been designed to support empathic responses is BATHE (Miller, 2004; Stuart & Lieberman, 2002), an acronym that offers a 5-part script for responding in situations in which a patient or family member is experiencing strong emotion and is possibly overwhelmed by current circumstances. Although this model offers a sequenced script (much like the SPIKES model), the emphasis of the person enacting BATHE should be on helping the other individuals to identify, express, and begin to gain an understanding of his/her emotions—the words and the order of the script are only a guide.

The BATHE process includes asking the other person for B—Background information ("What has been going on? What has upset you?"); exploring A—Affect (both affect as in emotion and affect as in "How has this affected you emotionally?"); inviting the person to identify one aspect of the problem or T—Trouble ("What troubles you the most about this situation?"); helping the other person focus attention on how she/he has been H—Handling the situation or responding emotionally and practically ("How have you been handling this diagnosis?"); responding with E—Empathy—means responding without trying to change or fix the situation or the emotional response of the patient ("Sounds like you've been working hard to keep things going;" "Seems like a very stressful time for you.").

Underlying both the framework of empathic opportunities and responses (Suchman et al., 1997) and BATHE (Stuart & Lieberman, 2002) is a relational quality of handing over the stage to patients, allowing them the space, and providing the mindful attention necessary to support and hold their emotions. Although BATHE, like the other models, was designed for clinicians, all of us may at some point be called upon to offer empathy during a challenging health situation. Remembering the key steps of the BATHE model can help us be present and supportive of others without trying to change or fix a situation whose outcome may be unforeseeable.

Now, examine a time when you received bad news, using Theorizing Practice 9.1 as a guide.

Theorizing Practice 9.1
Receiving Bad News

Think of a time when you received bad news. Identify whether this was an example of effective or ineffective communication. Use one or more of the protocols described in the chapter—SPIKES, COMFORT, or BATHE—to analyze this event and identify what was done well and what might have been missing. Pay attention to what was accomplished in terms of adapting the *process* of the communication, the *content,* and the *relational* messages to help you cope with the bad news. If the adaptation was inadequate, what could have been changed to improve it?

■ Chronic Illness and Family Caregiving

When the diagnosis is not terminal but is life changing, families are typically involved in making ongoing and progressive decisions in support of the person who is ill. Because of the vast advances in medicine in the last 50 years, many conditions that were once swiftly terminal are becoming chronic and in need of ongoing management at home. Although social support is covered elsewhere in this volume (see Chapter 10), the topic of communication through health challenges must necessarily include models of communication that involve families. This section discusses the *family systems* approach, the *family development spiral* model for understanding health transitions in the family setting, and the *family meeting* as a particular ritual facilitated and supported by one or more healthcare practitioners at a time of decision making.

Family Systems and the Family Life Cycle

Within the communication discipline, family communication is grounded in a relational perspective that emphasizes meaning as constructed *in between* people rather than *within* individuals (Bochner, 1978, 1984; Millar & Rogers, 1976; Rogers & Escudero, 2004). General systems theory (Sieburg, 1985), structural family therapy (Lannamann, 1989; Minuchin, 1974), and the work of Gregory Bateson (1972) and the Palo Alto Group (Watzlawick et al., 1967) provided a theoretical framework for understanding families as constituted through interaction, ritual, and storytelling. Parallel developments in psychology (Ackerman, 1966; Haley, 1963; Satir, 1967) perceived individual behavioral problems as being reflective of the family system in which the individual was embedded. The perspective that the health of the individual and the health of the family are interrelated is most evident in the specialty of family medicine, which is characterized by (1) a lifespan perspective on care and (2) the identification of the family rather than the individual as the context of care (a perspective that is also reflected in hospice and palliative care as a specialty).

The family development spiral proposed by Miller and Cohen-Katz (first published in Foster & Cohen-Katz, 2011) is a reformulation of the family life cycle model (Carter & McGoldrick, 1980, 1988, 1999) that maps out key moments of transition in the history of a family. It is a developmental model in that it begins with the family of origin, moves through the phases of "launching" and formulation of a new family unit, encompasses phases of different manners of parenting (including adoption, "aunt-ing" and "uncle-ing") as well as reevaluations of the "adult unit" of the family (including changes in sexual orientation, later life marriage, divorce, widowhood), and moves to shifting generational roles in which the younger generation is

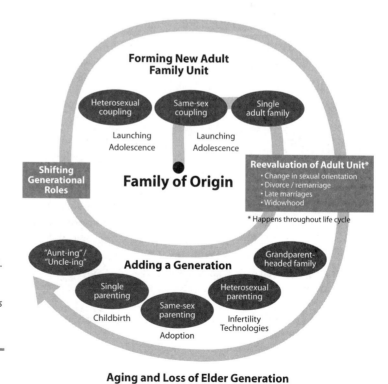

Source: Copyright 2010, Miller, W. L., & Cohen-Katz, J. L., published in Miller-Day, M. (2011). *Family communication, connections, and health transitions: Going through this together* (p. 228). New York, NY: Peter Lang.

Figure 9.1   Family Development Spiral

"launched" and a new family of origin begins. Although the concept of the family life cycle has been around for decades, the reformulation presented here responds specifically to critiques that the earlier models assumed heterosexuality, traditional gender roles, and reinforced dominant notions of a nuclear family that can no longer be assumed. The family development spiral aims to reflect a broad spectrum of family life, including same-sex marriages and parenting, multigenerational parenting, single-parent families, and informal caregiving relationships with children.

Implications of the family development spiral for communicating through health challenges are vast. First, understanding family from an inclusive, fluid, and developmental perspective can help health practitioners remember that many variations of family can and do exist. Second, there is often a reciprocal relationship between health challenges and transitions in family life—a couple divorces and an adolescent child shows signs of chemical dependency; a chronic illness diagnosis signals the shifting of a caregiving parent into a more dependent role; a couple struggles to become pregnant and seeks assistance with fertility treatments; a single parent finds herself caught between the needs of caregiving for an aging parent and raising children of her own and begins to gain weight and suffer from insomnia. A third implication is that health challenges and transitions of individuals come to be viewed within the context of a family, and practitioners can be more actively aware of the impact of family communication on the care and decision making of the patient. Indeed, it becomes difficult to perceive the patient without considering the network of family relationships surrounding him/her.

The Family Meeting

The family meeting is a communication format employed by a range of health practitioners, typically in an inpatient environment, such as a hospital or nursing home, during a time of health challenge or transition, such as a new diagnosis or a change in the patient's condition. The format of the meeting includes fairly predictable tasks, including setting the stage, joining with the family and building rapport, discovering goals for the meeting, facilitating discussion, brainstorming resources, developing a plan, and documenting and debriefing (McDaniel, Campbell, Hepworth, & Lorenz, 2005). At such times, multiple family members tend to be involved and invested in the care of the patient, and so the principal role of the practitioner is to serve as a facilitator of the meeting rather than as an advisor or decision maker. Although breaking bad news may be an instigating factor in the decision to hold a family meeting, many other contingencies may result in the need for the patient and family members to gather together with one or more members of a healthcare team in order to arrive at some consensus—decisions about hospitalization or transition to residential care, decisions about life-sustaining treatment or initiating hospice care, or simply gaining a better understanding about the wishes of the patient. The section that follows focuses on a particularly significant context for challenging health communication that often requires communication among family members—the end of life.

HCIA 9.1

Communication Challenges in Family Care

Katherine Miller

In 2004, we reached a painful and difficult decision. My parents could no longer live independently in their Florida condominium, thousands of miles away from their four daughters. Dad definitely didn't want to leave, but it was clear Mom could no longer care for him after his two strokes. They had to move closer to a daughter, and for reasons including climate and my somewhat flexible schedule as a college professor, I was that daughter. So, for more than seven years, I was a caregiver. However, I was also an academic who studied issues in health and family communication, so I decided to undertake research about the communication challenges involved in providing care for elderly parents.

I worked with graduate student colleagues (Jennifer Willyard, Martha Shoemaker, and Penny Addison) at Texas A&M University and at Arizona State University (Lauren Amaro) on a series of research projects considering questions of how caregivers define themselves in the caregiving role, how they interact with their parents, the challenges of accessing community resources, and—especially—how communication among siblings influences both decisions in the twilight of parents' lives and the ongoing experience

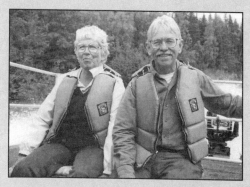

Courtesy of Katherine Miller, personal collection.

of providing care. Our joint research involved in-depth interviews with family caregivers from across the United States, and Lauren's dissertation considered responses to an online survey completed by family caregivers and one of their siblings. Here are just a few important takeaways from our work.

First, there is very rarely extensive—or even minimal—deliberation among family members about plans for late life caregiving. It's not a pleasant topic and neither parents nor children want to think about what could be difficult final years. So caregiving often begins with a crisis and decisions about caregiving are usually made by default. It's typically a daughter—often the one who is geographically closest or has an employment situation that will allow caregiving. But there is rarely any talk at all about how caregiving will work in the family and the roles that various siblings can play in the process.

Second, caregivers struggle with issues of identity—defining themselves in the midst of this new role. There are tensions that must be resolved as the parent and child roles are often reversed and as the caregiver finds she must develop a wide array of new competencies—everything from helping a parent with basic bodily functions to learning about Medicare policies to negotiating with an employer for time off. This new identity can, of course, lead to great stress, and the negative physical and mental outcomes of caregiving are well documented. The new identity can also be intensely rewarding as caregivers develop a new bond with their parents at the end of life.

(continued)

Third, communication among siblings matters a great deal during the years of caregiving. Relationships are sometimes strengthened as siblings share challenges, but they often deteriorate, especially if they were at all tenuous before. Communication challenges often center on the practical: Who will take Mom to the doctor? Can you come for a few weeks to give me a break? How will we pay for this? But the practical can bleed into relationships: Why do you get to make the decisions just because you're there? Why can't you respect the needs of my family? Could you just acknowledge everything I'm doing for our parents? It's a communicative quagmire that bridges the mundane activities of daily life and existential questions of mortality, morality, and family connection.

As Baby Boomers age and end-of-life care improves, more and more families will be placed in the position of providing long-term care for elderly parents. From our research and other scholarship investigating family communication in caregiving contexts, several practical suggestions are clear:

- Have the conversation. Talk with your parents about their care preferences. Talk with your siblings about your own needs and preferences. Make decisions before the crisis arises. No, it's not the most fun conversation to have, and it's probably not a topic for the Thanksgiving dinner table. But it's critical that the conversation happens.

- Recognize the complexity of caregiving and the need for collaboration. Caregiving involves a huge gamut of activities, depending on the needs of the elderly parent, and the tasks of caregiving change over the years. Caregiving might start out as helping with paying the bills and mowing the lawn and eventually turn into providing 24-hour hands-on care. Talk with your siblings about who can do what. Talk about living arrangements that would be acceptable to all family members. If you're a primary caregiver, be willing to cede control. And don't leave your parents out of these decisions.

- Say thank you. It's a simple thing, but scholarship in positive psychology shows us that expressing gratitude can be beneficial both for the giver and the recipient. Our research suggests that even a simple "Thanks for all you do," can make a difference, but it's even better if the gratitude acknowledges specific acts and the specialness of the individual. And, remember that gratitude is a two-way street. Caregivers should also acknowledge the contributions of other family members, creating a more positive family culture in the midst of stressful times.

QUESTIONS TO PONDER

1. Have your parents provided care for elderly family members? How are/were decisions made among siblings regarding care responsibilities?

2. What key issues will you consider when it's time to have "the conversation" with your own parents?

Sources: Amaro, L. (2014). *Dyadic outcomes of gratitude exchange between family members and their siblings.* Dissertation completed at the Hugh Downs School of Human Communication, Arizona State University. Miller, K., Shoemaker, M. M., Willyard, J., & Addison, P. (2008). Providing care for elderly parents: A structurational approach to family caregiver identity. *Journal of Family Communication, 8,* 19–43. Willyard, J., Miller, K., Shoemaker, M., & Addison, P. (2008). Making sense of sibling responsibility for family caregiving. *Qualitative Health Research, 18,* 1673–1686.

Communicating at the End of Life: Hospice and Palliative Care

Hospice and palliative care are currently conceived as closely intertwined models of care that share common values related to quality of life, management of pain, caring for the patient and family as a "unit of care," and "whole person" care that encompasses physical, emotional, spiritual, social, and psychological needs. The two fields of practice share different origins and orientations: hospice care originated in the United States as a primarily home-care/outpatient, nursing-oriented model, and palliative care emerged from the need for a medical specialty focused on the alleviation of suffering in the inpatient setting, particularly related to cancer treatment. Nevertheless, the two fields are now so closely related that they share a professional organization (the National Hospice Organization became the National Hospice and Palliative Care Organization in 2000), and many large hospitals have "hospice and palliative care" units that strive to establish continuity across the inpatient and outpatient care settings.

Unfortunately, one of the significant complexities of communication in the end-of-life context is *political* rather than *personal*—specifically, the ability of patients to access the level of care they need when they need it. Hospice care was added as a Medicare benefit in 1982, and although hospices initially resisted reimbursement structures as antithetical to its charitable foundations (Connor, 1998), Medicare ensured the ongoing financial support of hospice across the country. At the same time, it added a level of complexity and oversight that is not always compatible with the uncertainty of end-of-life prognoses and trajectories.

HCIA 9.2

Help(less): Caring for My Mother with Terminal Cancer

Marissa J. Doshi

On November 27, 2009, my mother, Bella, was diagnosed with stage III lung cancer. She died the following year—five days short of her 66th birthday. On learning that her case was diagnosed as terminal, I flew to Mumbai, India, from Texas and spent 48 hours with my mother before her death. Here, I recall and reflect on those 48 hours.

November 20, 2010

I'm on a plane to India. My mind wanders into its usual thought patterns: I'm going home! It's going to be much fun! A sudden bump jolts me back to reality: What am I thinking? This trip is not going to fun. My mama is dying. I'm going home to say goodbye.

November 21, 2010

My mother can no longer eat. A broken clothes hanger is being used as a makeshift IV drip stand. The oxygen tube in my mother's nostrils repeatedly pops out as the tape used to keep it in place keeps coming off. "The doctors just told us that oxygen and an IV drip were needed, not how to set up the equipment," my aunts explain. We don't know how to regulate the IV drip. We stop it when saline starts seeping out of my mother's skin.

Although we try to keep my mother comfortable, we are caring for her based on instinct rather than knowledge. I begin looking online for hospices in this city of 18 million. I'm

(continued)

appalled to find just one. When I bring up the issue with my father, he says, "That place is for those with nobody." My aunts and uncle chime in, saying that they would never support the decision of "abandoning" my mother in "that place." I don't want to force my dad to do anything that would make him feel like the right to care for his wife is being taken away from him, and right now, there does not seem to be a way to frame hospice as a useful alternative.

I feel helpless and angry. Where are the doctors? "I don't think the oncologist wants us calling him any more. He said he is busy with other patients," my dad says, his voice soft and trembling. The healthcare team abruptly cut off all contact once my mother's case was diagnosed as terminal.

November 22, 2010

My uncle and I go to a pharmacy to pick up an oxygen cylinder. We check the markings on the cylinder carefully to make sure it's full. After all, the only way of distinguishing between a full and empty cylinder is a single chalk mark—the full ones are labeled "F" and the empty ones, "E." Later that night, when we hook up the cylinder, we find out that it is empty. My dad manages to get another one from an NGO (nongovernmental organization). We got lucky; some days ago, we learned that people needing oxygen cylinders are often turned away because there is a shortage of cylinders. Socialites get first dibs on these cylinders for their oxygen parties, recreational events at which attendees inhale pure oxygen to increase energy levels or counteract the effects of breathing polluted air.

November 23, 2010

At 11:05 P.M., my mother passes away. She is in my arms. I hear her breathing slow down and the final gurgle with which she draws her last breath. Her moans stop. I don't cry. My dad is not at home—he has gone to pick up a back-up oxygen cylinder, hoping that my mother will last the night.

Moving Forward

Forced to cope with almost nonexistent hospice and palliative care services led me to realize the vulnerability that a poor healthcare system imposes on people, a vulnerability that cannot be overcome even with financial stability. Caring for my mother firsthand during her final hours led me to experience the desperation and fear that my father had to experience for the past year, as well as the physical and emotional toll experienced by primary caregivers. I struggled with the guilt and frustration that came from not being able to provide consistent or well-informed support to my parents, and for the first time, I truly understood the importance of emotional support for caregivers.

According to a 2011 report by the Indian Association of Palliative Care, only 2% of patients requiring palliative care receive it; my mother was not in that 2%. Still, in her last days, she was surrounded by the love of family and friends. This autoethnography points out various inadequacies in Mumbai's healthcare systems that need to change if dignified death is to become possible. The stigmatization of palliative care and hospice is internalized by caregivers like my father and adds to their emotional and physical strain. They feel and are viewed as guilty of shirking responsibilities and abandoning the patient if they rely on external support systems such as hospice. Further, by abruptly ending care for terminally ill patients, the medical community reduces the definition of "care" to "treatment." Patients' and caregivers' voices and emotions are silenced.

This autoethnography is not an argument for setting up hospice facilities in Mumbai that are identical to those in the West. Rather, my aim is to highlight the lack of support systems for the terminally ill and their caregivers in my city. My hope is that this work provides insight into the attitudes toward palliative care and hospice in Mumbai and explains in part how these attitudes impact terminally ill patients and their families. Understanding these attitudes is, I hope, the first step toward imagining and setting up support systems that allow a dignified death to become a realistic option for the terminally ill.

QUESTIONS TO PONDER

1. What are the cultural tensions highlighted in this story? How do these tensions influence the experience narrated here?

2. If you were asked to design an end-of-life care program for Mumbai, what would it look like? How could you strive for cultural sensitivity?

Source: Doshi, M. J. (2014). Help(less): An autoethnography about caring for my mother with terminal cancer. *Health Communication, 29,* 840–842. Reprinted by permission of the publisher (Taylor & Francis Ltd. http://www.tandfonline.com).

Most people know that in order to qualify for hospice care a patient's primary care physician must be willing to certify that the patient has six months or less to live. What is less commonly known is that a patient may be recertified for shorter periods of time following the initial six months if he/she is still living but has continued to decline in health. Because inappropriate billing of Medicare for services is fraudulent and comes with severe penalties for individual practitioners and hospice organizations, hospice continues to struggle with "late referrals" to hospice, when hospice is called to support a patient who has days or merely hours to live. With such little time, patients and families are scarcely able to benefit from the services that hospice can offer such as home-based nursing visits, medication management, volunteer services, and durable medical equipment coordination and delivery. The problem of late referral is further exacerbated by the reluctance that many physicians face in declaring their patient's condition to be terminal, and thus the problem persists despite the extraordinary and positive support that hospice typically provides.

Advance Care Planning

Advance care planning is an important focus of conversations related to end-of-life care that reflects all three of the complexities addressed in this text—*cultural, political,* and *personal.* Advance care planning may involve completing one or more documents that help individuals and family members make decisions about end-of-life care in advance of a health crisis and/or the individual's loss of capacity to make such decisions. Advance care planning may include any or all of the following:

1. Advance Directive or Living Will: a document that outlines the wishes of the individual with respect to life-sustaining treatment and/or withdrawal of support under specified circumstances that may occur in the future. To be effective as a legal document, the Advance Directive needs to conform to the requirements of the state in which it would be enacted. (See the Mayo Clinic website for additional information: http://www.mayoclinic.org/healthy-living/consumer-health/in-depth/living-wills/art-20046303)

2. POLST (Physician Orders for Life Sustaining Treatment): a document completed through consultation with a healthcare practitioner that provides guid-

ance for medical treatment in the event of a current health crisis. The POLST form and usage varies from state to state and is typically introduced to patients and family members by a healthcare practitioner during admission to a hospital or at the onset of a serious health threat. (See the national POLST website for more information: http://www.polst.org/)

3. DNR (Do Not Resuscitate) Order: like the POLST, this is a medical order that guides emergency medical care, but the DNR is relevant specifically to the event of heart or multisystem failure. The DNR ensures that the patient is not resuscitated and put on artificial support. (See the Cleveland Clinic website for more information: http://my.clevelandclinic.org/health/healthy_living/hic_Do_Not_Resuscitate_Orders_and_Comfort_Care)

4. Healthcare Proxy: the designation of a specific individual to make healthcare decisions on behalf of the person who is incapacitated. A healthcare proxy is often required as part of a state's regulations for an Advance Directive or Living Will. (see the American Bar Association website for more information: http://www.americanbar.org/groups/real_property_trust_estate/resources/estate_planning/living_wills_health_care_proxies_advance_health_care_directives.html)

5. Durable Power of Attorney for Healthcare: a legal document that assigns a Healthcare Proxy—a specific individual who is responsible for making legal decisions and taking action on behalf of the person who is incapacitated. (See the American Bar Association website for more information: http://www.americanbar.org/groups/real_property_trust_estate/resources/estate_planning/living_wills_health_care_proxies_advance_health_care_directives.html)

6. Ethical Will or Legacy Letter: outlines the values, life lessons, wisdoms, and hopes that a person wishes to communicate to future generations. Unlike other documents listed as part of advance care planning, the Ethical Will is not a legal document and does not relate to healthcare specifically, but may help family members understand and respond appropriately to the end-of-life wishes of their loved one. (See the Life Legacies website for more information: http://www.life-legacies.com/ethicalwills/)

In addition to the political complexities of the forms, which require adherence to state regulations and (often) the oversight of an attorney or medical professional, the stakes are high for healthcare organizations to be more proactive in supporting the completion of advance directives. The high costs of healthcare in the United States are mostly incurred in the last years of life, with those who reach 85 spending one-third of their lifetime expenditures after that age (Alemayehu & Warner, 2004). The question that remains to be addressed is to what extent these healthcare expenditures are improving quality of life versus merely extending life. A related question is whether, given open discussion and supported decision making, patients and family members would elect to undertake such medical intervention late in life.

Communication is essential to redirecting our cultural tendency to medicalize the end of life and, instead, to respond to the end of life with greater social support and emphasis on quality of life rather than quantity. Healthcare practitioners can play a significant role in initiating advance care planning discussions with patients prior to the onset of a health crisis (Rauscher & Nacinovich, 2012); however, research indicates that passive information sharing about advance directives does little to increase understanding and completion of advance directives (Tamayo-Velázquez et al., 2010). Conversations between practitioners and patients related to advance directives are most effective when enacted as part of an ongoing process of information sharing and decision making rather than as a one-time event (Bravo, Dubois, & Wagneur, 2008; Tamayo-Velázquez et al., 2010). Although most patients believe that it is appropriate for physicians to initiate conversations about advance care planning, research indicates that patients with advance directives tend to share them with family members rather than with their providers (Ozanne, Partridge, Moy, Ellis, & Sepucha, 2009). This tendency may well reflect the extent to which patients expect their providers to take the lead—if the physician does not raise the topic of end-of-life care, then they are not likely to do so either.

Family members play an essential role in advance care planning, particularly because they are typically most closely involved in caregiving and ensuring that the wishes of the patient are supported. Children of older adults are especially implicated in advance care planning and what Fowler, Fisher, and Pitts (2014) call planning for "future care needs" (p. 717)—a conversation that encompasses far more than advance care planning by including discussions of caregiving responsibilities, finances, options for residential care and so on. As their study demonstrates, the manner in which children of older adults initiate conversations can predict how supportive parents perceive that communication to be, and all communication efforts must be consciously adapted to the communicative and relational norms of the family. Furthermore, racial and ethnic norms differ regarding the appropriateness of advance care planning. For example, collectivist cultures that value family-oriented decision making over autonomy may not see the need for advance care conversations (Villagran, Wittenberg-Lyles, & Hajek, 2007), and historically disenfranchised groups may not want to involve healthcare professionals in such discussions for fear that their loved one may be abandoned and have care withdrawn prematurely.

Within the constellation of family relationships, spouses are most often involved in communication about end-of-life planning and are most commonly listed as healthcare proxy or surrogate within advance directives. One proposal for engaging a conversation with a spouse or partner is an innovative model called "The Five Wishes" (www.agingwithdignity.org) and adapts it to an interview format (Eckstein & Mullener, 2010). The article provides detailed prompts to help couples consider each of the following five questions:

1. The person I choose to make healthcare decisions when I can't make them for myself is:
2. My wish for the kind of medical care I want or do not want is:
3. My wish for how comfortable I want to be is:
4. My wish for how I wish people to treat me is:
5. My wish for what I want my loved ones to know is:

Advance care planning can do much to alleviate the stress and difficulty of navigating the end of life, particularly when it comes to making medical decisions and choices about how to spend that time. By making some of those decisions in advance of a terminal diagnosis, the hope is that individuals and families will be freer to engage in the more personal and relational activities of caring for and saying goodbye to one another. Consider how you might approach your own family members about these important conversations in Theorizing Practice 9.2.

Theorizing Practice 9.2
The Conversation Project

Visit the website for the Conversation Project (http://theconversationproject.org), a grassroots campaign whose goal is to assist the public in having conversations about wishes for end-of-life care. While reviewing the website, read through the steps outlined in the "Starter Kit." Considering the various perspectives and advice in this chapter, what communication tools do you imagine would be useful to you as you approach your own family members about having this important conversation?

Communication and Social Dying

> She was afraid that she would die as a number in some bed with strangers all around her. . . . She thought that they'd come in the next morning and realize that she had died. I didn't really do anything. I hadn't been in the room with someone who was dying before, and I didn't know what to do. All I knew to do was to be myself and give myself, to rub her hand or her forehead. (Shyanne, hospice volunteer, quoted in Foster, 2007, p. 153)

In this chapter, I have already discussed the complex communication tasks surrounding the breaking of bad news such as the delivery of a terminal diagnosis, which would transition a patient from curative to palliative (comfort) care, or transition him/her into hospice care if they have six months or less to live. What remains to be addressed is what happens after the diagnosis is made, when the patient exists in the liminal or threshold space (Turner, 1995) between living and dying. As discussed earlier in the chapter, a significant dimension of effectively negotiating bad news conversations consists of paying attention to the relational dimension of the messages rather than the content. Similarly, one of the consistent insights offered by hospice workers is that establishing a caring relationship is more important than trying to have the "right" conversations. Three themes emerged from stories of hospice patients (Foster, 2002): the most valuable end-of-life communication involves (1) focusing on the patient and family, (2) emphasizing the life of the patient rather than the impending death of the patient, and (3) being fully present and attending to the interaction. Of course, for family members close to the patient, there may be much need and benefit derived from enacting explicit conversations about the dying process (Keeley, 2007). However, because we live in a death-denying culture, many people are uncomfortable facing mortality and may avoid communicating with a terminally ill patient because they fear they may have to talk about death. Such avoidance may lead to additional pain and suffering of the patient associated with a state called *social death.*

End-of-life theorists have proposed that there can be a social death that precedes physical death by weeks, months, or even years (Lawton, 2000; Seale 1998). Although the term tends to be reserved for patients who experience extreme isolation and almost complete loss of social contacts as a consequence of their advanced illness and debilitation, most hospice patients experience some degree of social dying as a result of their changed health status, their decreasing mobility, and their increasing dependence on the assistance of others. I have proposed elsewhere (Foster, 2007, pp. 200–201) that the most important function of a hospice volunteer is to alleviate the pain associated with social dying. Although relationally focused communication from family members and health practitioners will also serve this function, the role of the visiting hospice volunteer is almost exclusively related to establishing and maintaining the social contacts of the hospice patient.

With this in mind, then, guidelines for communicating with patients who are facing life-limiting or terminal illness must be grounded in the assumptions of relational communication, which privileges presence, mutual influence, and implicit messages over information exchange. This is particularly important when people consider how many patients face the end of life with limited capacity to hold a "conversation" either because of advanced dementia or Alzheimer's disease, aphasia due to a stroke, or fatigue associated with advanced illness. As indicated in the vignette that began this section, an inability to engage in a conversation does not foreclose the capacity to communicate care and support. Nonverbal messages and a willingness to be present for the person who is dying are essential to communicating support.

HCIA 9.3

Personhood and Communication at the End of Life

Jillian A. Tullis

What makes a person a person? A beating heart? Brain function? Working lungs? The ability to eat and drink? The ability to think or have thoughts? What about the ability to communicate? These are the types of questions we ask when we talk about personhood. Usually we pose such questions at the beginning of life, especially when discussing the ethics of abortion or embryotic stem cell research, but these are important questions at the end of life as well.

Perhaps you remember the controversial case of Terri Schiavo, who at the age of 26, entered a persistent vegetative state after her brain was deprived of oxygen after losing consciousness, and remained so for the next 15 years. Terri Schiavo's husband and parents fought over whether or not to remove her life support. After legal battles, political fighting, and public protests, her husband was allowed to remove her feeding tube and 13 days later she died. Or maybe you're familiar with the more recent case of Brittany Maynard who had an inoperable brain tumor, and at the age of 29 decided to end her life under Oregon's Death with Dignity law. These high profile cases influence policies, legal precedents, laws, and public dialogues. Yet each day in hospitals, hospices, nursing homes, and even in our

(continued)

own homes, debates about personhood—or what makes a life—are taking place. These conversations, however, don't often make the evening news or the Yahoo! home page. Instead, loved ones make the agonizing decision to withdraw life support while huddled in a dimly lit hospital family room. Other times, conversations related to personhood occur while a terminally ill person receives hospice care in his/her home. No matter the setting where end-of-life communication takes place, concerns about personhood arise.

Philosopher Simone Evnine describes agency as one of the defining qualities of person-hood involving the ability to think, make plans, and take actions. While there are other charac-teristics of personhood, this essay focuses on agency because it is most closely connected to communication. As a researcher and a hospice volunteer, I have had opportunities to observe communication about personhood at the end of life, noting the ways in which agency is a critical component for maintaining a person's dignity and quality of life. These aspects of such difficult conversations are not easily recognizable, unless you know where to focus.

Consider the story of one of the first hospice patients I met when collecting data for my dissertation. Sonny was in his 70s and dying of chronic obstructive pulmonary disease, also known as emphysema, which makes it difficult and eventually impossible to breathe. He was living independently until his illness became terminal and then he moved in with his eldest daughter. I shadowed Allison, the social worker assigned to check on Sonny's mental well-being, and the three of us would talk about all kinds of topics, including politics, his love of horse racing, and his family. Our visits would sometimes overlap with visits from Sonny's nurse, Judy. The story below focuses on one such visit.

> Five months had passed since I started my research and Sonny was declining, losing more and more of his autonomy. Instead of taking his motorized scooter to get a sandwich at a shop down the street, he was staying home; it was even difficult to walk to the bathroom or to the refrigerator without his oxygen. One day, Sonny complained, which was unusual since he was always upbeat.
> "There's nothing more you can do for me. Except for this thing," he says, pointing to the nasal canula he took off a few minutes after Allison and I arrived. At first I feel a little hurt, but then taken aback.
> "What, you don't like us anymore, Sonny?" Judy says teasingly as she packs up her blood pressure cuff and stethoscope.
> "No, no, that's not what I mean," Sonny says flatly. "Going to the bathroom is a pain," he says, drawing out the word pain. He points toward the door leading to the main part of the house reminding us of the walk he must take to get to the toilet.
> Judy interrupts, "Well, do you have a urinal?"
> "Yeah. I use it at night."
> "What about your port-a-potty? Do you use that?" Judy asks, pointing to the bedside commode.
> "I don't want to have to clean that thing out," Sonny says with an aggravated tone.
> "Maybe you could have your daughter do it for you?"
> "I'm not going to have her do that," Sonny says, looking disgusted. "She works full time. I'm not going to ask her to do something like that."
> Judy's persistence is beginning to make me feel uncomfortable because with each question Sonny is getting more and more upset. Thankfully Allison interrupts and redirects the conversation to a less serious topic. A few minutes after Judy leaves, Allison returns to Sonny's original statement and says, "'There's nothing more we can do for you,' I've never heard you talk like that before. What did you mean?" This probing question from Allison allowed Sonny to clarify and articulate his frustrations about his decline and limitations after which he seemed relieved to get the matter off his chest.

Judy's initial offer to help is reasonable and probably what any of us would do, but rather than invite Sonny's input, it frustrated him. Not all complaints warrant solutions, perhaps especially for people who are dying. Sonny needed a sympathetic ear because sometimes comforting messages that acknowledge and sympathize are more beneficial. Asking Sonny what, if anything, his hospice team could do to help would put him in a better position to articulate his wishes and possibly act upon them, which are central tenants of agency.

Dependence on the medical system or a medical device is not easy for most people to accept, and it can make people feel helpless and frustrated. It is easy to overlook the more mundane aspects of personhood, but Sonny's story illustrates how limitations in physical space and movement, nonverbal cues (e.g., removing oxygen tubing to illustrate personal strength and control), and a patient's resistance to suggestions illustrate how personhood at the end of life is what makes a life simple, yet important.

QUESTIONS TO PONDER

1. Come up with your own definition of personhood. What does personhood mean to you?

2. How important is communication to your definition of personhood? If you couldn't communicate, would you want to continue living?

Source: Tullis, J. A. (2012). Personhood and communication at the end of life. *Journal of Medicine and the Person, 10,* 110–113.

■ Communication and Grief

As Bosticco and Thompson (2005) put it, most powerfully, "Grief, which is both a social and communicative process, is one of the most challenging and overwhelming circumstances an individual must face in life" (p. 257). Grief may accompany any change that radically alters people's sense of their life narrative or trajectory, and death is the most ubiquitous cause for grief. This final section of the chapter presents some of the conceptual frameworks and research findings related to grief, focusing on communicative and relational dimensions of grief, particularly within the context of the family.

The most widely recognized model related to grief and the end-of-life experience is Elizabeth Kübler-Ross's (1969) five stages—denial, anger, bargaining, depression, and acceptance. Possibly because they are so widely known, these stages have been parodied in popular culture and also criticized despite Kübler-Ross's clear framing of the model in her initial and subsequent publications. Thus it is important to recognize that the "stages" are not intended to be a comprehensive and exhaustive description of the psychology of death and dying, nor are they offered as a tool to predict the responses of those who face a terminal prognosis. Rather, they describe some of the common emotional responses that individuals experience when they face the prospect of dying, and, perhaps most importantly, the stages emphasize the diverse reactions that people may have and the importance of continuing to listen and remain accepting of those reactions. Possibly the most significant legacy of Kübler-Ross's work is that it has provided a basis for our culture to reflect upon and discuss the end of life to an extent that was not typical prior to the publication of her work.

Communication patterns within families are related to grieving and can predict how successfully grief is navigated with respect to levels of psychological distress (Carmon, Western, Miller, Pearson, & Fowler, 2010). Underlying these patterns are two cognitive orientations to communication within the family: *conformity orientation,* which describes the degree to which the family maintains shared norms, beliefs, and behaviors, and *communication orientation,* which describes the degree to which members of the family communicate openly with one another about a range of topics (Carmon et al., 2010). Research on individuals who experienced a bereavement of a family member in the last five years found that families with more open communication are more likely to experience positive personal growth as a consequence of the bereavement, which suggests there is a distinct advantage to communicating about death in ways that promote sensemaking and healing (Carmon et al., 2010).

However, bereavement events vary widely with respect to the closeness of the individual to the person who has died, the expectedness of the death, the age of the person who has died, and the circumstances of the death. Suicide and death of a child are two types of events that call for particular sensitivity and attention to sensemaking because, unlike the death of an elderly person from "typical" causes (regardless of how beloved that person is), suicide and the death of a child seem senseless and call into question our sense of the natural order of life (Powell & Matthys, 2013; Titus & de Souza, 2011). Although, as we have already discussed, communicating expressions of grief is essential to the process of sensemaking and healing, one of the complicating dimensions of bereavement due to suicide or the loss of a child is the high potential for silencing that grief due to cultural norms. As a cultural taboo, death by suicide often leaves family survivors with a sense of stigma that limits their capacity to speak freely about the event. Grieving parents may experience a similar sense of stigma in which their expressions of intense and/or extended grief are unwelcome. Further disorienting can be the different responses to grief within a family—ranging from dramatic expressions of emotion to restrained stoicism—which may cause additional distress if family members expected they would grieve in the same way (Titus & de Souza, 2011).

Maria Brann (2014) describes her experience of "disenfranchised grief" following the loss of her first pregnancy to miscarriage (p. 23)—that is, a grief that cannot be openly and publicly expressed and acknowledged. In Brann's case, the grief following her loss was exponentially intensified after a brutal experience of nonsupport from her health practitioner—a midwife whom Brann had selected because of her desire to receive empathetic and woman-centered care (p. 23). Seeking care two days after the beginning of the miscarriage, Brann and her husband met with the midwife after sitting for an hour in the waiting room surrounded by happy pregnant women. Expecting a warm embrace and concerned conversation about the miscarriage, Brann and her husband were met with a series of bewildering statements and questions from the midwife including a perfunctory, "How are you today? . . . You went to the hospital on Saturday, correct? . . . I think everything is returning to normal. Do you want to go back on birth control?" (pp. 20–21). Brann and her husband's direct requests for support were met by an offer to mail them a pamphlet on grieving that, almost predictably, never materialized.

Brann's (2014) analysis of the nonsupport she received holds important insights for what health practitioners and friends may do to respond to grief and counteract the disenfranchisement of those who suffer from extreme or stigmatized losses. First, recognizing that there is no time limit on grief and that gentle invitations to recall the loved one, express emotions about the event, and receive support are, for the most part, welcomed. Second, it is important to share information about processes of loss (e.g., what can happen physically during the dying process or what can happen to a woman's body during a miscarriage), as well as what to expect when grieving. Social support is constituted through a range of supportive activities. If unsure about how to respond, it can help to remember that providing needed information can be as comforting as offering emotional support, and those who are not adept at providing one may be able to offer the other rather than retreating from the bereaved person. Third, different kinds of support and communication are needed at different times. So, when in doubt, asking a person what she/he might want or need is preferable to making assumptions. Fourth, messages that disconfirm the loss, however well intentioned, are particularly distressing. As reported in many narratives of miscarriage (Silverman & Baglia, 2014), statements such as "it obviously wasn't meant to be" or "there must have been something wrong with the baby" or "at least you know that you can get pregnant" are particularly painful and result in the bereaved person becoming further isolated. Consider your own supportive responses in Theorizing Practice 9.3.

Theorizing Practice 9.3
Empathic Response

Recall the last conversation you had when someone was asking you to really listen to her or him (it need not be a health-related conversation). How well did you respond to the other person's emotional cues? Did you miss any opportunities to respond empathically? What made it easy/difficult for you to listen empathically?

▪ Epilogue

Although my partner Jay and I experienced intense grief and some examples of quite incompetent communication in the aftermath of the miscarriage described in the opening of this chapter, we were also very fortunate to have received significant support—from our practitioner Holly, from friends, and from family members. To conclude this chapter, I share a story from the early months after our daughter Aria was born, almost two years after our miscarriage.

We had travelled with our baby to a conference in Florida and were able to meet up for lunch with family friends who were seeing Aria for the first time. Carolyn, the wife of Jay's friend of 30 years, Joe, had brought an impressive array of dresses for Aria and clearly shared our joy at the arrival of this little person. What moved us most, however, was when Carolyn asked us about the miscarriage.

"We feel very lucky to have her," Jay remarked

"That's right. You lost one, didn't you?" Carolyn asked.

"Yes," I replied quietly, "In September two years ago."

Carolyn turned to Aria as she dandled her on her lap. "You might have had a big brother or a big sister."

I held my breath and shot a look at Jay who had already looked at me. In one astounding moment, Carolyn had validated our loss, named a secret and intimate thought that we (and possibly all bereaved parents) had experienced, and had done so in a manner that was poignant in the right way. Nothing more needed to be said.

■ Conclusion

Although others may have responded less positively to such a direct reference to a loss like this and may perceive it to be tactless, for us, in that context, it was perfect and we remain grateful for her genuine expression of confirmation and support. When facing a difficult conversation related to health challenges, the capacity to be present, genuine, and expressive of support is an essential component of the journey to healing.

Discussion Questions

1. What is the most challenging health situation that you have faced—either your own situation or that of someone close to you? What made it challenging? What do you recall about the communication surrounding that situation?

2. When you hear that someone you know is experiencing a health challenge, what are your immediate thoughts and feelings? What is your own sense of how well you tend to respond in that situation?

3. Have you or someone close to you ever received bad news from a health practitioner? What do you remember about the communication of that news and how well it was communicated? If you were to write the script of that event using the principles presented in this chapter, what would you be sure to include?

4. Having read the chapter, what do you understand to be the similarities and differences between hospice and palliative care? How might you initiate a conversation with a loved one about how they imagine they would like their care to be handled in the case of a terminal illness?

5. Responding to another person's grief can be extremely challenging. Given what you have read in this chapter, what will you be sure to remember when you learn that someone has received bad news about their health or experienced a significant loss?

NOTES

[1] Foster, E. (2010). My eyes cry without me: Illusions of choice and control in the transition to motherhood. In S. Hayden & L. O'Brien Hallstein (Eds.), *Contemplating maternity: Discourses of choice and control* (pp. 139–158). Lanham, MA: Lexington Press. Reprinted with permission.

[2] When I originally published this narrative, I used the title "technician" to describe the role of the women who conducted the prenatal ultrasound examinations that were a focus of the story. I have since learned (Foster & McGivern, 2014) that "medical sonographer" is the preferred title of the profession, because it emphasizes the skill and expertise required to perform the exams. The term "technician" is often employed in a hospital environment to emphasize these workers' lower place on the medical hierarchy.

[3] The term "elderly primigravida" is an archaic medical label used to designate a female patient over the age of 35 who is pregnant for the first time.

[4] In this chapter, I use the term "practitioner" to indicate that many professional care providers in the healthcare context may be involved in helping patients to navigate challenging health situations. I refer to specific health professions (physicians, nurses, and social workers) only when necessary.

REFERENCES

Ackerman, N. (1966). *Treating the troubled family.* New York, NY: Basic Books.

Alemayehu, B., & Warner, K. E. (2004). The lifetime distribution of healthcare costs. *Health Services Research, 39,* 627–642.

Austin, J. L. (1983). *How to do things with words.* London, UK: Oxford University Press.

Baile, W. F., Buckman, R., Lenzi, R., Glober, G., Beale, E. A., & Kudelka, A. P. (2000). SPIKES—a six-step protocol for delivering bad news: Application to the patient with cancer. *The Oncologist, 5,* 302–311.

Bateson, G. (1972). *Steps to an ecology of mind.* New York, NY: Ballantine.

Bochner, A. P. (1978). On taking ourselves seriously: An analysis of some persistent problems and promising directions in interpersonal research. *Human Communication Research, 4,* 179–191.

Bochner, A. P. (1984). The functions of communication in interpersonal bonding. In C. Arnold & J. Bowers (Eds.), *The handbook of rhetoric and communication* (pp. 544–621). Needham Heights, MA: Praeger.

Bosticco, C., & Thompson, T. L. (2005). Narratives and story telling in coping with grief and bereavement. *OMEGA—Journal of Death and Dying, 51,* 1–16.

Brann, M. (2014). Nine years later and still waiting: When health care providers' social support never arrives. In R. E. Silverman & J. Baglia (Eds.), *Communicating pregnancy loss: Narrative as a method for change* (pp. 19–31). New York, NY: Peter Lang.

Bravo, G., Dubois, M., & Wagneur, B. (2008). Assessing effectiveness of interventions to promote advance directives among older adults: A systematic review and multi-level analysis. *Social Science and Medicine, 67,* 1122–1132.

Buckman, R. (1984). Breaking bad news: Why is it still so difficult? *British Medical Journal, 288,* 1597–1599.

Buckman, R., Tulsky, J. D., & Rodin, G. (2011). Empathic responses in clinical practice: Intuition or tuition? *Canadian Medical Association Journal, 183,* 569–571.

Burgoon, J. K., Stern, L. A., & Dillman, L. (1995). *Interpersonal adaptation: Dyadic interaction patterns.* New York, NY: Cambridge University Press.

Carmon, A. F., Western, K. J., Miller, A. N., Pearson, J. C., & Fowler, M. R. (2010). Grieving those we've lost: An examination of family communication patterns and grief reactions. *Communication Research Reports, 27,* 253–262.

Carter, B., & McGoldrick, M. (Eds.) (1980). *The family lifecycle: A framework for family therapy.* New York, NY: Gardener Press.

Carter, B., & McGoldrick, M. (Eds.). (1988). *The changing family lifecycle: A framework for family therapy.* New York, NY: Gardener Press.

Carter, B., & McGoldrick, M. (1999). *The expanded family lifecycle: Individual, family and social perspectives.* Needham Heights, MA: Allyn & Bacon.

Connor, S. R. (1998). *Hospice: Practice, pitfalls, and promise.* Washington, DC: Taylor & Francis.

Eckstein, D., & Mullener, B. (2010). A couple's advance directives interview using the Five Wishes questionnaire. *The Family Journal: Counseling and Therapy for Couples and Families, 18,* 66–69.

Foster, E. (2002). Lessons we learned: Stories of volunteer-patient communication in hospice. *Journal of Aging and Identity, 7,* 245–256.

Foster, E. (2007). *Communicating at the end of life: Finding magic in the mundane.* Mahwah, NJ: Erlbaum.

Foster, E. (2010). My eyes cry without me: Illusions of choice and control in the transition to motherhood. In S. Hayden & L. O'Brien Hallstein (Eds.), *Contemplating maternity: Discourses of choice and control* (pp. 139–158). Lanham, MA: Lexington Press.

Foster, E., & Cohen-Katz, J. (2011). Caring for the family: Teaching systems and cycles in a family medicine residency program. In M. Miller-Day (Ed.), *Family communication, connections, and health transitions* (pp. 321–348). New York, NY: Peter Lang.

Foster, E., & McGivern, J. (2014). A story we can live with: The role of the sonographer in the diagnosis of fetal demise. In R. E. Silverman & J. Baglia (Eds.), *Communicating pregnancy loss: Narrative as a method for change* (pp. 75–87). New York, NY: Peter Lang.

Fowler, C., Fisher, C. L., & Pitts, M. J. (2014). Older adults' evaluations of middle-aged children's attempts to initiate discussion of care needs. *Health Communication, 29,* 717–727.

Goldsmith, J., Ferrell, B., Wittenberg-Lyles, E., & Ragan, S. (2013). Palliative care communication in oncology nursing. *Clinical Journal of Oncology Nursing, 17,* 163–167.

Goldsmith, J., Wittenberg-Lyles, E., Villagran, M., & Sanchez-Reilly, S. (2008, November). *Communicating emotional support when breaking terminal bad news using the SPIKES Model: Fourth year medical student encounters.* Paper presented at the Annual Meeting of the National Communication Association.

Haley, J. (1963). *Strategies of psychotherapy.* New York, NY: Grune & Stratton.

Hochschild, A. R. (2003). *The managed heart: Commercialization of feeling* (2nd ed.). Berkeley: University of California Press.

Holman Jones, S. (2005). (M)othering loss: Telling adoption stories, telling performativity. *Text & Performance Quarterly, 25,* 113–135.

Kaplan, M. (2010). SPIKES: A framework for breaking bad news to patients with cancer. *Clinical Journal of Oncology Nursing, 14,* 514–516.

Keeley, M. (2007). *Final conversations: Helping the living and the dying talk to one another.* St. Louis, MO: VanderWyk & Bernham.

Kübler-Ross, E. (1969). *On death and dying: What the dying have to teach doctors, nurses, clergy, and their own families.* New York, NY: Scribner.

Lannamann, M. (1989). Communication theory applied to relational change: A case study in Milan systemic family therapy. *Journal of Applied Communication Research, 17,* 71–91.

Lawton, J. (2000). *The dying process: Patients' experiences of palliative care.* London, UK: Routledge.

McDaniel, S., Campbell, T. L., Hepworth, J., & Lorenz, A. (2005). *Family-oriented primary care* (2nd ed.). New York, NY: Springer-Verlag.

Millar, F. E., & Rogers, L. E. (1976). A relational approach to interpersonal communication. In G. E. Miller (Ed.), *Explorations in interpersonal communication* (pp. 87–104). Beverly Hills, CA: Sage.

Miller, W. (2004). The clinical hand: A curricular map for relationship-centered care. *Family Medicine, 3,* 330–335.

Minuchin, S. (1974). *Families and family therapy.* Cambridge, MA: Harvard University Press.

Narayanan, V., Bista, B., & Koshy, C. (2010). "BREAKS" Protocol for breaking bad news. *Indian Journal of Palliative Care, 16,* 61–65.

Ozanne, E. M., Partridge, A., Moy, B., Ellis, K. J., & Sepucha, K. R. (2009). Doctor–patient communication about advance directives in metastatic breast cancer. *Journal of Palliative Medicine, 12,* 547–553.

Pineau, E. (2000). Nursing mother and articulating absence. *Text & Performance Quarterly, 20,* 1–19.

Pollock, D. (1999). *Telling bodies performing birth.* New York, NY: Columbia University Press.

Powell, K. A., & Matthys, A. (2013). Effects of suicide on siblings: Uncertainty and the grief process. *Journal of Family Communication, 13,* 321–339.

Rauscher, J., & Nacinovich, M. R. (2012). Concerns and wishes—Communication of advance care planning. *Journal of Communication in Healthcare, 5,* 1–2.

Rogers, L. E., & Escudero, V. (2004). Theoretical foundations. In L. E. Rogers & V. Escudero (Eds.), *Relational communication: An interactional perspective to the study of process and form* (pp. 3–21). Mahwah, NJ: Erlbaum.

Satir, V. (1967). *Conjoint family therapy.* Palo Alto, CA: Science and Behavior Books.

Seale, C. (1998). *Constructing death: The sociology of dying and bereavement.* Cambridge, UK: Cambridge University.

Shanahan, M. K. (2000). *Your over 35 week-by-week pregnancy guide: All the answers to all your questions about pregnancy, birth, and your developing baby.* Roseville, CA: Prima.

Shetty, A. A., & Shapiro, J. (2012). How to break bad news—tips and tools for resident physicians. *Journal of Medical Education Perspectives, 1,* 20–24.

Sieburg, E. (1985). *Family communication: An integrated systems approach.* New York, NY: Gardener Press.

Silverman, R. E., & Baglia, J. (Eds.) (2014). *Communicating pregnancy loss: Narrative as a method for change.* New York, NY: Peter Lang.

Spry, T. (2000). Tattoo Stories: A postscript to Skins. *Text & Performance Quarterly, 20,* 84–96.

Stuart, M. R., & Lieberman, J. A., III. (2002). *The fifteen-minute hour: Practical therapeutic interventions in primary care* (3rd ed.). Philadelphia, PA: Saunders.

Suchman, A. L., Merkakis, K., Beckman, H. B., & Frankel, R. (1997). A model of empathic communication in the medical interview. *Journal of the American Medical Association, 277,* 678–682.

Tamayo-Velázquez, M., Simón-Lorda, P., Villegas-Portero, R., Higueras-Callejón, C., García-Gutiérrez, J., Martínez-Pecino, F., & Barrio-Cantalejo, I. (2010). Interventions to promote the use of advance directives: An overview of systematic reviews. *Patient Education and Counseling, 80,* 10–20.

Titus, B., & de Souza, R. (2011). Finding meaning in the loss of a child: Journeys of chaos and quest. *Health Communication, 26,* 450–460.

Turner, V. (1995). *The ritual process: Structure and anti-structure.* Hawthorne, NY: Aldine De Gruyter.

VandeKieft, G. K. (2001). Breaking bad news. *American Family Physician, 64,* 1975–1978.

Villagran, M., Goldsmith, J., Wittenberg-Lyles, E., & Baldwin, P. (2010). Creating COMFORT: A communication-based model for breaking bad news. *Communication Education, 59,* 220–234.

Villagran, M., Wittenberg-Lyles, E., & Hajek, C. (2007, November). *The impact of communication, attitudes, and acculturation on advance directives decision making.* Paper presented at the annual meeting of the National Communication Association, Chicago, IL.

Watzlawick, P., Beavin, J. H., & Jackson, D. D. (1967). *The pragmatics of human communication.* New York, NY: Norton.

Wittenberg-Lyles, E., Goldsmith, J., & Ragan, S. (2010). The COMFORT initiative: Palliative nursing and the centrality of communication. *Journal of Hospice and Palliative Nursing, 12,* 282–292.

Wittenberg-Lyles, E., Goldsmith, J., Parker Oliver, D., Demeris, G., & Rankin, A. (2012). Family communication in oncology care. *Seminars in Oncology Nursing, 28,* 262–270.

Wittenberg-Lyles, E., Goldsmith, J., Richardson, B., Hallett, J. S., & Clark, R. (2013). The practical nurse: A case for COMFORT communication training. *American Journal of Hospice and Palliative Care, 30,* 162–166.

10

Communicating Health and Connection in Supportive Communities

Jill Yamasaki

Charlie is a 9-year-old decorated USAG Level 5 gymnast who, with his 20 Mile Athletic Center teammates from Parker, Colorado, is favored to repeat last year's team championship and win the individual all-around title at this year's Valeri Liukin Invitational outside of Dallas. He isn't nervous—he says he never gets nervous—and he isn't arrogant or smug. When the crowd gasps at his effortless handstand on the high bar—the only one performed by a gymnast at that level— or 20 Mile parents cheer wildly when he's called to the winners' podium eight times, Charlie simply raises his hand in a gymnast's salute and steps back to rejoin his team. "Charlie is a good person because he's nice and he cares about his teammates and he's a really good gymnast," say his teammates. "Charlie is so awesomely humble, even when he's flashing a #1," echo their parents.

It's only before he collects his medals and is crowned both all-around and team champion that Charlie's gentle demeanor cracks. His face scrunched in distress, he walks up to his dad and, with a quiver in his low voice, says, "Those boys over there are laughing at me. They're making fun of my head." His dad, who has had this conversation with Charlie more times than he can count, kneels to Charlie's level and puts his hands on his shoulders. "Forget about them. You know what you need to do? You need to do what Peyton did last week," he says, referring to famed quarterback Peyton Manning's response to critics who had long questioned his ability to win cold-weather games. "Tell them to shove it where the sun don't shine." Charlie smiles widely, and a teammate's dad pats him on the back. "And then flash them that smile from the top of the podium."

As you can tell from the story and see in the pictures (on the next page), Charlie is a healthy, strong, bald young boy who has alopecia areata. Alopecia areata is a common autoimmune skin disease that results in the loss of scalp and body hair. It usually starts with one or more small, round, smooth patches on the scalp and can progress to total scalp hair loss (alopecia totalis) or complete body hair loss (alopecia universalis). Charlie has had no hair or eyebrows since he was diagnosed with alopecia totalis at

251

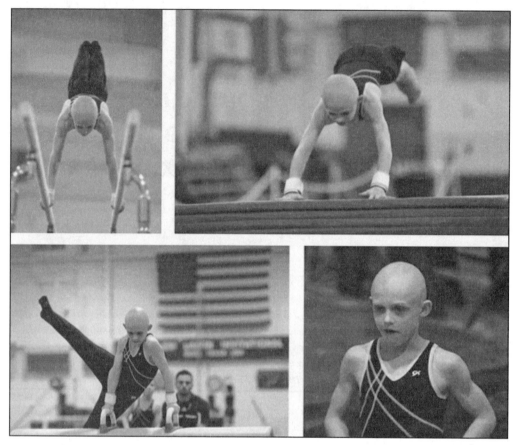

Courtesy of Josh Dieringer.

age 8. Although it is not a painful or life-threatening condition, alopecia areata is unpredictable with no known cure. And, as you can imagine, it can be incredibly traumatic and emotionally challenging for the 6.5 million men, women, and children who live with it in the U.S. alone. Fortunately, as you will learn in this chapter, Charlie and his family are thriving with support from meaningful relationships fostered in his close-knit gymnastics and alopecia areata communities.

Our health, well-being, and general quality of life are embedded in the structure and content of our relational lives (Goldsmith & Albrecht, 2011). Each of us belongs to a number of different communities based on factors such as location, demographics, and interests. Along with family, formal education, and various forms of media, it is within these communities that we construct our health beliefs, obtain our health information, and feel the social pressures that reinforce or undermine our health behaviors. Consider your own membership in various communities based on your age, language, friendships, family, year in school, abilities, hobbies, gender, neighborhood, and religion, and then consider which of these influence your physical, mental, and emotional health in positive or negative ways. Which are most salient and why?

By defining ourselves—or being defined by others—as healthy or unhealthy, we may affiliate with particular communities (Geist-Martin, Ray, & Sharf, 2011). Strangers who encounter Charlie may be surprised to know he is a budding, accomplished gymnast. They see his hairless head, missing eyebrows, short stature, and pale skin and often assume he is gravely ill or strangely different. In restaurants, it is not uncommon for well-meaning adults to offer him encouraging words or to pay for his family's meal; on the playground, kids sometimes point, smirk, or laugh at him. As part of the 20 Mile community, though, coaches, parents, and teammates see Charlie as an athletic, muscular kid who is determined, kind, soft-spoken, and one of them.

I weave Charlie's story throughout this chapter to illustrate how he draws support and increased courage from his close-knit gymnastics community to accept himself and advocate for others. I begin by examining the various conceptualizations of community, noting that regardless of type or attribute, communities emerge through communication. Then, I consider the complexities of supportive communication for improving the well-being of people perceived to be in need, including the availability of support through social networks and community connections. Finally, I explore the ways community resources (or lack of resources) influence the health and well-being of its members, emphasizing an appreciative and imaginative approach of citizen inclusivity and capacity.

Conceptualizing Community

Charlie's parents first noticed his uneven hairline around Christmas when he was 7. At the time, they thought it was just a very bad haircut, but soon they noticed three large bald circles at his part, around one of his ears, and in the back at his neck. His pediatrician diagnosed him with alopecia areata, explaining that it was very common in kids and would likely come and go throughout his life. Charlie and his parents were relieved to hear it likely wouldn't get any worse. Although they didn't know the cause, they were confident his hair would grow back in six months without treatment.

Earlier that fall, Charlie's aunt encouraged him to enroll in a beginner boys' gymnastics class at 20 Mile, where her daughter tumbled after school. Charlie had been scaling countertops and high ledges since he could walk, and he mastered the monkey bars as a toddler. In his first day at the gym, Coach JR pulled Charlie's mom aside and asked whether Charlie wanted to join the pre-team, the first step toward competitive gymnastics. Charlie did, and, within a week, Coach JR invited him to join the Level 4 competition team for the upcoming season. Charlie was ecstatic to be part of the team, especially because he got his own locker. He began competing a month before that fateful Christmas. Charlie and his teammates practice 12 hours per week year-round and travel nationally for meets every November through April.

Community is a word that often connotes good feelings but is bandied about in so many ways that its definition has become blurry. We talk about the gay community, the African American community, the Washington Park (substitute the name of your own local neighborhood) community, the recovery community, the long-term care community, the animal rescue community, and the online gaming community. It's clear from these examples that members of a community may not know one another, live near one another, or even have much in common with one another. Regardless, communities are ultimately social accomplishments that simultaneously emerge from and are maintained by communication (Rothenbuhler, 1991, 2001). Members of a community create and sustain shared cultural meanings through a common set of customs, rituals, rules, language, and other communicative practices (Adelman & Frey, 1997; Geist-Martin et al., 2011). In this way, communities actively participate in the creation and perpetuation of culture. This perspective implies that the emotional connection, interdependence, and mutual influence inherent in supportive communities are performances of the various cultural conceptions (e.g., of health, aging, disease, pain) that shape the values and behaviors of community members (Rothenbuhler, 1991).

Communication scholars have primarily conceptualized community by focusing on four general attributes: physical, support, influence, and meaning making (Underwood & Frey, 2008). Each of these attributes is grounded in social interaction, and all of them may overlap. Consider Charlie's gymnastics community, for example. His gym, 20 Mile Athletic Center, is a physical place where gymnasts, coaches, and families share a sense of belonging, participate in established routines, and identify as 20 Mile Strong. A brief examination of these intersecting attributes will help lay the foundation for the remainder of this chapter.

Popular definitions of community usually incorporate the notion of a geographically bounded place, particular group, or virtual site. Health scholars study physical locations ranging from geographic areas, such as food insecurity in rural America (Ramadurai, Sharf, & Sharkey, 2012), to specific cities, such as healthcare in New Orleans before and after Hurricane Katrina (Rudowitz, Rowland, & Shartzer, 2006), to built environments, such as the illicit use of ADHD medications on a college campus (DeSantis, Webb, & Noar, 2008). A second set of health-related studies focuses on organized groups, such as Dancing Wheels, a modern dance company that integrates professional stand-up and sit-down (wheelchair) dancers (Quinlan & Harter, 2010), or PAWS Houston, a volunteer-driven nonprofit organization dedicated to preserving the human–animal bond between patients and their personal pets during long periods of hospitalization (Yamasaki, in press). Online communities, including Facebook (Wright, 2012), CaringBridge (Anderson, 2011), and various health-related forums (Tanis, 2008), have generated increased interest, as well. Importantly, the shared experience of place, including relational connections with others and an emotional bond to places and things (Altman & Low, 1992), also figures into community members' interpretations of and commitment to their physical site or group.

Relatedly, psychological belonging, social bonding, and emotional aid comprise the support attribute of community (Underwood & Frey, 2008)—or what Peter Block (2008) deems the *structure of belonging*. In their seminal work on communal life in a residential facility for people with AIDS, Adelman and Frey (1997) detail the everyday communicative practices that symbolically construct health and community, such as house governance, bereavement rituals, and formal and informal supportive conversations. Other studies examine how stories of identity, history, and possibility moderate between physical places and feelings of belonging to create a sense of community and well-being for residents (Kim & Ball-Rokeach, 2006; mcclellan, 2011; Nowell, Berkowitz, Deacon, & Foster-Fishman, 2006).

The collective stories circulating within community also serve to regulate social order, inspire collective action, and justify behavioral norms—all influence attributes identified by scholars as an inherent feature of community life (Underwood & Frey, 2008). In his ethnography of a cigar shop, for example, Alan DeSantis (2002, 2003) identifies recurring prosmoking arguments that the regular patrons share to (1) refute the findings of the medical establishment, (2) shield them from the impact of antismoking messages, and (3) relieve their anxiety created by smoking. This sense of us versus them is also evident in a study that explores how elderly residents story prior personal and professional experiences to (1) make sense of assisted living and (2) cope with membership in a community comprised of diverse interests, backgrounds, and impairments to ultimately enjoy their lives within the facility (Yamasaki & Sharf, 2010).

Finally, members communicate shared beliefs, attitudes, and values—meaning-making attributes (Underwood & Frey, 2008)—that shape the identity and ideology of a community. To illustrate, a growing number of studies have explored imaginative alternatives to the dominant narrative of decline that largely shapes the ways we envision old age in retirement and long-term care communities (Biggs, Bernard, Kingston, & Nettleton, 2000; Yamasaki, 2009; Yamasaki, 2013). In these communities, shared narratives of possibility, growth, and humanity in late life contribute to greater well-being and quality of life. Theorizing Practice 10.1 asks you to consider how community exists—or is lacking—in your own neighborhood.

Theorizing Practice 10.1
Who Are the People in Your Neighborhood?

Read the following selection from Peter Lovenheim's (2010, pp. xv–xviii) *In the Neighborhood: The Search for Community on an American Street, One Sleepover at a Time*, and consider your own neighborhood. What barriers, if any, separate you from your neighbors, and what inventive ways could bring you closer?

> *It was a calamity on my street, in a middle-class suburb of Rochester, New York, that got me thinking about this. . . . My neighbor had shot and killed his wife, and then himself. Their two young children had run screaming into the night.*
>
> *Though the couple—both physicians—had lived on our street for seven years, my wife and I hardly knew them. We'd see them jogging together. Sometimes our children would carpool. Some of the neighbors attended the funerals and called on relatives. Someone laid a single bunch of yellow flowers at the family's front door, but nothing else was done to mark the loss. Within weeks, the children had moved with their grandparents to another part of town. The only indication that anything had changed was the FOR SALE sign on the lawn.*
>
> *A family had vanished, yet the impact on our neighborhood was slight. How could that be? Did I live in a community or just in a house on a street surrounded by people whose lives were entirely separate? Few of my neighbors, I later learned, knew each other more than casually; many didn't know even the names of those a few doors down.*
>
> *Why is it that in an age of cheap long-distance rates, discount airlines, and the Internet, when we can create community anywhere, we often don't know the people who live next door?*
>
> *It was not a fluke that the neighbors involved in the shooting were physicians; many of the people who live on my street are physicians, business owners, and other professionals. I understood that as busy people they valued their privacy; for many, privacy was one of the reasons they had moved here. Indeed, the physical design of our street promoted this. Lots were wide; outdoor activity, if any, occurred in backyards. And as in many suburban*

(continued)

neighborhoods, there was no public space to congregate. In short, despite its being upscale, my street reflected the reality on many streets in America today: people were cordial, but they liked their privacy and went about their lives largely detached from those living around them.

What would it take, I wondered, to penetrate the barriers between us? I thought about childhood sleepovers and the insight I used to get from waking up inside a friend's home. More recently, my family and I had done summer house exchanges with families in Europe— they stayed in our house while we stayed in theirs. After living in these strangers' homes— waking in their beds, fixing meals in their kitchens, and walking in their neighborhoods—we had a strong sense of what their lives were about, something that would have been impossible to achieve just through conversation.

But would my neighbors let me sleep over and write about their lives from inside their houses? In fact, they did, and the understanding I gained—and the lasting connections that were made—validated my hunch that sleeping over would be essential. . . . Eventually, I met a woman living three doors away who was seriously ill with breast cancer and in need of help. She had recently divorced and had two young daughters. My goal shifted: could we build a supportive community around her—in effect, patch together a real neighborhood?

This is the story of my journey.

■ Communicating Support

Only three months after his initial diagnosis, Charlie's bald spots started increasing in size. His parents could no longer cover them with creative styling, so they decided it was time to shave his head. The decision was extremely traumatic for all of them, but especially for Charlie. He wanted to look "normal" and didn't realize the cover-up job no longer looked good. Fortunately, his parents were able to time the decision with Charlie's first out-of-state meet in Las Vegas. Coach JR convinced Charlie to shave the sides and spike the hair on top into a "faux hawk" by doing the same with his own hair. His teammates loved Charlie's new look, which helped ease Charlie into eventually shaving his entire head. He wore a hat to school, but Coach JR wouldn't let him wear one to the gym. When Charlie's parents asked whether he could wear a cap to practice, Coach JR said, "No, you don't need that, Charlie. Just shave it off. It'll be cool." Charlie did, and the gym became the one place he felt comfortable going bald. Everyone accepted him. Once his hair fell out completely and a specialist diagnosed him with alopecia totalis, most of them even rubbed his head for good luck before meets. "That's my lucky head!" exclaims Coach Wes when people inquire about Charlie. "Many people ask if he has cancer, but nope, he's completely healthy. Just built like a BULL."

Supportive communication can buffer our stress and help us cope in the midst of life-altering health experiences. Health problems, by their very nature, increase uncertainty. They disrupt the predictability of our lives and often force us to redefine who we are. As Charlie struggled with his changing appearance, his coaches' ongoing encouragement illustrates what countless scholars have long argued: Communication is central to improving the well-being of people in need. Evidence demonstrates that supportive communication promotes psychological and physical health by (1) providing health-relevant information, (2) motivating healthy behavior, (3) promoting self-esteem and self-care, and (4) reducing emotional distress (MacGeorge, Feng, & Burleson, 2011).

Social Support

Albrecht and Adelman (1987) first conceptualized social support as communication that reduces uncertainty and increases perceptions of personal control. Research demonstrates that people cope best when they feel informed, actively involved, and valued (e.g., Metts & Manns, 1996). However, scholars have since recognized that reducing uncertainty may be impossible or even undesirable (such as telling people how long they have to live) in some situations (e.g., Babrow, Hines, & Kasch, 2000; Brashers, Neidig, & Goldsmith, 2004). Charlie and his parents, for example, now know alopecia areata is highly unpredictable and cyclical. The disease course is different for every person, and hair can grow back in or fall out again at any time. Charlie currently has no scalp hair, but it could grow back at some point or his alopecia totalis could eventually progress to alopecia universalis. Given the nature of Charlie's condition, the social support he receives through meaningful relationships at the gym plays an important role in strengthening his confidence and self-acceptance in the face of these unknowns.

Social support encompasses the verbal and nonverbal assistance, comfort, or advice we give to others or seek and receive during difficult times. Some commonly recognized types of social support include *informational support* (e.g., giving advice or sharing information), *instrumental support* (e.g., assisting with tasks or providing resources), *appraisal support* (e.g., offering new perspectives), *esteem support* (e.g., enhancing self-worth and feelings about abilities, attributes, or accomplishments), and *emotional support* (e.g., expressing care, empathy, and acceptance). People prefer different types of support—problem-focused or emotion-focused—under different circumstances, including the nature or status of the problem, the recipient's own needs and resources, the provider's expertise, and the quality of information or aid received (Goldsmith & Albrecht, 2011, p. 340).

While enacted (i.e., received) support has been linked to improved health and overall well-being (Goldsmith & Albrecht, 2011; MacGeorge et al., 2011), the perception that people are (or would be) available to offer needed support may be even more beneficial (Haber, Cohen, Lucas, & Baltes, 2007; McDowell, & Serovich, 2007; Reinhardt, Boerner, & Horowitz, 2006). Research with family caregivers, for example, illustrates the negative costs—or social support burden—associated with seeking, maintaining, and receiving social support (Wittenberg-Lyles, Washington, Demiris, Oliver, & Shaunfield, 2014). Support that is not perceived as helpful or supportive may increase the recipient's stress and anxiety, as could having to ask for help or relinquish control in order to please others. During her 15-month-old daughter's nine-week ordeal with septic shock, Sherianne Shuler (2011) realized "there are plenty of ways to offer well-meaning but ineffective support" (p. 199), including vague offers (e.g., "let us know what we can do to help"), emotionally draining visits (e.g., having to support or entertain visitors), and an overwhelming number of calls and visits in the first days that drop to very few in later weeks when the family is still trying to cope.

Support Groups

Sometimes people would rather receive social support from individuals who are outside their circle of family or friends (i.e., weak ties versus strong ties). Weak-tie support is sometimes perceived as more useful than strong-tie support because it can offer diverse points of view and information, present less risk when disclosing information, offer more objective feedback, and require less role obligation than support provided from close personal relationships (Wright & Miller, 2010). Support groups are particularly popular ways to find and receive weak-tie support. Support groups exist for people with similar difficult circumstances (e.g., illness, trauma, addiction, stigma, loss) to come together for mutual information and support. They may utilize a number of face-to-face formats, from informal self-help groups moderated by a volunteer peer facilitator to treatment groups guided by a trained professional, or take place entirely online. Some meet daily (e.g., Alcoholics Anonymous), some form organically (e.g., a group of patients receiving chemotherapy in the same room at the same time on a weekly or monthly basis), and some even comprise annual family vacations. For example, dozens of free residential summer camps create communities that foster camaraderie, possibility, inclusivity, and fun for seriously ill children and their families. Some of these better-known camps include the Hole in the Wall Gang Camp (http://www.holeinthewallgang.org), Camp Sunshine (http://www.campsunshine.org), The Rainbow Connection Camp (http://www.rccamp.org), and Camp Good Days and Special Times (http://campgooddays.org).

Clearly, support groups offer many advantages. Hearing similar stories and feelings from people who share the same challenges and experiences helps members validate and normalize their own experiences and feelings. They realize they are not alone, feel a sense of belonging, and often feel better about themselves when they are able to reciprocate support to other members of the group. Members also benefit from the collective expertise of people with firsthand information who can offer relevant problem-focused support in constructive and meaningful ways. And, as weak-tie support, members can feel supported—and, importantly, heard—without the risk of potentially damaging close personal relationships.

Computer-mediated support groups can be especially beneficial for people coping with health-related stigma, such as addiction (e.g., Jodlowski, Sharf, Haidet, Nguyen, & Woodard, 2007), eating disorders (e.g., Yeshua-Katz & Martins, 2013), or mental illness (e.g., Vayreda & Antaki, 2009). In addition to convenience, online interactions offer increased anonymity and a reliance on verbal messages (i.e., postings) rather than visual social cues (i.e., sex, race, age, etc.). These features tend to promote increased self-disclosure and a willingness to discuss sensitive topics without the embarrassment of revealing personal information to strangers in face-to-face encounters (Wright, 2016; Wright, Johnson, Bernard, & Averbeck, 2011; Wright & Rains, 2013). Theorizing Practice 10.2 helps you familiarize yourself in with some of the online support programs available to individuals with alopecia areata and their families.

Theorizing Practice 10.2
Seeking Support and Creating Community

The National Alopecia Areata Foundation (NAAF; http://www.naaf.org) support program offers a number of different ways to create a sense of community among individuals with alopecia areata and their families:

1. Members-only message boards where individuals living with alopecia areata can seek, share, and respond to personal stories, questions, advice, and encouragement.

2. Face-to-face support groups across the world with a common mission to provide individuals with alopecia areata, their families, and their friends a safe, comfortable, and trusting environment in which to share their personal experiences.

3. *Alopecia Areata News*, a quarterly newsletter written for the alopecia areata community by parents, fundraisers, researchers, doctors, supporters and more.

4. *Helping Hearts through Hands*, a pen-pal program that connects people who have or know people with alopecia areata and want to share their experiences and gain support from others like them.

5. An annual four-day family conference for people of all ages who have alopecia areata or care about people who do.

6. Extensive online presence, including the website, Twitter, Facebook, and YouTube.

If you or a loved one were diagnosed with alopecia areata, which of the above would most appeal to you? Would your answer be different two years after diagnosis? How would your participation change over time?

HCIA 10.1

Online Social Support for Recovering Addicts

Kevin B. Wright

One of the main ideas that drew me to the study of health communication is the notion that people can improve their mental and physical health by interacting with others during times of stress and crisis. Few problems are more stressful than health issues, particularly if a person is facing a stigmatized health condition. Health-related stigma may make it difficult for individuals to seek social support from others, especially when the stigma is linked to negative personal behaviors, such as drug use, or behaviors that are viewed as within a person's control, such as the ability to stop using drugs any time.

Thankfully, people who seek support for stigmatized health concerns often experience positive health outcomes, even when the support they receive comes from people they may not know well. In fact, close friends and family members often have difficulty providing adequate support to someone who is addicted to drugs. They may engage in problematic behaviors such as: not talking about the problem, talking about the problem too much, enabling the addict, using social control strategies (e.g., hiding money or car keys from the addict), or providing unwanted advice. These communication problems can be attributed to their lack of personal experience with or understanding of addiction.

Heroin addiction is a good example of a stigmatized illness, and the stigma associated with heroin use and dependency can actually prevent people who are addicted from getting the proper support and treatment they need to recover from this problem. Still, people can and do recover from drug addiction, although it typically requires a period of detoxification to get through the physical dependence to the addictive substance. After detoxification, people need many years of social support to learn new ways to cope with their problems without relying on drugs. The social support an addict receives is important to the recovery process, and it has been linked to positive mental and physical health outcomes,

(continued)

such as reduced stress, increased quality of life, reduced depression, shorter hospital stays, reduced incidents of stress-related illness, and reduced relapse rates.

In recent years, more and more people are seeking social support online via online support communities and social networking sites such as Facebook. More than 36 million Americans currently use some type of health-related online support community, and this number is projected to grow in the coming years. Although the people that an individual may encounter in an online support community are likely strangers, at least at first, they are also more likely to share many similarities with the addict. Each member of the community can understand what another person is feeling, recognize common triggers or situations that lead a person to engage in drug use, and also understand what it is like to live with the stigma of drug addiction. Moreover, they are less likely to judge each other since they share a common addiction, and it is very unlikely that people within the online support community will know members of an addict's close friend and family network. So, it is often less risky to communicate about problems such as drug addiction within this type of environment.

A variety of research studies, including some of my own, have found that the support that drug addicts find in online communities is often perceived as more helpful and satisfying than the support that an addict can obtain from his or her closer network ties (i.e., close friends and family members). Much of the research suggests that the support that people obtain in online communities is as good as, and in some cases better than, the support people receive from closer ties. In addition, the support people receive online is linked to the same positive health outcomes (e.g., reduced depression, lower morbidity and mortality rates, etc.) as support obtained in the face-to-face world.

However, using online support communities to overcome a serious problem like drug addiction is not without its problems. Ultimately, an addict has to cope with his or her addiction in the face-to-face world. I like to think of online support communities as an important resource for people with health concerns, but it is only one of many resources that a person can use. Certainly, consulting with medical professionals and finding ways to better communicate about stigmatized health issues with closer ties can provide benefits to people struggling with addiction. Through online interactions with other addicts, people can realize that they do not need to feel ashamed of their problems. In addition, community members may emphasize the importance of medical treatment, using the community for ongoing support and information, and the need to continue repairing the close relationships that were damaged by the addictive behavior.

QUESTIONS TO PONDER

1. What stigmas do you associate with heroin use? What other types of health conditions are stigmatized?

2. What types of communication problems might people living with these conditions experience with their friends and family members?

3. How might online support communities make it easier to communicate and obtain support for these health concerns?

4. What problems might occur within online support communities that may limit the positive effects of the social support a person may potentially obtain?

5. Can you think of other advantages to using these communities for people facing health concerns?

Source: Wright, K. B., & Rains, S. (2013). Weak-tie support network preference, stigma, and health outcomes in computer-mediated support groups. *Journal of Applied Communication Research, 41*, 309–324.

■ Community Connections and Capacities

A year after Charlie's diagnosis, a mutual friend approached his parents at church and offered to introduce them to Anne Trujillo, a longtime news anchor at Channel 7 in Denver who was coming to terms with her own recent diagnosis. "Of course, I notice everyone's hair now. I see plenty of men who have had some hair loss. People don't think twice about that. They do when it comes to women," she said in a personal message posted on social media. "We women judge ourselves harshly. This is a message to women: Let's be more supportive of one another. Now I have an opportunity, with my job, to be able to say it out loud." Anne, who wears hair extensions, found it liberating to go public after months of viewer speculation regarding her changing appearance. "I can see how people would want to stay home and hide, but I've done enough crying," said Anne.

"I'm getting comfortable with the idea of being a role model. As an adult, I can deal with this. I'm okay. I'm not panicked anymore." The following year, she and Charlie, now friends, appeared together in a televised public service announcement. The PSA aired regularly on Channel 7 throughout September, a month dedicated to national alopecia areata awareness.

That same September, the National Alopecia Areata Foundation (NAAF) teamed up with Major League Baseball to LOOK AT US! The Colorado Rockies agreed to hold an Alopecia Awareness Night, and Charlie's mom persuaded her company to donate 250 game-day tickets for the 20 Mile team to sell as a fundraiser. "Being completely bald at 8 years old is extremely traumatizing and can severely affect a child's self-esteem," explained his mom.

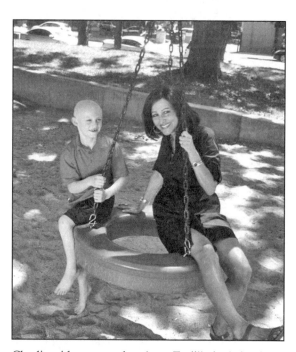

Charlie with news anchor Anne Trujillo in their televised PSA. (Courtesy of Josh Dieringer.)

"Without the strong support and acceptance of Charlie's teammates and gym family, we're not sure how he would have gotten through that first year. Since gymnastics has been such an integral part of Charlie's success in dealing with this disease, I want the team booster club to benefit from the proceeds while bringing awareness to a cause that's very close to our family."

20 Mile families united to sell the tickets. Many posted Facebook pleas to their own friends and family. "We're still looking for people to buy Rockies tickets to support Matt's gymnastics team AND to raise money for the National Alopecia Areata Foundation," wrote one teammate's mom. "Alopecia areata is an autoimmune disease that one of Matt's teammates, Charlie, has. But, you'd NEVER know it 'cause he's not letting it stop him ROCK the gymnastics world." Coach Wes posted a similar message: "Some fundraising mixed with a little fun. Help our little dudes

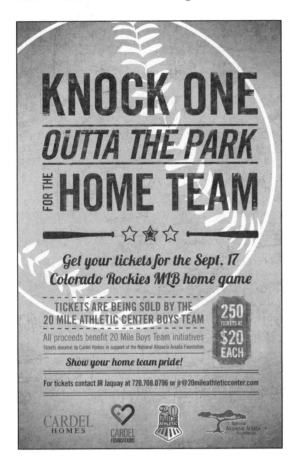

raise awareness and some extra cash for their upcoming season. Charlie's family is trying to bring awareness and support not only to the National Alopecia Areata Foundation, but for our own little man Charlie who rocks a bald head better than anyone I know! We're a pretty fun crowd to mingle with so DO IT!" They sold all 250 tickets, and the 20 Mile coaches, gymnasts, families, and friends enjoyed a night out together in support of Charlie and the NAAF community.

Supportive interactions occur within networks of relationships that weave individuals into groups and communities (Putnam & Feldstein, 2003). Our social networks are composed of individuals—from families, friendships, and formal organizations (e.g., school, work, clubs, religious groups, etc.)—with whom we have social ties (weak or strong) and from whom we receive social support on a personal level. They are dynamic, meaning our affiliations within these networks can—and usually do—change over time (Abramson, 2013). As we've learned in this chapter, our physical and mental health is influenced by our connections to others. In addition to our own social networks, we have (or may lack) resources and social connections within our larger communities. Putnam (2000) describes these connections, as they occur in political, civic, social, religious, and workplace participation, as *social capital*. Social capital refers to the features of social life—networks, norms, and trust—that facilitate cooperation and coordination for mutual benefit.

Consider Charlie's story, for example, and the ways his family's web of social networks mobilized with the greater community to raise awareness for alopecia areata and funds for his gymnastics team. First, a friend at church introduced Charlie and his parents to Anne Trujillo, who had only recently been diagnosed with alopecia and wanted to use her position as a news anchor to bring awareness to the condition. To do so, she invited Charlie to partner with her in a public service announcement that would be televised throughout September, deemed National Alopecia Areata Awareness Month. As part of that initiative, Major League Baseball teamed up with the National Alopecia Areata Foundation (NAAF), and the Colorado Rockies agreed to donate a portion of one game's proceeds to the cause. Charlie's mom, in recognition of the support he receives from gymnastics in coping with the condition, arranged for

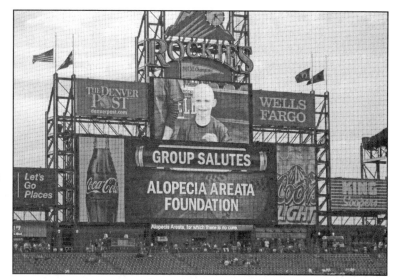

The Colorado Rockies and NAAF honored Charlie and others living with alopecia during the game. (Courtesy of Josh Dieringer.)

her company to donate game-day tickets to his team at 20 Mile, who then rallied their own social networks to buy tickets. In the end, 250 people attended the game in support of Charlie and his family, 20 Mile gymnastics, and the NAAF.

Community Connections

Community connectedness is a significant focus of study for health communication scholars. Tomison (1999) defines community connectedness as a strong sense of identity or feeling of belonging to the community; good relationships with neighbors, friends, and/or family; and a number of links with people or groups from outside the individual's immediate group. Indeed, the availability of formal and informal social support between and among friends, family members, acquaintances, neighbors, and even strangers indicates connections to the community and offers profound consequences for physical and mental well-being (Albrecht & Goldsmith, 2003). In particular, dense support networks—those in which relational partners are closely linked through multiple roles and more likely to presume the reciprocation of future supportive behavior—most often facilitate supportive communication and provide a sense of attachment to the wider community (Goldsmith & Albrecht, 2011).

Communities high in social capital generally include high civic engagement, member participation in voluntary activities, and high levels of trust and norms of mutual aid between its members (Putnam, 2000). Putnam distinguishes between two types of social capital: bonding and bridging. *Bonding social capital* is formed of strong ties among family members and close friends, while *bridging social capital* comprises overlapping networks of weaker ties, such as neighbors, acquaintances, and coworkers. Bridging social capital is harder to create than bonding social capital, but it is essential for healthy public life (Putnam & Feldstein, 2003). Ultimately, communities as a whole benefit most when social networks are diverse, inclusive, tie together organizations, and span other communities (Flora, 1998).

Just as the Internet has proven beneficial for the provision of weak-tie social support (Wright, 2009, 2016; Wright et al., 2011), it also has potential for strengthening social capital. Some studies demonstrate that teenagers and college students who use social network sites report higher social capital in both their online and school relationships (Ahn, 2012; Ellison, Steinfield, & Lampe, 2007). Other studies conducted with adults find that heavy Internet users with bridging ties have higher social engagement, use the Internet for social purposes, and participate more often in local meetings and events than heavy Internet users with no bridging ties (Kavanaugh, Reese, Carroll, & Rosson, 2005; Mesch & Talmud, 2010). Combined, such research suggests that the Internet—in the hands of bridging individuals—is a tool for enhancing social relations, increasing information exchange, and strengthening face-to-face interactions, all of which help to build both bonding and bridging social capital in communities (Kavanaugh et al., 2005).

Still, researchers have determined that weak social ties at the expense of meaningful relationships can be just as harmful as other well-established risk factors to health, including alcoholism, obesity, and smoking (Holt-Lunstad, Smith, & Layton, 2010; Steptoe, Shankar, Demakakos, & Wardle, 2013; Szalavitz, 2013). These profound consequences have compelled some experts to deem social isolation a public health issue in need of interventions (Nutt, 2016). And, while the Internet may offer hundreds of Facebook friends or Instagram followers, the quality—rather than quantity—of close relationships may ultimately matter more for happiness, health, and well-being. Satisfying friendships, according to communication scholar Bill Rawlins, embody three common expectations: someone to talk to, someone to depend on, and someone to enjoy (Beck, 2015; see also Rawlins, 2009). Social media may help us maintain many friendships at a superficial level, but we need meaningful connections to thrive.

Community Capacities

Community connectedness is linked to the health of community members and to the health of the community itself. Indeed, our individual behaviors, social relationships, and physical environments are all closely related to our local community ties. Communities that have a variety of health-related resources, high levels of reciprocal trust among their members, and meaningful social ties generally face lower numbers of health-related barriers and are better able to sustain the health of their members (Dutta, 2008). Community ties also serve as communicative links for providing health information to community members and reinforcing health-enhancing behaviors through community networks. According to Cannuscio, Block, and Kawachi (2003), communities with high levels of social capital are better equipped to protect the health of their members, including those who are socially isolated, and are more effective in responding to external health threats. Individuals who feel part of a healthy community are likely to see that they can contribute something worthwhile to that community, as well, thereby creating a cycle of positive support and enhanced community life (Tomison, 1999).

John Kretzmann and John McKnight—cofounders and codirectors of the Asset-Based Community Development (ABCD) Institute at Northwestern University—have long observed that many experts approach the social health problems of communities through a negative conceptual framework focused on deficits, problems, and needs. From this perspective, institutional services provide solutions that put community members in the role of dependent clients. Kretzmann and McKnight (1993; see also McKnight & Block, 2010) offer an alternative influential model that acknowledges the existence of problems but emphasizes the capacities, gifts, and assets of community residents. These residents include not only individuals but also local institutions, such as schools, hospitals, and libraries, and voluntary citizen associations, such as churches, sports leagues, and clubs. Kretzmann and McKnight, as well as Putnam, offer a perspective of community health that is premised on genuine, internal empowerment of residents, trusting that they can mobilize the resources necessary to handle the problems they face. This perspective incorporates partnership, largely within but also with entities outside of the community, such as universities, government agencies, and public health professionals. To that end, the ABCD Institute works with community-building leaders to support community-based efforts to rediscover local capacities and to mobilize citizens' resources to solve problems. What would those efforts look like or entail for you? See Theorizing Practice 10.3 to assess the needs and capacities of your primary physical community.

Theorizing Practice 10.3
Assessing Your Community

- Identify your primary physical community. This may be your former or current neighborhood, university campus, dormitory, and so on.

- List the social health problems, needs, and deficits of your community.

- Now think about your community in terms of its capacities, assets, and gifts. Who are the constituent members, local institutions, and voluntary associations that can be mobilized to help with social health concerns?

- How do you fit into this picture?

Source: Geist-Martin, Ray, & Sharf, 2011, p. 346

HCIA 10.2

Transforming Needle Park to Promote Urban Health

Gary L. Kreps

Marvin Gaye Park (MGP), in the inner-city, Anacostia neighborhood of Washington, DC, was named in honor of the great R & B singer Marvin Gaye who grew up nearby. More than 600 low-income, predominantly African American families live in the park's adjacent neighborhoods. When the city closed a nearby methadone clinic in 2008, hundreds of addicts were drawn to the park, which became known popularly as "Needle Park" due to rampant drug use within its borders. The growing drug trade, violence, and deterioration of the park

(continued)

environment discouraged parents from allowing their children to play in the park, limiting opportunities for youth physical activity. This limitation on physical activity disproportionately affecting low-income, inner-city, minority youth can lead to obesity, diabetes, heart disease, and other serious health problems.

In response, volunteers, led by the National Recreation and Park Association (NRPA), worked with recreational equipment corporations, city agencies (such as local police, the park authority, and the Mayor's office), local organizations, and community members to drive out the drug trade and clean up the park. They removed more than 3.5 million pounds of trash, 9,000 hypodermic needles, and 78 abandoned cars from the park. A new playground area was built, including swing sets and modern playground activity stations. A special safety surface throughout the play area and park benches around the perimeter completed the installation. There also was landscaping work done to the park, as well as lights, fences, and other improvements added to make the park more attractive for youth recreational activities. The renovation represented a significant environmental change for the community served by the park.

I directed a research team to assess the influences of the environmental changes to the park on youth physical activity. Our team was interested in the role of communication in reducing health inequities, such as profoundly negative health outcomes that harm at-risk populations, referred to as health disparities research. Our work was grounded in the Ecological Theory that describes how environmental factors can facilitate or discourage health behaviors, a serious issue in many inner-city neighborhoods where there are limited safe and suitable recreational facilities available. The research team conducted observational research at MGP as well as in a comparison park, Oxon Run Park (ORP) located in a nearby urban community. A specific area within ORP was selected for observation based on its comparable size and location to MGP in order to simulate baseline physical activity levels prior to the renovation of MGP. The physical activity of area youth from 6 to 14 years of age was measured at the two sites using direct field observations.

The second site, ORP, was chosen as a comparison park because it simulated the approximate size and type of playground area at MGP prior to renovation, although it does not have all the debris that was part of the old Needle Park. The community where ORP is located is demographically similar to the MGP neighborhood, where almost all the residents are African American, and the proportion of families living below the poverty line is 32%. The comparison park's observation area has no equipment, as was the case with MGP pre-renovation. However, ORP is located in a safer area, which is to say that it had no community reputation as being unsafe, or did not demonstrate being inhabited by drug dealers or drug users. In many ways, ORP is a very conservative comparison area for this study, since it is much cleaner and safer than the old MGP area.

The results of the study showed that implementation of environmental changes to park facilities at MGP resulted in dramatically increased youth physical activity. The data showed significant differences between the renovated park and the comparison park in terms of youth physical activity rates and intensity. In contrast to the comparison park, where very few visitors and minimal physical activity were observed, a sizable number of youth visited the renovated park. Most of the youth visitors to the park actively engaged in physical activity (76.7%), and used the park equipment (62.6%) for a fair amount of time, an average of 25 minutes.

The CDC recommends that youth engage in one hour of aerobic physical activity per day, with three of those days including bone-strengthening activities such as jumping rope or running and three of those days including muscle strengthening activities such as gymnastics or pushups. Considering the fact that youth in this study spent more than 75% of their time (approximately 18 minutes per visit) participating in physical activity, the renovated park is likely to help youth achieve recommended levels of physical activity to promote their health.

QUESTIONS TO PONDER

1. How does the physical environment that surrounds where you live influence your health beliefs and health behaviors? What is a specific example?

2. In what ways do you think your own living environment is similar to or differs from that of the residents of the MGP neighborhood? What environmental factors may lead to exercise-related health disparities for inner-city, low income, and minority youth?

3. Focus on one or two of the specific environmental factors leading to exercise-related health disparities you've just identified in #2 above. How could these issues be re-designed or re-considered in order to encourage youth physical activity?

4. Why is community participation in urban redesign an important part of health promotion?

5. What implications can be drawn from this study about other applications of environmental design to promote health?

Source: Kreps, G. L., Villagran, M. M., Trowbridge, J., Baldwin, P., Barbier, Y., Chang, A., Jun, J., Tucker, M., Saxton-Ross, A., & Friedman, S. (2013). Evaluation of the influence of an urban community park revitalization on African-American youth physical activity. In M. J. Dutta & G. L. Kreps (Eds.), *Reducing health disparities: Communication interventions* (pp. 209–225). New York, NY: Peter Lang.

▪ Epilogue

Today, Charlie is 12 years old, a Level 8 gymnast, and a confident 6th grader in the third year of his new school. His classmates have accepted his appearance without question and, on the class's YouTube Fridays, they marvel at the 20 Mile videos uploaded by his coaches and teammates' parents. "The kids at my old school teased me a lot, so I always wore a hat because it bothered me," says Charlie. "But now I like being bald. No one has said anything mean here. Not one." He stops to watch himself perform on rings, then shrugs and nods thoughtfully. "This is who I am. I hope I always stay this way."

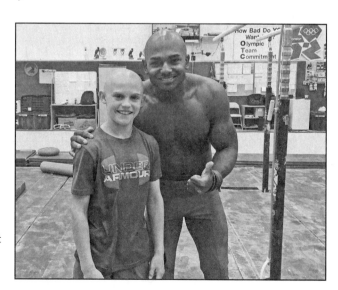

Charlie with U.S. Olympic gymnast John Orozco. (Courtesy of Josh Dieringer.)

■ Conclusion

Social support, social ties, and meaningful social roles are associated with better physical and mental health for people of all ages (Goldsmith & Albrecht, 2011). Our communities—whether conceptualized by physical, support, influence, and/or meaning-making attributes—emerge through communication and help shape our health-related values and behaviors. When illness or difficult conditions disrupt the predictability of our lives and force us to redefine who we are, supportive communication helps us manage uncertainty and more effectively cope. Social support encompasses the verbal and nonverbal assistance, comfort, or advice we give to others or seek and receive from close, casual, formal, and informal ties. These social ties comprise various social networks that, when combined with community resources and capacities, facilitate the cooperation, coordination, and imagination needed for supportive communities that are healthy and connected.

Discussion Questions

1. What does *community* mean to you? How would you characterize the different ones to which you belong?

2. Describe the different types of social support and give an example of each from your own experiences.

3. What is the difference between weak-tie and strong-tie support? Where do the people in your life fit? When and why would you seek support from some instead of others?

4. Pick a cause that's important to you and imagine a way to support it. What social connections could you call upon in the interrelated networks comprising your personal relationships and community resources? How could you coordinate them for mutual benefit?

REFERENCES

Abramson, T. A. (2013). The ties that bind. In J. M. Blanchard (Ed.), *Aging in community* (pp. 211–216). Chapel Hill, NC: Second Journey Publications.

Adelman, M. B., & Frey, L. R. (1997). *The fragile community: Living together with AIDS.* Mahwah, NJ: Erlbaum.

Ahn, J. (2012). Teenagers' experiences with social network sites: Relationships to bridging and bonding social capital. *The Information Society: An International Journal, 28,* 99–109.

Albrecht, T. L., & Adelman, M. (1987). Communicating social support: A theoretical perspective. In T. L. Albrecht & M. Adelman (Eds.), *Communicating social support* (pp. 18–39). Newbury Park, CA: Sage.

Albrecht, T. L., & Goldsmith, D. J. (2003). Social support, social networks, and health. In T. L. Thompson, A. M. Dorsey, K. I. Miller, & R. Parrott (Eds.), *Handbook of health communication* (pp. 263–284). Mahwah, NJ: Erlbaum.

Altman, I., & Low, S. M. (Eds.) (1992). *Place attachment. Human behavior and environment: Advances in theory and research* (Vol. 12). New York, NY: Plenum.

Anderson, I. K. (2011). The uses and gratifications of online care pages: A study of Caring-Bridge. *Health Communication, 26,* 546–559.

Babrow, A., Hines, S., & Kasch, C. (2000). Illness and uncertainty: Problematic integration and strategies for communicating about medical uncertainty and ambiguity. In B. B. Whaley (Ed.), *Explaining illness: Messages, strategies, and contexts* (pp. 41–67). Mahwah, NJ: Erlbaum.

Beck, J. (2015, Oct. 22). How friendships change in adulthood. *The Atlantic*. Retrieved from http://www.theatlantic.com/health/archive/2015/10/how-friendships-change-over-time-in-adulthood/411466/?utm_source=pocket&utm_medium=email&utm_campaign=pockethits

Biggs, S., Bernard, M., Kingston, P., & Nettleton, H. (2000). Lifestyles of belief: Narrative and culture in a retirement community. *Ageing & Society, 20,* 649–672.

Block, P. (2008). *Community: The structure of belonging*. San Francisco, CA: Berrett-Koehler Publishers.

Brashers, D. E., Neidig, J. L., & Goldsmith, D. J. (2004). Social support and the management of uncertainty for people living with HIV or AIDS. *Health Communication, 16,* 305–331.

Cannuscio, C., Block, J., & Kawachi, I. (2003). Social capital and successful aging: The role of senior housing. *Annals of Internal Medicine, 139,* 395–400.

DeSantis, A. D. (2002). Smoke screen: An ethnographic study of a cigar shop's collective rationalization. *Health Communication, 14,* 167–198.

DeSantis, A. D. (2003). A couple of white guys sitting around talking. *Journal of Contemporary Ethnography, 32,* 432–466.

DeSantis, A. D., Webb, E. M, & Noar, S. M. (2008). Illicit use of prescription ADHD medications on a college campus: A multi-methodological approach. *Journal of American College Health, 57,* 315–324.

Dutta, M. J. (2008). Culture, social capital, and health. *Communicating health: A culture-centered approach* (pp. 205–219). Cambridge, UK: Polity Press.

Ellison, N. B., Steinfield, C., & Lampe, C. (2007). The benefits of Facebook "friends": Social capital and college students' use of online social network sites. *Journal of Computer-Mediated Communication, 12,* 1143–1168.

Flora, J. L. (1998). Social capital and communities of place. *Rural Sociology, 63,* 481-506.

Geist-Martin, P., Ray, E. B., & Sharf, B. F. (2011). *Communicating health: Personal, cultural, and political complexities*. Long Grove, IL: Waveland Press.

Goldsmith, D. J., & Albrecht, T. L. (2011). Social support, social networks, and health: A guiding framework. In T. L. Thompson, R. Parrott, & J. F. Nussbaum (Eds.), *Handbook of health communication* (2nd ed., pp. 335–348). Mahwah, NJ: Routledge.

Haber, M. G., Cohen, J. L., Lucas, T., & Baltes, B. (2007). The relationship between self-reported received and perceived social support: A meta-analytic review. *American Journal of Community Psychology, 39,* 133–144.

Holt-Lunstad, J., Smith, T. B., & Layton, J. B. (2010). Social relationships and mortality risk: A meta-analytic review. *PLOS Medicine, 7*(7), e1000316.

Jodlowski, D., Sharf, B. F., Haidet, P., Nguyen, L. C., & Woodard, L. D. (2007). "Screwed for life": Examining identification and division in addiction narratives. *Communication & Medicine, 4,* 15–26.

Kavanaugh, A. L., Reese, D. D., Carroll, J. M., & Rosson, M. B. (2005). Weak ties in networked communities. *The Information Society: An International Journal, 21,* 119–131.

Kim, Y-C., & Ball-Rokeach, S. J. (2006). Community storytelling network, neighborhood context, and civic engagement: A multilevel approach. *Human Communication Research, 32,* 411–439.

Kretzmann, J. P., & McKnight, J. L. (1993). *Building communities from the inside out: A path toward finding and mobilizing a community's assets*. Skokie, IL: ACTA Publications.

Lovenheim, P. (2010). *In the neighborhood: The search for community on an American street, one sleepover at a time*. New York, NY: Perigee.

MacGeorge, E. L., Feng, B., & Burleson, B. (2011). Supportive communication. In M. L. Knapp & J. A. Daly (Eds.), *Handbook of interpersonal communication* (4th ed., pp. 317–354). Thousand Oaks, CA: Sage.

mcclellan, e. d. (2011). Narrative as vernacular rhetoric: Understanding community among transients, tourists, and locals. *Storytelling, Self, Society, 7,* 188–210.

McDowell, T. L., & Serovich, J. M. (2007). The effect of perceived and actual support on the mental health of HIV-positive persons. *AIDS Care, 19,* 1223–1229.

McKnight, J., & Block, P. (2010). *The abundant community: Awakening the power of families and neighborhoods.* San Francisco, CA: Berrett-Koehler Publishers.

Mesch, G. S., & Talmud, I. (2010). Internet connectivity, community participation, and place attachment: A longitudinal study. *American Behavioral Scientist, 53,* 1095–1110.

Metts, S., & Manns, H. (1996). Coping with HIV and AIDS: The social and personal challenges. In E. B. Ray (Ed.), *Communication and disenfranchisement: Social issues and implications* (pp. 347–364). Mahwah, NJ: Lawrence Erlbaum.

Nowell, B. L., Berkowitz, S. L., Deacon, Z., & Foster-Fishman, P. (2006). Revealing the cues within community places: Stories of identity, history, and possibility. *American Journal of Community Psychology, 37,* 29–46.

Nutt, A. E. (2016, January 31). Loneliness grows from individual ache to public health hazard. *The Washington Post.* Retrieved from https://www.washingtonpost.com/national/health-science/loneliness-grows-from-individual-ache-to-public-health-hazard/2016/01/31/cf246c56-ba20-11e5-99f3-184bc379b12d_story.html

Putnam, R. D. (2000). *Bowling alone: The collapse and revival of American community.* New York, NY: Simon & Schuster.

Putnam, R. D., & Feldstein, L. M. (2003). *Better together: Restoring the American community.* New York, NY: Simon & Schuster.

Quinlan, M. M., & Harter, L. M. (2010). Meaning in motion: The embodied poetics and politics of Dancing Wheels. *Text & Performance Quarterly, 30,* 374–395.

Ramadurai, V., Sharf, B. F., & Sharkey, J. R. (2012). Rural food insecurity in the United States as an overlooked site of struggle in health communication. *Health Communication, 27,* 794–805.

Rawlins, W. K. (2009). *The compass of friendship: Narratives, identities, and dialogues.* Thousand Oaks, CA: Sage.

Reinhardt, J. P., Boerner, K., & Horowitz, A. (2006). Good to have but not to use: Differential impact of perceived and received support on well-being. *Journal of Social and Personal Relationships, 23,* 117–129.

Rothenbuhler, E. W. (1991). The process of community involvement. *Communication Monographs, 58,* 63–78.

Rothenbuhler, E. W. (2001). Revising communication research for working on community. In G. J. Shepherd & E. W. Rothenbuhler (Eds.), *Communication and community* (pp. 159–179). Mahwah, NJ: Erlbaum.

Rudowitz, R., Rowland, D., & Shartzer, A. (2006). Health care in New Orleans before and after Hurricane Katrina. *Health Affairs, 25,* w393–w406.

Shuler, S. (2011). Social support without strings attached. *Health Communication, 26,* 198–201.

Steptoe, A., Shankar, A., Demakakos, P., & Wardle, J. (2013). Social isolation, loneliness, and all-cause mortality in older men and women. *Proceedings of the National Academy of Sciences of the United States of America, 110,* 5797–5801.

Szalavitz, M. (2013, March 26). Social isolation, not just feeling lonely, may shorten lives. *Time.* Retrieved from http://healthland.time.com/2013/03/26/social-isolation-not-just-feeling-lonely-may-shorten-lives/

Tanis, M. (2008). Health-related on-line forums: What's the big attraction? *Journal of Health Communication, 13,* 698–714.

Tomison, A. (1999). *Creating the vision: Communities and connectedness.* Invited address to the OzChild Child Exp, 22 April, 1999, Melbourne.

Underwood, E. D., & Frey, L. R. (2008). Communication and community: Clarifying common discourse across a scholarly community. In C. S. Beck (Ed.), *Communication yearbook 31* (pp. 370–418). Mahwah, NJ: Routledge.

Vayreda, A., & Antaki, C. (2009). Social support and unsolicited advice in a bipolar disorder online forum. *Qualitative Health Research, 19,* 931–942.

Wittenberg-Lyles, E., Washington, K., Demiris, G., Oliver, D. P., & Shaunfield, S. (2014). Understanding social support burden among family caregivers. *Health Communication, 29,* 901-910.

Wright, K. (2012). Similarity, network convergence, and availability of emotional support as predictors of strong-tie/weak-tie support network preference on Facebook. *Southern Communication Journal, 77,* 389–402.

Wright, K. B. (2009). Increasing computer-mediated social support. In J. C. Parker & E. Thorson (Eds.), *Health communication in the new media landscape* (pp. 243–266). New York, NY: Springer.

Wright, K. B. (2016). Communication in health-related online social support groups/communities: A review of research on predictors of participation, applications of social support theory, and health outcomes. *Review of Communication Research, 4,* 65–87.

Wright, K. B., Johnson, A. J., Bernard, D. R., & Averbeck, J. (2011). Computer-mediated social support: Promises and pitfalls for individuals coping with health concerns. In T. L. Thompson, R. Parrott, & J. F. Nussbaum (Eds.), *Handbook of health communication* (2nd ed., pp. 349–362). Mahwah, NJ: Routledge.

Wright, K. B., & Miller, C. H. (2010). A measure of weak-tie/strong-tie support network preference. *Communication Monographs, 77,* 502–520.

Wright, K. B., & Rains, S. A. (2013). Weak-tie support network preference, health-related stigma, and health outcomes in computer-mediated support groups. *Journal of Applied Communication Research, 41,* 309–324.

Yamasaki, J. (2009). Though much is taken, much abides: The storied world of aging in a fictionalized retirement home. *Health Communication, 24,* 588–596.

Yamasaki, J. (2013). The poetic possibilities of long-term care. In L. M. Harter & Associates, *Imagining new normals: A narrative framework for health communication* (pp. 107–124). Dubuque, IA: Kendall/Hunt Publishing Company.

Yamasaki, J. (in press). The communicative role of companion pets in patient-centered critical care. *Patient Education and Counseling.*

Yamasaki, J., & Sharf, B. F. (2010). Opting out while fitting in: How residents make sense of assisted living and cope with community life. *Journal of Aging Studies, 25,* 13–21.

Yeshua-Katz, D., & Martins, N. (2013). Communicating stigma: The pro-ana paradox. *Health Communication, 28,* 499–508.

11

Communicating through Health Campaigns and Entertainment-Education

Katherine A. Foss

Cecelia, eight months pregnant with her first baby, was driving in her car with her best friend, Kristi, a mother of three small children. Cecelia was asking Kristi her advice about breastfeeding. Cecelia had read online and in expectant mother books that breastfeeding is healthier for both mother and baby. She had even recently watched an episode of Modern Family, and the fact that Gloria had chosen to breastfeed impressed her. But Cecelia wanted to get her best friend's first-hand take on breastfeeding: what the experience is really like and how she can succeed at it.

Approximately 77% of American women intend to breastfeed, yet only 37.7% are exclusively nursing at three months ("Breastfeeding Report Card," 2014). This disparity is problematic, given the extensive health benefits of breast milk for children, which increase with duration.[1] Even with public health campaigns promoting breastfeeding, initiation and duration rates have fallen short of national objectives laid out by United States Department of Health and Human Services (U.S. Department of Health and Human Services, 2011). Just as troubling, many women do not reach their personal breastfeeding goals, likely due to the cultural climate that has normalized commercial formula feeding as the dominant means of feeding a baby ("Breastfeeding and the Use of Human Milk," 2005; Stuebe, 2014). Thus, breastfeeding advocates, including myself, have sought new ways to encourage women to breastfeed. One site is entertainment television, which has offered somewhat positive, but limited, messages about breastfeeding, with very few breastfeeding women of color (Foss, 2013). My research in this area prompted an informal discussion with Dan O'Shannon, a coproducer on the television sitcom *Modern Family*. I asked if he could help promote breastfeeding, particularly for Latina women, by showcasing breastfeeding with the character Gloria, a Colombian woman who is part of the main cast. To my surprise, the 2012–2013 season involved Gloria's pregnancy and birth. And, as I had suggested, Gloria breastfed the baby, with multiple references about breastfeeding included throughout the remainder of the season.

273

As this example demonstrates, media can convey prosocial messages, offering representations that model healthy behaviors. These messages can be casual and isolated or part of formal health campaigns. This chapter provides an overview of the use of media in traditional campaigns, as well as an in-depth look at one area that straddles formal campaigns and prosocial messages through entertainment-education. While overlap certainly exists between traditional approaches and more entertainment-centered campaigns in design and theories, they each have unique strengths and drawbacks, depending on the intended audiences and desired outcomes.

■ Traditional Health Campaigns

Traditional health campaigns strategically disseminate messages in order to effect change in health knowledge, attitude, and or behavior. Rogers and Storey (1987) defined the tenets of a campaign, explaining that "(1) A campaign intends to generate specific outcomes or effects (2) in a relatively large number of individuals, (3) usually within a specific period of time and (4) through an organized set of communication activities" (p. 821). Aktin and Rice (2012) refined this definition, stating that campaigns are "purposive attempts to inform or influence behaviors in large audiences within a specified time period using an organized-set of communication activities . . . to produce noncommercial benefits to individuals and society" (p. 3). In other words, campaigns use carefully constructed messages that are widely disseminated to change the knowledge level, attitude, and/or behavior of the targeted population in a specific time frame through means that can be measured and evaluated (Atkin & Salmon, 2010; Backer, Rogers, & Soporty, 1992; Rogers & Storey, 1987). In campaigns, media outlets play an important role in conveying messages to the public, working to inform, persuade, model healthy behaviors, and shape perception of cultural norms (Wakefield, Loken, & Hornik, 2010).

HCIA 11.1

The *Go Sun Smart* Story:
Fighting Skin Cancer on the Ski Slopes

Peter A. Andersen ■ David B. Buller ■ Barbara J. Walkosz
Michael D. Scott ■ Gary R. Cutter ■ Mark B. Dignan

People love the sun. They flock to the beach, lay out by a pool, and pursue outdoor activities such as hiking, running, golfing, or skiing that are most fun in the gorgeous sunshine. But the bright sun has a dark side: skin cancers, largely caused by excessive time in the sun and sun burning. According to the American Cancer Society, skin cancer is the most common cancer, exceeding all other types. Furthermore, one type of skin cancer, melanoma, is among the most deadly.

Here in the new millennium people know about sun protection at beaches and pools. But some of the most dangerous solar radiation takes place at high altitudes above the protective layer of the atmosphere. People associate solar radiation with heat, but heat has little impact on the amount of radiation or on sun burning. Employees and guests at ski resorts are complacent about sun protection and even consider the raccoon look from sun burning around ski goggles as a status symbol.

This is the story of Go Sun Smart, a worksite wellness program designed and implemented by our team of health communication researchers, endorsed by the National Ski Areas Association (NSAA), and funded by the National Cancer Institute (NCI). For the past 20 years, our team has implemented and tested a sun safety campaign at more than 300 ski resorts in North America. Our goal has been to examine and reduce the risk for skin cancer among people who work and recreate at high altitude ski resorts.

First, we sought the endorsement of the NSAA in Lakewood, Colorado, the primary professional association for ski resorts in North America and for the nearly 200,000 part- and full-time workers at the resorts. Getting NSAA support was important, since it was the primary channel for disseminating information to the ski and snowboard industry, and our gateway to the resorts. We presented to NSAA a persuasive case detailing the level of risk for skin cancer and showed that an on-site wellness program not only could reduce this risk but also might reduce potential liability issues and lawsuits against the resorts. Moreover, a sun safety campaign was consistent with other industry campaigns on avalanche safety, altitude sickness, helmet safety, and frostbite.

Our ambitious goal was to change the sun safety behavior of an entire industry, including nearly 200,000 employees and more than 20 million annual skiers and snowboarders. We conducted employee focus groups at 26 ski resorts to understand employees' attitudes and behaviors about their work, risk-taking tendencies, and sun protection attitudes.

For more than a year, our team met and designed materials that were (1) entirely based on communication theory, (2) delivered in channels to maximize exposure and repetition, (3) geared to ski employees and guests, and (4) created with vivid high sensation messages that would appeal to ski employees and guests.

Our multimedia campaign employed both traditional and new media that focused on a single theme, "Use sunscreen, sunglasses, and a hat," the primary behaviors needed to avoid sunburning at high altitude. The campaign featured vivid, artistic posters, as well as a website (www.gosunsmart.com), content for employee newsletters, brochures, window decals,

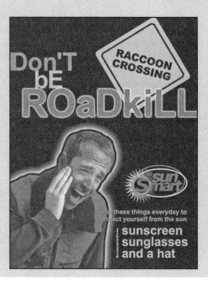
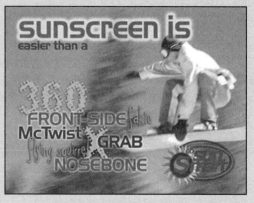

(continued)

buttons, water bottles, emails, table tents, and several employee training modules. Materials were distributed throughout the resorts.

Our evaluation showed that ski employees at resorts randomly assigned to our campaign were significantly more aware of the importance of sun safety than the employees at resorts serving as a control group. More than 85% of employees at the campaign resorts remembered receiving one of our sun safety messages. Most pleasing was a 14% reduction in sunburning at resorts that received the Go Sun Smart campaign. Additionally, research showed an even stronger long-term effect of the campaign into the summer, where employees at resorts exposed to our campaign engaged in more sun safety, had fewer sunburns, and were more likely to talk to their families about sun safety than employees at resorts that did not get our program. Evidence also showed that guests engaged in more sun safety behavior when they encountered more Go Sun Smart sun safety messages, and parents at Go Sun Smart resorts were persuaded to take more sun safety precautions with their kids at ski school than parents at resorts that did not get the Go Sun Smart program. Moreover, the resorts that did not get the Go Sun Smart program received it in the second year with results virtually identical to the original studies.

Subsequently, the Go Sun Smart program was expanded in a national dissemination project to more than 300 NSAA resorts across North America. Study results showed that this dissemination project was very successful, while sun safety messages that were not from the Go Sun Smart campaign had no effect, indicating that a program based on communication theory was essential for the effectiveness of the campaign.

QUESTIONS TO PONDER

1. Can you think of a health campaign or message that made you think or behave differently? What do you think made it successful for you?

2. The Go Sun Smart campaign focused on one theme disseminated through various media to resort employees and guests. Think about a health issue important to you and design a campaign using some of the key ideas from this program. What is your message? Who is your audience? How and through what channels will you disseminate your message?

Sources: Andersen, P. A., Buller, D. B., Voeks, J. H., Walkosz, B. J., Scott, M. D., Cutter, G. R., & Dignan, M. B. (2008). Testing the long-term effects of the Go Sun Smart Worksite Health Communication Campaign: A group-randomized experimental study. *Journal of Communication, 68,* 447–471. Buller, D. B., Andersen, P. A., Walkosz, B. J. Scott, M. D., Cutter, G. C., Dignan, M. B., Kane, I. L., & Zhang, X. (2012). Enhancing industry-based dissemination of an occupational sun protection program with theory-based strategies employing personal contact. *American Journal of Health Promotion, 26,* 356–365. Scott, M. D., Buller, D. B., Walkosz, B. J., Andersen, P. A., Cutter, G. R., & Dignan, M. (2008). Go Sun Smart. *Communication Education, 57,* 423–433. Walkosz, B. J., Buller, D. B., Andersen, P. A., Scott, M. D., Dignan, M. B., Cutter, G. R., & Maloy, J. A. (2008). Increasing sun protection in outdoor recreation: A theory-based health communication program. *American Journal of Preventive Medicine, 34,* 502–509.

Campaigns vary in their intended purposes, depending on: (1) whether the idea or behavior is "new" to the population, (2) how much information is currently available as a result of past campaigns, and (3) the extent of audience resistance to adopting the healthier behavior. Some campaigns have been used to introduce a fresh idea or create awareness of a newly identified health behavior, risk, or new immunization options, such as the 2006 "One Less" campaign for the vaccine Gardasil, protecting against the human papillomavirus (HPV) (Grantham, Ahern, & Connolly-Ahern, 2011). Formal campaigns have also been effective in changing attitudes or perceptions about health topics, like perceptions of the risk of sun exposure and the need for protection (Buller et al., 2012; Robinson, Rigel, & Amonette, 1997; Walkosz et al., 2008). Other campaigns are preventive, encouraging behavior change that will result in improved health long-term, as in promoting breastfeeding or reducing hypertension (Haroon, Das, Salam, Imdad, & Bhutta, 2013; Imdad, Yakoob, & Bhutta, 2011; Roccella, 2002). Finally, many health campaigns aim to discourage unhealthy behaviors, as illustrated with anti-tobacco efforts or HIV prevention and other sexual responsibility messages (Graves, Sentner, Workman, & Mackey, 2011; LaCroix, Snyder, Huedo-Medina, & Johnson, 2014; Pierce, Macaskill, & Hill, 2002; Worden & Flynn, 2002).

Theories Commonly Used in Health Promotion

Effective campaigns draw from established theoretical models. Theories provide foundations for campaigns, establishing precedents for how or why certain behavior can be affected (Fishbein & Cappella, 2006). Some communication theories help to explain how people's attitudes toward healthy behaviors impact their willingness to change their own behaviors. *The Health Belief Model* suggests that for change to occur, people must first view themselves as at risk for the unhealthy consequence, believe that modifying their behavior will reduce the risk, and believe that the benefits outweigh the difficulties in overcoming barriers and other downsides to modifying the behavior (Becker, Maiman, Kirscht, Haefner, & Drachman, 1977; Janz & Becker, 1984; Pechmann, 2001). This model also considers social events and other cues to action that may increase the likelihood of adopting the behavior (Janz & Becker, 1984). The Health Belief Model is particularly helpful in using beliefs to predict the adoption of preventive behaviors, such as immunization rates, health screenings, and positive lifestyle choices, or the likelihood of participating in risky behaviors, like tanning or tobacco use (Carpenter, 2010; Greene & Brinn, 2003; Janz & Becker, 1984; Kim, Ahn, & No, 2012).

Other theories focus more on people's cognitive processing. Bandura (1977a) first posited that people learn through direct experience or by viewing the experiences of others (modeling). Called the social learning theory, and later renamed *social cognitive theory (SCT)*, Bandura explained that the extent to which people learn and then model behavior is influenced by the appeal or attraction of the person doing the behavior, the apparent reward of the behavior, a person's ability to remember and then replicate the behavior, and the degree of motivation to make the change (Bandura, 1977a). The adoption of healthier behavior depends on perceived risk of not changing behavior, self-efficacy (the extent to which people believe they can do the behavior), the ability to change, and perceptions of the source's credibility (Bandura, 1977b).

As Cecelia and Kristi continued their car ride, Kristi talked about her experiences with breastfeeding and shared her opinions openly with Cecelia. Kristi is currently breastfeeding her six-month-old daughter. She breastfed her oldest until he was eighteen months old and her middle child until he was nearly three. Kristi told Cecelia that breast milk has the right amount of nutrients to help the baby grow (confirming what Cecelia had read in an online article). Kristi also talked about how breastfeeding made her feel as "one" with her baby; it really created a close, natural bond that she thinks wouldn't happen with bottle feeding. She also said that it's cheaper than buying formula, and it's easier because there are no bottles to wash or nipples to sterilize. She beamed with enthusiasm about how much she enjoyed breastfeeding each of her children.

As Kristi shared her advice and experiences, Cecelia admired her best friend's love for her children and allegiance to keeping them healthy. Cecelia was deep in thought as to whether she could do the same thing. She expressed her concerns to Kristi, who reassured her and emphasized the importance of having help and support. Kristi recommended taking a breastfeeding class at the hospital, utilizing the lactation consultants, and looking into La Leche League. She then described some of her challenges with breastfeeding—her second child was tongue-tied. She also experienced mastitis and clogged ducts. Kristi encouraged Cecelia to set small goals for herself and to ask for assistance. With Kristi's guidance, Cecelia was determined to make it work but unsure about what breastfeeding would really be like.

The theory of planned behavior stems from Fishbein and Ajzen's (1975, 2011) *theory of reasoned action* and emphasizes the role that intention to modify behavior plays in the desired outcome (Madden, Ellen, & Ajzen, 1992). According to this theory, factors that affect intention—and, ultimately, the desired behavior change—include individuals' feelings toward the desired behavior, behavioral control, self-efficacy, and individuals' perceptions of how the health behavior is regarded within their social group (Ajzen, 2005; Madden et al., 1992). These factors influence intention, which influences whether or not the desired behavior will be achieved. Building on the theory of planned behavior, Fishbein (2000) developed the *integrative model of behavioral prediction,* which suggests that if no environmental obstacles exist, it is very likely that people's commitment to the behavior with the abilities and tools required for the behavior will result in the desired behavior (Fishbein, 2000; Fishbein & Cappella, 2006). These theories are helpful for understanding how to design campaigns that appeal to individuals' intention and commitment to change an unhealthy behavior, for example, persuading smokers to quit (Fishbein & Cappella, 2006).

Since many health campaigns use fear appeals to persuade audiences, the *Extended Parallel Process Model* (*EPPM*) was developed to explain the potential influence of such appeals (Witte, 1992). This model explains when and how fear appeals may be effective. Specifically, the EPPM proposes that how people perceive a message (as "perceived efficacy," as a "perceived threat," or as nonthreatening) impacts the extent to which they are prompted to modify their behavior and the type of behavior they are likely to adapt (Witte, 1992, p. 338). If people perceive the situation as dangerous, yet have trust in their ability to control the situation, they are likely to assume a protective position, with positive behavioral change (Witte, 1992). Conversely, if the threat is perceived as high, but self-efficacy is low, people are more likely to act defensively, with maladaptive or coping behaviors (Witte, 1992). Thus a more effective fear message personalizes the risk and provides clear ways to avoid the risky or dangerous behavior, thereby encouraging adaptive, rather than maladaptive, behavior changes (Witte, 1992). While fear appeals can be effective, Murray-Johnson and Witte (2003) caution that they should only be used for "target audience members who can easily perform the recommended response (possess response efficacy), but do not recognize either the severity of the health threat or perceive that the threat will only impact others, not themselves" (p. 478). Messages can be one-sided, showcasing the favorable attributes of the desired behavior or two-sided, in which downsides of the desired behavior are addressed and countered.

Theories that outline media's effects are also useful in message design and dissemination. Fishbein and Yzer (2003) argued for the application of primary theory in health promotion, stating that media's ability to stimulate similar thoughts about a topic can help reinforce the connection between beliefs about desired behaviors and, therefore, help achieve the desired effects. Other theories of health promotion and media effects will be discussed later in this chapter.

Designing Effective Health Campaigns

One aspect of breastfeeding that worried Cecelia was pumping. How would she be able to do that at work? As a regional manager for a chain of clothing stores, she needed to drive (at times quite a distance) to meet with each store's manager. How would having to pump affect the nature of her job? She knew that, legally, her employer had to provide time and space for pumping. Cecelia just had to figure out how to make it work. For Cecelia, pumping involved planning and thinking ahead. She would have to make sure she carried a cooler with her, so she could put her breast milk in it and schedule in pumping breaks as if they were business meetings. Perhaps she could ask her female coworkers how they fit pumping into the job. Maybe she could also look online to see how other working mothers handled pumping. She knew it was worth it; she merely had to figure out the logistics.

Television's modeling of breastfeeding can help normalize the activity, as demonstrated with the example from *Modern Family*. That said, breastfeeding promotion poses challenges. Campaigns have successfully convinced most people of breast milk's value, as even college students and others without children note its health benefits (Kavanagh, Lou, Nicklas, Habibi, & Murphy, 2012). Yet, most people are uncomfortable seeing breastfeeding and with breastfeeding in public (Li et al., 2004). Furthermore, promotion efforts have persuaded 77% of women to attempt to breastfeed, yet the duration is short, demonstrating the cultural lack of breastfeeding support and the complex array of factors that determine success ("Breastfeeding Report Card," 2014). In other words, to be truly effective in raising breastfeeding initiation and duration rates, campaigns need to not only encourage positive attitudes toward breastfeeding but also address obstacles like short maternity leaves, fear of scrutiny for nursing in public, physiological barriers like nipple pain and thrush, and the importance of having social and emotional support. Cultural sensitivity is also important, as certain groups have historically held different beliefs and attitudes toward breastfeeding and breast milk. For example, one study of breastfeeding attitudes in six Native American communities found that solid food was introduced much earlier than the American Academy of Pediatrics (AAP) recommends (Horodynski, Calcatera, & Carpenter, 2012). Such knowledge could be used to specifically tailor messages to the Native American community.

Traditional health campaigns tend to follow the same general approach and procedure. This overview draws from existing literature on campaign design (Atkin & Freimuth, 2012; Atkin & Salmon, 2010; Hornik, 2002; Rogers & Storey, 1987; Snyder & Hamilton, 2002; Wright, Sparks, & O'Hair, 2012). This process can vary, but generally adheres to the following steps:

1. Conduct audience analysis research using focus groups, surveys, and other means to understand the target audience, their behaviors and habits, mediated exposure and other factors that may influence the structure and effectiveness of the campaign. Existing data on the target population may also be used. Who has been targeted in previous campaigns? Who is most at risk for the behavior? Who is at moderate risk? The intended population could be clustered by inter-sections of age, race, sex, socioeconomic status, geographic region, lifestyle, occupation, or other factors that especially place them at risk for unhealthy behaviors. Campaigns may also target leaders in the community or primary institutions or policy makers. This information will help define the parameters of the campaign, including the specific target, media outlets, message construc-tion, and evaluation means. For example, to increase breastfeeding rates cam-paign designers would first determine whether to target subpopulations of women of childbearing age or aim to influence the general public or policy makers' awareness and attitudes toward breastfeeding. Breastfeeding initiation and duration rates, any community resistance to breastfeeding, and past and existing campaign efforts would be researched to better understand the cultural climate and target audience.

2. Determine the desired outcome of the campaign with clear and realistic goals. This outcome may occur in terms of awareness of an issue or innovation, change in attitudes, and/or change in behavior. This outcome should be mea-surable, not abstract. For breastfeeding, objectives may be to raise intention, initiation, or duration or may be attitudinal—with the goal of increasing awareness of breastfeeding benefits, bolstering support for breastfeeding, or increasing comfort levels of the general public.

3. Identify the outlets for the campaign's messages. Using a multimedia approach can increase exposure and reinforce the message for greater effects. The media channels should fit with the demographics and media consumption of the intended group, as well as work within the budget, time frame, and geographic span of the campaign. Media channels may include social media and other websites, radio and television programs, billboards, posters, fliers, newspapers, and other venues. Breastfeeding campaigns intended for teenaged mothers would likely utilize social media, whereas messages aimed at persuading grandmothers to support their daughters' breastfeeding efforts might be placed in women's magazines or on television.

4. Create the campaign's messages, with sensitivity to social, economic, political, environmental, and cultural contexts. These messages should be engaging and easy to understand for the intended population. Common health campaign messages attempt to persuade audiences with threats of enforcement (i.e., fines for not wearing seat belts), the introduction of information and/or services to help modify the behavior (i.e., smoking cessation supplies), and the use of role models or testimony to showcase the new behavior. The creation of effective appeals in breastfeeding campaigns is tricky. In developed countries, most breastfeeding campaigns have emphasized breastfeeding benefits, rather than highlighting the risks of not breastfeeding (Stuebe, 2009). On the other hand,

campaigns in developing countries often use risk and fear appeals to promote breastfeeding, which helps explain why these campaigns have generally been more effective in raising rates (Imdad et al., 2011).

5. Pretest the campaign messages using interviews, focus groups, or surveys with participants from the intended audience to ensure that the messages are clear, easy to understand, culturally appropriate, and salient. Revise the campaign messages as needed. For a campaign designed to raise college students' comfort with breastfeeding, researchers would pretest the campaign messages to determine whether the message is clear, easy to comprehend, and persuasive with this intended audience.

6. Conduct the campaign within a predetermined time frame.

7. Evaluate the effectiveness of the campaign using outcomes as well as interpretive research. The evaluation measure should reflect the media channel and intended audience. To assess exposure, people can look at TV ratings, reviews of YouTube videos or web pages, clicks, "Likes", or Shares in social media. Surveys or focus groups can be used to determine consumer awareness, knowledge, and the extent to which intention and behavior were affected by the message. The campaign as a whole can also be evaluated as a model for future campaigns.

8. After the conclusion of the campaign, surveys and point-of-referral monitoring can determine long-term effects in the maintenance phase of the campaign. Long-term effects on breastfeeding rates, for example, can be measured by examining initiation and duration rates in the years following the campaign for the subpopulation targeted.

Campaigns that yield more success share common traits. Effective campaigns tend to draw from proven social scientific theories, use evaluative techniques in the planning stages of the campaign, and set clear and realistic objectives for the campaign's outcome. For example, the *1% or Less* campaign to promote healthy eating by selecting lower fat milk has had great success in decreasing fat consumption, likely because of its clear, instructive message (drink 1% or skim milk), and goals that are relatively easy to achieve (Maddock et al., 2007; Reger, Wootan, Booth-Butterfield, & Smith, 1998). Those campaigns that disseminate messages across media platforms, paired with interpersonal components also tend to be more successful (Backer, Rogers, & Sopory, 1992). Campaign messages must be culturally sensitive and resonate with the intended audience enough to counter audience resistance to the desired changes (Murray-Johnson & Witte, 2003; Salmon & Atkin, 2003). The Florida *Truth* campaign illustrated the importance of understanding the intended audience and using a multiplatform approach. This anti-tobacco campaign in the late 1990s depended on feedback from teenagers during the creation of the messages, developed clever and engaging ads that appealed to teenagers, and then was disseminated during popular teen programming and other audience-specific outlets (Bauer, Johnson, Hopkins, & Brooks, 2000; Hicks, 2001). Because of these strategies, the *Truth* campaign significantly decreased adolescent intention to smoke and smoking prevalence (Bauer et al., 2000; Hicks, 2001). It should be noted that certain types of messages typically have better results. Campaigns that incorporate enforcement, like fines or other penalties, produce more dramatic outcomes than other message strategies (Snyder & Hamilton, 2002).

Creating campaigns for developing countries includes an additional set of challenges. The environment, sanitation and local resources, nutrition, and general health must be considered (Rice & Foote, 1989). And, just as important, researchers need to understand the targeted population, including its cultural beliefs and attitudes (Audet et al., 2012). Power dynamics in individual households and the community as a whole, child care practices, religion, language, and other factors may also influence access to the population, the ability to (and outlets for) disseminating campaign messages, reception of the campaign, and its effectiveness (Rice & Foote, 1989). Culturally sensitive campaigns have helped to increase condom use and other HIV prevention measures, reduce childhood morbidity from malaria and diarrheal-related illness, heighten vaccination rates for preventable diseases, and improve health in numerous other ways in developing countries (Fewtrell et al., 2005; LaCroix et al., 2014; Sweat, Dennison, Kennedy, Tedrow, & O'Reilly, 2012; Terlouw et al., 2010).

Of course, some groups of people are particularly resistant to the messages of health campaigns. This resistance is often reinforced through counter-messages that dissuade consumers from modifying behavior, reassuring them that the risks are exaggerated or worth the benefit. For example, DeSantis and Morgan (2003) explained how a popular cigar magazine used seven distinctive strategies to challenge antismoking campaign messages and retain their loyal customers. These strategies included distinguishing cigars from cigarettes (minimizing the risk and addictive properties of cigars), suggesting "health benefits" of cigar smoking, and selectively questioning the medical research demonstrating the harmful effects of cigars (DeSantis & Morgan, 2003). Such counter-messages can be difficult to overcome through traditional health campaigns, as you'll see in Theorizing Practice 11.1.

Theorizing Practice 11.1
Increasing Seat Belt Use—Campaign (In)effectiveness

What makes some campaigns successful, while others yield only minimal effects? While nearly 85% of Americans routinely wear seat belts now, this was not always the case ("CDC Study Finds," 2011). In 1981, only 11% of people buckled up ("Achievements in Public Health," 1999). Seat belt laws and informative campaigns helped to change the cultural climate—but not without resistance. Indiana passed a law mandating seat belt use in 1985, which went into effect in July 1987. News coverage about the law, paired with a multimedia campaign, attempted to inform residents and persuade them to use seat belts. Messages were distributed through public service Announcements (PSAs) in television, radio, newspapers, and billboards, as well as through community organizations. In August 1987, 811 people were surveyed about the campaign and their seat belt use. Although 64% reported awareness of the campaign, even recalling slogans, exposure to the messages did not significantly impact seat belt use, even for the most influential medium (radio). Researchers noted very little variance due to the campaign messages and determined that personal factors had more influence. Overall, they concluded that the campaign had minimal effects on seat belt usage.

And yet, only five years later, the Click It or Ticket seat belt campaign in North Carolina was considered a great success. An extensive campaign was launched in fall 1993, with a follow-up period in the summer of 1994. These media messages warned people about citations for not buckling up and aired in conjunction with strict enforcement of seat belt violations. Police officers set up checkpoints for seat belt usage, giving almost 60,000 citations for non-seat belt use. Overall, the campaign increased seat belt use from 64% up to 70%. A dramatic reduction in serious motor vehicle injuries and fatalities was also noted. The campaign was considered effective enough that other states initiated their own Click It or Ticket campaigns, helping to raise seat belt rates nationwide ("*Announcement:* Click It or Ticket Campaign," 2015).

Both campaigns targeted the general adult public, combined legislation and mediated efforts, and attempted to modify the same behavior, with vastly different results. While the two campaigns were relatively close in time, seat belt use had already begun to climb by the early 1990s, when the North Carolina study took place. The campaign structure also differed. Gantz, Fitzmaurice, and Yoo (1990) describe how the Indiana campaign's time frame was not well defined, whereas the North Carolina campaign had clearly defined periods of media distribution and enforcement. Furthermore, while the Indiana campaign occurred with the law, enforcement was not used as a persuasive strategy for behavior change, nor were the citations for not buckling up heavily publicized. In North Carolina, on the other hand, the slogan Click It or Ticket directly used enforcement to encourage seat belt use, paired with very public checkpoints with fines for incompliance.

Consider these two studies and answer the following questions:

1. How do seemingly minor differences impact the effectiveness of a campaign?

2. What other health behaviors work well with enforcement messages?

3. How does context influence campaign design and effectiveness?

Source: Based on research by Gantz, Fitzmaurice, & Yoo, 1990; Williams, Wells, & Reinfurt, 2002.

HCIA 11.2

The Power of Storytelling to Improve Health Outcomes

Meghan Bridgid Moran ■ Sheila Murphy
Joyee S. Chatterjee ■ Lauren B. Frank ■ Lourdes Baezconde-Garbanati

Think back to high school when you had to learn facts about science, math, history, and English. Can you remember the atomic weight of potassium or the date that the Spanish Civil War began? Now think back to the fairy tales you heard as a child. Can you remember what made Pinocchio's nose grow, or what kind of slipper Cinderella wore? If it was easier for you to remember the details of Pinocchio's and Cinderella's stories, you are not alone! People are often better able to remember information when it is presented to them in the form of a story or, more precisely, a *narrative*. Narratives or storytelling are increasingly being used to communicate important health information and to persuade people to adopt healthy behaviors.

Research indicates that there are three main reasons why narrative communication is effective at educating and persuading audiences. First, narratives facilitate *identification* with the characters in the story. Identification is when audiences feel similar to, feel like they know, like, or want to be like a character. If you've ever tried to dress or act like a character in a movie, or felt as though the main character in your favorite book was just like you, we would say you identified with that character. Narratives also produce a state of *transportation*—or immersion—into the story. If you've ever been so engrossed in a favorite novel or TV show that a friend had to call your name three times before he/she got your attention, you were transported into the story. Finally, narratives produce a wide range of *emotions*

(continued)

that facilitate persuasion and keep us engrossed in the story. Whether you're laughing, crying, or trembling with fear, narratives have a special ability to make us *feel*. Together, identification, transportation, and emotional response make people more likely to remember the information being conveyed to them and to be persuaded by the story's message.

Even though a lot of research has demonstrated that narratives can be effective at increasing knowledge and promoting behavior change, most health information continues to be communicated in a traditional non-narrative format, using statistics, facts, and figures. Additionally, previous studies have not directly compared the same information communicated in a narrative versus a non-narrative film. To address this gap, our interdisciplinary team of researchers conducted a randomized study to see whether a narrative or a non-narrative format would communicate identical information more effectively.

To conduct this study, we worked with professional filmmakers to create two films—one narrative and one non-narrative—each containing identical information about cervical cancer prevention, detection, and treatment. The narrative film was called *The Tamale Lesson*. It followed the Romero family as they prepared for their daughter's Quinceañera (special 15th birthday celebration, marking transition into womanhood for Latina girls). At the start of the film, the viewers learned that the oldest daughter, Lupita, had been diagnosed with HPV (Human Papillomavirus that causes cervical cancer); subsequently, the women in the family discussed cervical cancer prevention and detection as they prepared tamales for the party. The non-narrative film, *It's Time*, featured identical information about cervical cancer, but was presented in a traditional format featuring doctors, experts, and patients sharing factual information. We chose to focus on cervical cancer because even though it is highly preventable through regular Pap tests and the HPV vaccine, about 4,000 women in the U.S. die from it every year. Additionally, there are significant ethnic and racial disparities in cervical cancer morbidity and mortality: Hispanic and African American women are more likely than non-Hispanic white women to be diagnosed with and die from cervical cancer.

Once the films were complete and pretested with focus groups, we conducted a study with African American, Mexican American, and non-Hispanic white women. These participants completed a baseline survey and then viewed either the narrative or the non-narrative film. Next, the participants completed additional surveys two weeks and six months later, and we compared changes between the women who saw *The Tamale Lesson* and women who saw *It's Time*.

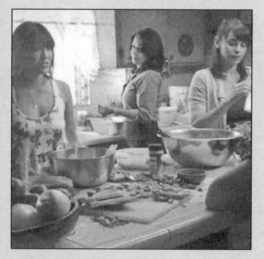

The Tamale Lesson.

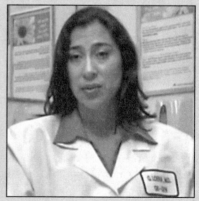

It's Time.

Our findings indicate that while both films produced positive changes in knowledge, attitudes, and behavior, the narrative film was more effective than the non-narrative film. Specifically, women who viewed *The Tamale Lesson* remembered more of the facts presented in the film and had more positive attitudes towards Pap tests. Most importantly, women who viewed *The Tamale Lesson* were more likely to have gotten or made an appointment for a Pap test! We also compared the film's effect by ethnic group and found that *The Tamale Lesson* worked particularly well with Mexican American and African American women. This may be because these women also exhibited higher levels of identification, transportation, and emotion in response to the film.

The results of this study add to a growing body of evidence that supports the use of narrative as an effective way of communicating health information. Our study found that narrative was particularly effective at reducing existing health disparities and getting the target audience to engage in the desired health behavior. So, if you need to communicate important health information to someone, consider how it can be effectively conveyed in the form of a story!

QUESTIONS TO PONDER

1. Recall a story in which you identified with a character, felt transported, or felt strong emotions in response to events in the story. What was that experience like?

2. Think of specific books, TV shows, movies, or other story forms that communicate health information. Which of these are most effective at increasing knowledge, changing attitudes, or prompting behavior change? Why?

3. Have you ever learned something or made a healthy behavior change in response to a story that communicated health information? What do you think made the story effective?

Sources: Baezconde-Garbanati, L., Chatterjee, J. S., Frank, L. B., Murphy, S., Moran, M. B., Werth, L. N., Zhao, N., Amezola de Herrera, P., Mayer, D., Kagan, J., & O'Brien, D. (2014). *Tamale Lesson*: A case study of a narrative health communication intervention. *Journal of Communication in Health Care, 7*, 82–92. Murphy, S. T., Frank, L. B., Chatterjee, J. S., Moran, M. B., Zhao, N. & Baezconde-Garbanati, L. (2015). Comparing the relative efficacy of narrative vs non-narrative health messages in reducing health disparities using a randomized trial. *American Journal of Public Health, 105*, 2117–2123.

Entertainment-Education

As the example at the beginning of the chapter illustrates, there are other means to influence health behavior in a population. One solution to the lack of effectiveness for some traditional campaign approaches is the use of entertainment-education (E-E). Also called edu-tainment or prosocial entertainment, this approach combines narrative storytelling and entertainment programming to distribute health messages through such outlets as radio, television, songs, YouTube, and so forth. Media scholars Singhal and Rogers (1999) defined E-E as "the process of purposely designing and implementing a media message both to entertain and to educate, in order to increase audience members' knowledge about an educational issue, create favorable attitudes, and change overt behavior" (p. 9). The intended outcome is often twofold: positively impact individual knowledge and behavior, as well as improve the cultural climate to become more conducive to the desired behavior (Singhal & Rogers, 1999). Again, with *Modern*

Family as an example, creating positive representations of breastfeeding through favorite characters encourages women to breastfeed and, at the same time, helps to normalize breastfeeding so the general public supports breastfeeding-friendly practices.

Such outlets can directly target an audience and complement or compensate for inadequate health education. Many teenagers already get their information about sex from watching television (Brown & Keller, 2000). Obviously, not all of this information is positive or even accurate. Messages that encourage sexual responsibility embedded in the stories of popular TV shows can help counter the mixed interpretations of popular media and the ineffectiveness of abstinence-only education (Stanger-Hall & Hall, 2011). Entertainment-education can also reach audiences with low literacy rates or those individuals who may otherwise tune out other forms of health messages. And, with the oversaturation of messages in our increasingly fragmented media landscape, it can be difficult for public health advocates to break through the media clutter to reach the targeted group (Sherry, 2002).

The Impact of Entertainment on Society

Media messages can have dramatic effects on how we think and act. Indeed, it has been well established that entertainment media impacts consumers' knowledge, behavior, and perceptions of the world—even without a strategic plan to influence perception or behavior. Consider teenagers and sexual responsibility, for example. Scholars have noted the effects of the popular MTV reality programs *16 & Pregnant* and *Teen Mom,* two shows that document the real-life experiences of teenagers as they become young parents. Kearney and Levine (2014) determined a positive correlation between airdates of these programs and Internet activity: Google searches and Tweets for "birth control" significantly increased after episodes of the shows aired. Furthermore, Kearney and Levine (2014) argued that teenage birthrates declined in geographic areas with heavy viewership of these programs, a finding that was disputed by McKinney (2015). Indeed, not all effects noted have been positive. Martins and Jensen (2014) found that, compared to non-viewers, adolescent fans of these shows were more likely to envy teenage parents, rather than recognize teen pregnancy as a hardship. Consider the popular sitcom *Friends* and condom efficacy in Theorizing Practice 11.2.

Storied messages in film, television, print, and other media channels teach us about health, affecting our choices and behavior. For example, physicians describe learning from medical dramas while in medical school. In her memoirs of her experiences at Harvard Medical School, Dr. Ellen Lerner Rothman (1999) recollected that she and her classmates identified with the characters in the long-running TV medical drama *ER,* especially the fictional medical students and residents, and used the program to reinforce knowledge of clinical procedures and vocabulary:

> Through the *ER* physicians, residents, and medical students, my classmates and I explored who we wanted to be and what we were afraid we might become. We developed a paradigm for how we wanted to respond to our patients and explored how we would feel if we were unable to uphold it. (p. 26)

Entertainment can also be used to help students understand material in a classroom setting. For example, Østbye, Miller, and Keller (1997) reported using the medi-

Theorizing Practice 11.2
Friends and Condom Efficacy

The seventh season of the hit television show *Friends* ended with the cliff-hanger of the character Rachel Green's surprise pregnancy. For the first few episodes of the next season, fans anxiously eagerly waited to learn who fathered the fictional child, which was revealed in the second episode. In the following episode, aptly labeled "The One Where Rachel Tells Ross," Rachel informs the baby's father, another main character, Ross, of her pregnancy. Ross becomes bug-eyed and speechless, prompting Rachel to ask if he is okay.

Ross: Yeah, I need uh . . . I'm just—I don't know—I don't understand, umm, how this happened? We-we used a condom.

Rachel: I know. I know, but y'know condoms only work like 97% of the time.

Ross: What? What? What?!! Well they should put that on the box!!!

Rachel: They do!

Ross: No they don't!!! [He runs to the bedroom to check and returns with his box of condoms.] Well they should put it in huge black letters!!!!

Rachel: Okay Ross, come on let's just forget about the condoms.

Ross: Oh well I may as well have!

Rachel: Listen, y'know what? I was really freaked out too when I found out . . .

Ross: Freaked out? Hey no, I'm not freaked out! I'm indignant! As a consumer!

Later in the episode, Ross calms down and runs into his friends, Joey and Phoebe. He repeats the condom failure rate, stating, "But hey, in my defense I, I just found out condoms are like only 97% effective."

"What?" Joey exclaims, pulling out a large string of condoms.

The episode concludes with Rachel's first ultrasound. With Ross at her side, they learn that the baby is healthy and developmentally on track.

Friends fans remember this story line as a touching episode that added yet another twist in the on-and-off again relationship of Ross and Rachel. But this narrative served a greater purpose, as the episode was part of a national E-E campaign. Within four weeks of the episode airing, researchers had interviewed 506 teenagers, asking them about the information conveyed in the story line, inquiring whether or not they had discussed Rachel's pregnancy with an adult, and questioning the participants' beliefs in condom efficacy (Collins et al., 2003). Of those surveyed, 65% of participants recalled that pregnancy was due to condom failure. Furthermore, those who discussed the episode with an adult reported learning more about sexual risk than those who did not.

Think about the design of this study. What factors of this campaign made it particularly effective? Consider the program choice, delivery of the message, the message, and the evaluation measure (phone interviews with teenagers). Now think about genre—what are the advantages of using a sitcom for an entertainment-education campaign? What are the drawbacks? What other health issues could be addressed in this program?

Source: Based on research by Collins, Elliott, Berry, Kanouse, & Hunder, 2003.

cal drama *ER* to teach students with little background in health about medicine. Viewers learn medical terminology and concepts from watching fictional television (Gauthier, 1999). In fact, Davin (2004) found that people were more likely to believe the information conveyed in fictional television than in health documentaries. Entertainment narratives can also help those with serious health conditions. Sharf and Freimuth (1993) described how a story line in the show *Thirtysomething* followed a main character, Nancy Krieger Weston, as she experienced ovarian cancer, from diagnosis through treatment. An audience study using this story line found that many viewers learned new information about cancer from the story line, applied the illness narrative to their own social networks, and took action by engaging in preventive screenings (Sharf, Freimuth, Greenspon, & Plotnik, 1996).

Celebrities play an integral role in society, often more influential than political figures, war heroes, and other leaders (Brown & Fraser, 2004). Celebrities have such influence that their endorsements of products and social issues can yield dramatic results (Brown & Fraser, 2004). Following media coverage of former First Lady Nancy Reagan's mastectomy, women were 25% less likely to undergo breast-conserving surgery (Nattinger, Hoffman, Howell-Pelz, & Goodwin, 1998). In the 1990s, after Magic Johnson announced that he was HIV positive, people who felt more emotional involvement with the basketball player were more likely to show concern about HIV/AIDS and had greater intention to practice sexual responsibility (Brown & Basil, 1995). Cram and colleagues (2003) found that the number of colonoscopies jumped significantly in the month after Katie Couric led a colorectal cancer awareness campaign on the *Today Show*. And Dean (2016) detailed how Angelina Jolie's celebrity status increased online health information seeking following her disclosure that she had tested positive for the mutated BRCA1 gene and undergone a preventative double mastectomy.

And yet, the extent to which viewers are influenced by entertainment can be problematic, particularly when story lines offer inaccurate portrayals. For example, in the 1990s, a study of cardiopulmonary resuscitation (CPR) depictions in popular medical dramas revealed that television significantly overrepresented its success rate of CPR and minimized long-term risks associated with the practice (Diem, Lantos, & Tulsky, 1996). Therefore, carefully planned campaigns are important to ensure the delivery of accurate information. Importantly, while both prosocial entertainment and formal campaigns aim to disseminate messages that benefit society, they are not interchangeable.

History of Entertainment-Education

The use of storytelling to inform or persuade is and always has been an integral part of culture (Singhal & Rogers, 1999). However, educational narratives in newer technology began with radio programs in Britain and Jamaica in the 1950s (Singhal & Rogers, 1999). In the late 1960s, a Peruvian telenovela that featured a strong, independent seamstress, led to a surge in the sales of Singer sewing machines (Singhal & Rogers, 1999). Noticing this correlation, Miguel Sabido, a television writer-director-producer in Mexico, mapped out a deliberate strategy for implementing and measuring the impacts of education messages in entertainment media (Singhal & Rogers, 1999). Over the next 10 years, Sabido created a series of soap operas that promoted prosocial issues, with his persuasive messages stemming from psychological theories

(Sabido, 2004). These programs successfully boosted literacy rates, improved family planning methods, and positively impacted other behaviors addressed in the narratives (Sabido, 2004). Sabido's methodology was then utilized in numerous other E-E campaigns (Poindexter, 2004).

Campaigns in Developing Countries

A majority of E-E campaigns are implemented in developing countries, in which low literacy rates and access to education inhibit accurate knowledge about healthy behaviors (Beck, 2004; Singhal & Rogers, 2004). Campaigns have used theatrical performances, radio and television spots, print, and other media to convey messages on a variety of health and social concerns. In more recent years, campaigns have been implemented on HIV/AIDS prevention and awareness. For example, in the early 2000s, India's National AIDS Control partnered with several other organizations, including India's national television service, to implement an extensive E-E campaign on sexual responsibility (Sood, Shefner-Rogers, Sengupta, 2006). Over a little more than a year, the popular serial detective television drama *Jasoos Vijay* included four 30-minute episodes about antidiscrimination and HIV prevention (Sood et al., 2006). These efforts were paired with a series of nine, 1-minute public service announcements (PSAs) that aired on TV and radio, and a traveling reality TV show addressing teenagers about sexual health (Sood et al., 2006). This campaign was widely successful in increasing knowledge about sexual responsibility. Surveys of more than 4,000 participants indicated that those people exposed to the campaign messages were twice as likely to be aware of sexually transmitted infections (Sood et al., 2006). This campaign also helped to counter misperceptions and stigma about HIV/AIDS, yet yielded limited effects on condom-use behavior (Sood et al., 2006).

In Tanzania, radio soap operas have been used to increase knowledge and preventative behavior. For example, Vaughan, Rogers, Singhal, and Swalehe (2000) found that people exposed to the health messages reported fewer sexual partners and were more likely to use condoms. Mahoney and Bates (2013) reported that people in Botswana who listened to radio messages about HIV prevention showed lowered perceptions of stigma toward those who are HIV positive. Yet, overall knowledge was not increased (Mahoney & Bates, 2013).

Campaigns have been used to address other issues as well. For example, in the 1990s, the Soul City Institute for Health and Development Communication was created in South Africa, with the purpose of utilizing media for health education (Usdin, Singhal, Shongwe, Goldstein, & Shabalala, 2004). As part of this project, an E-E television series, *Soul City,* was created. Each season of the show highlighted a different health issue, including HIV prevention in regard to maternal and child health, land and housing reform, tuberculosis, tobacco control, and domestic violence (Usdin et al., 2004). One crucial component of the campaigns was to change the cultural climate. For example, with domestic violence, story lines emphasized the community's responsibility in speaking up about suspected abuse (Usdin et al., 2004). An advocacy campaign ran parallel to the E-E story lines, urging government officials to implement the Domestic Violence Act (DVA), recently approved legislation that had yet to be carried out (Usdin et al., 2004). The overall campaign was a success. Viewers of the television program were much more likely to perceive ill treatment as abuse and significantly less likely to view domestic violence as a "private" matter (Usdin et al., 2004). Moreover, the campaign sparked public discussion of abuse, led to an increase in support for abuse victims, and helped with the implementation of the DVA (Usdin et al., 2004). The *Soul City* project demonstrates the importance of community-level approaches in E-E campaigns, paired with advocacy for political action. See Theorizing Practice 11.3 for yet another example.

Theorizing Practice 11.3
Bringing Breastfeeding to Haiti

In 1987, fewer than 1% of the women in rural Haiti exclusively breastfed their babies (Gebrian, 2014). As Huffman, Zehner, and Victora (2001) have demonstrated, low breastfeeding rates can have a devastating impact on the health of babies and small children in developing countries. By the 1990s, The Haitian Health Foundation (HHF), led by Dr. Bette Gebrian, the public health director, created an extensive campaign designed to appeal to people in the villages, reestablishing breastfeeding as the normal means of feeding babies. To begin, Gebrian and her team had to counter a widespread belief in the villages that babies should not drink colostrum (the first breast milk, which is heavy in fat and nutritious properties that boost the immune system). Instead, newborns were fed a purgative, while the precious colostrum was thrown out. This practice contributed to high infant mortality rates and little breastfeeding success.

Thus, to increase breastfeeding rates in the villages, HHF workers first had to persuade villagers that newborns need colostrum, not the purgative. The health educators created an easy-to-remember slogan, which became widely known. Next, the HHF team worked with local health workers to educate them on the importance of breastfeeding and provided breastfeeding tools, including nursing bras and cups to express milk. Incentives and praise for women who exclusively breastfed were also created and communicated. Health practitioners made home visits to provide proper support and education for new mothers. But the health educators did not only speak with women about breastfeeding. Recognizing the importance of men in the villages, the health practitioners educated all members of the community on the need for breastfeeding. The support role was also recognized—fathers received T-shirts when their partners achieved six months of breastfeeding.

By 2010, a cultural transformation had occurred. Eighty percent of the women were exclusively breastfeeding. Along with the health practitioners, women in the community educated and supported each other with breastfeeding. Dr. Gebrian attributes much of the success of this campaign to the involvement of the community, the use of relevant, easy-to-understand slogans and examples, and the abundant lactation and emotional support for the breastfeeding mothers. Without understanding the familial structure and the reasons for not breastfeeding, the Haitian Health Foundation likely would not have succeeded in significantly increasing breastfeeding rates.

Based on what you've learned about this case, discuss the role that community support plays in changing health knowledge, attitudes, and behavior:

1. How can entertainment-education help with cultural transformation?

2. Think about how E-E can be used to normalize healthy choices while reeducating people with accurate information. How could Dr. Gebrian's approach be applied to breastfeeding in the United States?

Source: Based on research by Gebrian, 2014.

Campaigns in the United States

E-E campaigns have also become increasingly popular in the United States. For example, in the 1980s, drinking and driving had become recognized as a national issue of concern. Researchers at the Centers for Health Communication initiated the Harvard Alcohol Project, introducing the concept of the "designated driver" to American audiences—a notion borrowed from Scandinavia (Winsten, 1993). As part of its comprehensive strategy, the research team worked with television executives to promote the concept of the designated driver through their programming, with numerous television series addressing drinking and driving (Winsten, 1993). In addition to the fictional narratives, TV networks aired PSAs about designated driving and national organizations, professional sports leagues, major corporations, and police departments endorsed the concept of the designated driver (Winsten, 1994). Studies demonstrated that this campaign was widely effective in disseminating the concept of the "designated driver." Within two years, national surveys indicated that most people were familiar with the campaign (Winsten, 1994). Soon after, the term "designated driver" was officially entered into the dictionary, marking the pervasiveness of this campaign (Winsten, 1994). This campaign was not only successful in its intended purpose, it also solidly established that American entertainment could be effectively used as a prosocial tool.

Similarly, in the late 1990s, researchers at the Henry J. Kaiser Foundation worked with writers on the television medical drama *ER* to create informative story lines about emergency contraception and HPV—two new concepts at the time (Brodie et al., 2001). Surveys before and after the episodes aired showed a striking difference in the viewers' knowledge about these health issues. After the story line on emergency contraception, viewers' knowledge increased by 17% (Brodie et al., 2001). Furthermore, for those surveyed about HPV, 32% of participants reported that they had learned about it from the *ER* story arcs (Brodie et al., 2001).

E-E campaigns have also been used to reinforce behavior that has been known to be beneficial for decades. For example, Glik et al. (1998) created a campaign to remind consumers of the importance of immunizations. To ensure accuracy in the messages about immunizations, scripts were provided for people in the television industry, describing true stories about immunizations (Glik et al., 1998). During the 1996–1997 season, eight popular television programs included story lines about vaccinations, including *ER*, *7th Heaven*, and *Frasier* (Glik et al., 1998). Other programs featured immunization posters as part of the permanent set (Glik et al., 1998). Because of the success of embedded messages promoting immunizations in fictional programs, Glik and colleagues (1998) concluded that this approach was effective in educating viewers about the benefits of immunizations and saved millions of dollars in advertising.

The popularity of adolescent dramas in the 1990s, with programs like *My So-Called Life*, *Beverly Hills 90210*, and *Buffy the Vampire Slayer*, broadened opportunities for education through entertainment. Many of these shows routinely storied prosocial issues, including teen pregnancy, bullying, addiction, and body image. Advocacy groups also partnered with television writers to create scripts that deliberately aimed to change attitudes or behavior. To increase awareness about sexual health for teenagers, Members of the Media Project, an advocacy group, used television messages to inform teenagers about sexuality and reproductive health (Folb, 2000). With support from the Media Project, the television program *Felicity* addressed date rape in a two-part episode and provided a date rape hotline at the end of the show (Folb, 2000). After the program aired, more than 1,000 people called the hotline (Folb, 2000). Another *Felicity* episode provided information on safe sex and birth control (Folb, 2000). An informal survey indicated that 58% of viewers reported that the program was informative and 86% agreed that teenagers get useful information about birth control from television programs (Folb, 2000).

Other campaigns have raised awareness about HIV and pregnancy. In 2008, researchers at the Kaiser Family Foundation worked with writers of the television program *Grey's Anatomy* to educate viewers on the low risk of an HIV-positive mother transmitting the virus to her unborn child (Rideout, 2008). Surveys indicated a significant increase in knowledge about transmission following the episode, jumping from only 15% who knew the risk to 61% (Rideout, 2008). Perceptions of pregnancy for HIV-positive women also became much more positive after the show (Rideout, 2008). Education entertainment can also impact health prevention. For example, Whittier, Kennedy, St. Lawrence, Seeley, and Beck (2005) found that viewers in the targeted group of an *ER* story line about syphilis were significantly more likely to report intention to get screened for the disease, as well as to encourage others to undergo testing.

Overall, from the campaign examples, we know that E-E campaigns have been implemented globally and locally, on a numerous issues, through various media. Campaign success depends on consumers' prior knowledge and attitudes about the issue, if people believe change is necessary and attainable, and the extent to which the community and cultural climate is conducive to change. How and why change may occur will be discussed in the next section. Before continuing, however, take a moment to engage with Theorizing Practice 11.4.

Theorizing Practice 11.4
Analyzing Antisocial Messages

In the episode "The Instincts" of crime drama *Criminal Minds*, the FBI profilers determine that a deranged woman has been kidnapping children and feeding them only breast milk, causing them to starve to death. This negative message portrayed breastfeeding as deviant and potentially deadly, particularly for older children.

Since not every television producer or writer aims to create prosocial messages, one struggle for public health advocates is overcoming negative or antisocial health messages in popular culture. For example, fictional story lines that imply the dangers of vaccines might hinder pro-immunization campaigns. We regularly encounter such antisocial messages, which may convey false information or damaging representations about certain health issues or behaviors.

1. Think about your favorite fictional television program. What are the common themes in the show?

2. Does this program cover health issues (i.e., teenage pregnancy and safer sex, organ donation, immunization, etc.)? If so, how are these issues covered? Who experiences the health issue?

3. Would you consider the health messages to be positive or negative? How might these messages impact the audience?

4. Now, modify the message to be prosocial. What would you need to fix? How would this change impact the overall story line

Entertainment-Education Theories

Theoretical justifications explain how and why E-E campaigns may impact audiences. Many E-E campaigns draw from the same theories as more traditional health campaigns. *Social cognitive theory* (SCT) helps explain how E-E can promote change through narratives that model the benefits of healthy behavior, while highlighting the risk of negative behavior (Bandura, 2004). In this way, characters, through modeling, "serve as transmitters of knowledge, values, cognitive skills, and new styles of behavior" (Bandura, 2004, p. 78). SCT also sheds light on why story lines, more than other types of health messages, can be particularly persuasive. In health promotion campaigns, resistance to the health message often occurs, hindering the desire to change (Bandura, 1977b). Entertainment-education can help overcome resistance to change, as the appeal of favorite characters and the suspension of disbelief that accompanies fiction can help reduce counterarguments to modifying behavior (Bandura, 2004; Slater & Rouner, 2002).

As Cecelia is searching online, she comes across an article about breastfeeding portrayed on-screen. She scrolls down to see if she recognizes any of the TV shows or movies, or if she resonates with any of the characters. She comes across an episode of The Office, *which she had seen when it originally aired—Dwight offers to help Pam (who can't find her breast pump) express her milk. Not funny, thought Cecelia. But, she did think about what she would do if she forgot her pump, and she made a mental note to learn about alternatives. Manual expression seemed tricky, but definitely an option in a pinch.*

Slater and Rouner (2002) use a modification of another cognitive theory, the *Elaboration Likelihood Model* (ELM) to demonstrate the effects of E-E, incorporating the mediating effects of *absorption*—the extent to which viewers feel involved in the storylines—and *identification,* in which "an individual perceives another person as similar or at least as a person with whom they might have a social relationship" (Slater & Rouner, 2002, p. 178). These factors help reduce resistance and counterarguing (Slater & Rouner, 2002). Stronger identification with a celebrity or fictional character leads to a higher adoption rate of the celebrity's modeled behavior (Brown & Fraser, 2004). For example, if people like Sofia Vergara (Gloria on *Modern Family*), they are more likely to choose behaviors modeled by her—either as herself or her featured character. If Gloria breast-feeds, her fans are more likely to breastfeed. Therefore, the integration of celebrities can significantly impact the effectiveness of the E-E campaign (Brown & Fraser, 2004).

Related to identification, the *parasocial interaction theory* also provides insight into how and why E-E campaigns help with resistance. A term coined by Horton and Wohl (1956), parasocial interaction states that people identify with characters and even form relationships with them (Brown & Fraser, 2004; Sood, 2002). Moyer-Gusé (2008) built upon the ELM, concept of identification and parasocial interaction theory, to create the *entertainment overcoming resistance model.* This approach states that entertainment features, including parasocial interaction, identification, one's enjoyment of a program, and the viewer's perceived similarity/identification, help to reduce resistance to health messages in a narrative (Moyer-Gusé, 2008).

Cultivation theory, developed by Gerbner and Gross (1976), also helps to explain the influence of television on normalizing beliefs. In the 1970s, Gerbner demonstrated that television impacts the way in which people perceive the world (Gerbner & Gross, 1976). Specifically, cultivation theory states that heavier viewers of television hold a mediated view of reality. That is, they tend to see the world as it is portrayed on television (Gerbner & Gross, 1976). While this theory is often associated with skewed perception of violence, in health communication, it also broadly explains how a mediated reality constructs a view of the world, normalizing certain behaviors, like bottle-feeding infants, while making other behaviors seem abnormal or deviant. For example, if African American characters always choose bottles for their babies, these narratives normalize this behavior. Heavier viewers may then perceive bottle-feeding as the norm for African American mothers. This theory then demonstrates the importance of addressing cultural norms to impact individual behaviors.

The Obstacles of Entertainment-Education

The appeal of E-E can also serve as a drawback. The audience may miss the message or disregard it because of its placement in entertainment (Piotrow & de Fossard, 2004). Viewers may quickly forget the message or not understand its meaning (Brown & Walsh-Childers, 2002). Viewers may trivialize an issue, particularly for a comedic program (Moyer-Gusé & Nabi, 2011). For example, if viewers dislike the characters involved in a story line, they may be less likely to heed its message. In a study of the impact of humorous pregnancy story lines on perceptions of safer sex, Moyer-Gusé and Nabi (2011) noted a gender difference in participant responses. They speculated that the male participants' general dislike for the show (*The O.C.*) resulted in a boomerang effect, in which the E-E message causes participants to have less favorable attitudes or decrease in the intended behavior because of the message (Moyer-Gusé & Nabi, 2011). Furthermore, narratives may reinforce norms and stereotypes, even when the intention is to counter them. For example, in an E-E study designed to challenge stereotypes about obese people, Gesser-Edelsburg & Endevelt (2011) found that the audience interpreted the message as perpetuating "thinness ideals," instead of challenging hegemonic norms.

Access to media producers can also be an issue for scholars and public health advocates who wish to create E-E campaigns. As Poindexter (2004) explained, to get a message on U.S. television, people must consider the network owners and managers, television producers, and the scriptwriters. Therefore, utilizing entertainment television can be nearly impossible without the connections and financial resources to bypass the gatekeepers.

There can also be problems in the way in which the campaign is carried out. If the E-E program contains too much entertainment, without adequate information, viewers may not receive the intended message (Piotrow & de Fossard, 2004). For example, Moyer-Gusé, Mahood, and Brookes (2011) found that viewers perceived the negative consequences of sexual irresponsibility to be less severe when they were presented in a humorous situation. Likewise, if the program is too information-heavy and lacks entertainment, the audience will likely decrease (Piotrow & de Fossard, 2004). Issues with credibility and viewer relevance can also hinder the message (Piotrow & de Fossard, 2004). Finally, if the campaign drastically counters cultural norms or expectations, the program may be censored or pulled from the air (Piotrow & de Fossard, 2004). Because fictional television relies on advertisers, embedded controversial health messages can result in losses in sponsorship (Brown & Walsh-Childers, 2002). For example, in 1972, *Maude* producer Norman Lear chose to have the lead character in *Maude* have an abortion after the Population Institute encouraged television executives to address the problem of overpopulation and birth control in their programs (Montgomery, 1989). Because of the controversial story line on abortion, Lear received numerous letters from outraged fans and the CBS network lost advertisers (Montgomery, 1989). When the network aired reruns of the two "abortion" episodes in the following summer, no commercials aired during either program, causing a significant financial loss to CBS (Montgomery, 1989).

Many of these concerns can be remedied with the careful research, planning, and implementation of E-E campaigns. Awareness of potential cultural resistance to change can help researchers to address barriers in the message creation. The selection of the appropriate television program can help with the fit of the health message within the narrative. Pairing an E-E campaign with grassroots advocacy can boost overall changes in attitudes in behavior, as demonstrated with the *Soul City* project (Usdin et al., 2004). Such an approach could be an effective means to influence more women to breastfeed, taking the next step to the casual conversation and portrayal in *Modern Family.*

Designing Entertainment-Education Campaigns

As discussed earlier, traditional health campaigns have and can effectively convey breastfeeding's benefit. However, conventional campaigns have yet to produce a cultural climate that is supportive of breastfeeding, in which a mother nursing her baby in a restaurant does not have to worry about public stares or a rude manager requesting her to "cover up" or leave the premises (despite laws protecting her right to breastfeed anywhere, any time). E-E campaigns could help transform cultural attitudes by modeling breastfeeding and appropriate reactions to breastfeeding. In addition to *Modern Family*, breastfeeding is commonplace in contemporary television, depicted in the sitcoms *Friends* and *Mad about You*, and more recently *Parenthood* and *The New Normal*, as well as in other genres. Characters assume that new mothers will breastfeed, as story lines involve common concerns of nursing mothers (i.e., latching, others' discomfort, returning to work). E-E campaigns could expand these narratives to include more women of color, as with Gloria in *Modern Family*, showcase older babies breastfeeding to model longer duration, and address breastfeeding obstacles that have not been covered, like mastitis, paired with a solution. Viewers then would not only learn about overcoming challenges but also identify with the characters' experiences with breastfeeding. For example, new mothers might feel for Julia in *Nip/Tuck* as she struggles to latch on her new baby and then rejoice when she finally succeeds. Such character identification is difficult to mimic in conventional campaigns.

As with traditional health campaigns, most E-E campaigns follow a somewhat standard procedure. These campaigns can be local—targeted to one village or geographic area—or national, and can utilize a single medium, such as radio, recorded music, or television, or appear across platforms. Live theatrical performances that dramatize an issue of concern can also be used to inform or persuade audience members (Glik, Nowak, Valente, Sapsis, & Martin, 2002; Singhal, 2004). The placement of the campaign, time frame for the dissemination, narrative structure, and evaluation devices depend on the target audience, potential sites of resistance, prior knowledge of the health issue, and overall purpose of the campaign. To be effective, a campaign must also be culturally sensitive to social norms (Piotrow & de Fossard, 2004).

Campaigns that use entertainment-education can be implemented in a number of ways, but typically follow a similar design:

1. *Designing the Campaign.* First, an advocacy group approaches media producers about embedding a prosocial message in their media products. An alternative path is that the television producers or writers develop a prosocial story line in their programs (which may or may not be part of a formal campaign). Either way, the messages must be well researched, with a solid understanding of the characters, story arcs, themes, and genres of the media product. It may not be effective to include a prosocial message about domestic violence in a sitcom, for example. Yet, this issue may be appropriate for a crime drama or soap opera.

2. *Creating the Message.* Next, television writers work with experts on the issues to create a story line that accurately conveys the prosocial message, while preserving the integrity of the show. This message has to be direct enough to influence viewers, but not so distracting that it takes away from the show's narrative. As demonstrated in the *Friends'* condom efficacy study, statistics can be used sparingly to support the overall message.

3. *Conveying the Message.* The episode(s) with the prosocial story line airs. It may occur in a single episode or over a season.

4. *Evaluation.* In a formal campaign, the effectiveness of the message must be measured. Depending on the popularity of the E-E program, participants can be randomly recruited. Otherwise, people can be recruited by their viewing status. Depending on the issue, participants may fill out a preliminary survey prior to exposure. Following the airing of the message(s), surveys, interviews, or focus groups can be conducted to assess the impact of the campaign. This stage may be performed in multiple intervals.

5. *Follow-up.* Often, follow-up surveys or interviews may be conducted to determine the long-term effects of the health messages. This approach can also be used to confirm behavior changes. In this stage, researchers review the campaign, noting strengths and obstacles. They may also plan for a second campaign.

As with traditional health campaigns, the design and implementation of E-E campaigns may vary, depending on past campaigns, knowledge of the target audience, and the availability of media outlets. Moreover, E-E campaigns contain the additional challenge of embedding messages into entertainment media. When executed well, viewers absorb the message as part of a show's narrative, without overtly recognizing the message itself. For example, with the condom efficacy story line in *Friends*, most viewers were able to recall the rate of condom effectiveness, yet were unaware that the message was deliberately embedded as part of a campaign. This tricky balance is unique to E-E and raises the question of negotiation: How do you get your message across without preaching to the audience or undermining the characters or the program itself?

■ Epilogue

After Cecelia gave birth to her baby, she was excited to breastfeed. Her best friend's influence, her breastfeeding class, and the positive viewpoints she had read in books, in magazines, and online had convinced her it was the right and best thing to do. Although she had come across negative portrayals of breastfeeding (e.g., Dwight's comments in The Office*), the negative messages didn't derail her determination. With the help of a lactation consultant at the hospital and her partner's support, Cecelia worked through the challenging early days and was able to meet her breastfeeding goals.*

■ Conclusion

Health promotion is carried out in many different ways, depending on the health issue, audience, and theoretical models used. Traditional health campaigns have been quite effective in disseminating information and, depending on the behavior, impacting lifestyle changes. As demonstrated with breastfeeding promotion, some campaigns fall short, particularly when the healthy behavior may face cultural resistance. Theoretical models in health promotion help explain variances in campaign effectiveness and help researchers improve campaign design. In addition, entertainment-education has and can also be used to reach difficult audiences, convey information, and model healthy behaviors. Thinking of the anecdote in this chapter, entertainment-education may be the way to normalize breastfeeding, paving the way for higher initiation and duration rates. With traditional or entertainment-education campaigns, careful research and planning, cultural sensitivity, appropriate message design, and selected channels increase the likelihood of campaign success.

Discussion Questions

1. Think about two or three specific health campaigns that are particularly memorable to you. Which one do you feel was most effective and why?

2. What are the advantages to using entertainment to disseminate messages? What are the disadvantages?

3. Based on the examples in this chapter, and perhaps your own experiences as well, how do you think E-E programs in developing countries differ from those in the United States and other developed countries?

4. Imagine you are designing an E-E campaign to encourage children to exercise more frequently. What television program(s) would you select for your message? Why? Discuss how you might insert your health message into the narrative. What theory would support your campaign?

5. How do you think technology will impact the future of health promotion? How can emerging technologies be utilized for entertainment education?

NOTE

[1] Breastfed babies have lower risks of infectious disease, leukemia, allergies, dental and vision problems, skin issues, asthma and other respiratory issues, autism, and obesity (Caplan, Erwin, Lense, & Hicks, 2008; Gillman et al., 2001; McCrory & Layte, 2012; Odijk et al., 2003; Owen, Martin, Whincup, Smith,

& Cook, 2006; Palmer, 1998; Pratt, 1984; Sonnenschein-van de Voort et al., 2012; Verhasselt, 2010; Wright et al., 1998). Children who were breastfed also perform better cognitively, scoring higher on intelligence quotient and achievement tests (Jacobson, Chiodo, & Jacobson, 1999; Oddy, Li, Whitehouse, Zubrick, & Malacova, 2011; Quigley et al. 2012).

REFERENCES

Achievements in public health, 1900–1999 motor-vehicle safety: A 20th century public health achievement. (1999, May 14). *Morbidity and Mortality Weekly, 48*(18), 369–374. Retrieved from http://www.cdc.gov/mmwr/preview/mmwrhtml/mm4818a1.htm

Ajzen, I. (2005). *Attitudes, personality, and behavior* (2nd ed.). Milton-Keynes, UK: Open University Press/McGraw-Hill.

Announcement: Click It or Ticket Campaign. (2015, May 15). Centers for Disease Control and Prevention. *Morbidity & Mortality Weekly Report.* Retrieved from http://www.cdc.gov/mmWr/preview/mmwrhtml/mm6418a7.htm

Atkin, C., & Rice, R. (2012). Theory and principles of public communication campaigns. In R. E. Rice & C. K. Atkin (Eds.), *Public communication campaigns* (4th ed., pp. 3–20). Los Angeles, CA: Sage.

Atkin, C., & Salmon, C. (2010). Communication campaigns. In C. R. Berger, M. E. Roloff, & D. R. Ewoldsen (Eds.), *The handbook of communication science* (2nd ed., pp. 419–436). Thousand Oaks, CA: Sage.

Atkin, C. K., & Freimuth, V. S. (2012). Formative evaluation research in campaign design. In R. Rice, R. & C. Atkin (Eds.), *Public communication campaigns* (4th ed., pp. 53–68). Newbury Park, CA: Sage.

Audet, C. M., Matos, C. S., Blevins, M., Cardoso, A., Moon, T. D., & Sidat, M. (2012). Acceptability of cervical cancer screening in rural Mozambique. *Health Education Research, 27,* 544–551.

Backer, T. E., Rogers, E., & Sopory, P. (1992). *Designing health communication campaigns: What works?* Newbury Park, CA: Sage.

Bandura, A. (1977a). *Social learning theory.* Englewood Cliffs, NJ: Prentice-Hall.

Bandura, A. (1977b). Self-efficacy: Toward a unifying theory of behavioral change. *Psychological Review, 84,* 191.

Bandura, A. (2004). Social cognitive theory for personal and social change by enabling media. In A. Singhal, M. J. Cody, E. M. Rogers, & M. Sabido (Eds.), *Entertainment-education and social change: History, research, and practice* (pp. 75–96). Mahwah, NJ: Erlbaum.

Bauer, U. E., Johnson, T. M., Hopkins, R. S., & Brooks, R. G. (2000). Changes in youth cigarette use and intentions following implementation of a tobacco control program: Findings from the Florida Youth Tobacco Survey, 1998–2000. *JAMA, 284,* 723–728.

Beck, V. (2004). Working with daytime and prime-time television shows in the United States to promote health. In A. Singhal, M. J. Cody, E. M. Rogers, & M. Sabido (Eds.), *Entertainment-education and social change: History, research, and practice* (pp. 207–224). Mahwah, NJ: Erlbaum.

Becker, M. H., Maiman, L. A., Kirscht, J. P., Haefner, D. P., & Drachman, R. H. (1977). The Health Belief Model and prediction of dietary compliance: A field experiment. *Journal of Health and Social Behavior, 18,* 348–366.

Breastfeeding and the use of human milk. (2005). American Academy of Pediatrics Section on Breastfeeding. *Pediatrics, 115,* 496–506.

Breastfeeding Report Card—United States, 2014. (2014). Centers for Disease Control and Prevention. Retrieved from http://www.cdc.gov/breastfeeding/pdf/2014breastfeedingreportcard.pdf

Brodie, M., Foehr, U., Rideout, V., . . . Altman, D. (2001). Communicating health information through the entertainment media. *Health Affairs, 20,* 192–199.

Brown, W. J., & Fraser, B. P. (2004). Celebrity identification in entertainment-education. In A. Singhal, M. J. Cody, E. M. Rogers, & M. Sabido (Eds.), *Entertainment-education and social change: History, research, and practice* (pp. 97–116). Mahwah, NJ: Erlbaum.

Brown, J. D., & Keller, S. N. (2000). Can the mass media be healthy sex educators? *Family Planning Perspectives, 32,* 255–256.

Brown, J. D., & Walsh-Childers, K. (2002). Effects of media on personal and public health. In J. Bryant, & D. Zillmann (Eds.), *Media effects: Advances in theory and research* (2nd ed., pp. 453–488). Mahwah, NJ: Erlbaum.

Brown, W. J., & Basil, M. D. (1995). Media celebrities and public health: Responses to Magic Johnson's HIV disclosure and its impact on AIDS risk and high-risk behaviors. *Health Communication, 7,* 345–370.

Brown, W. J., & Fraser, B. P. (2004). Celebrity identification in entertainment-education. In A. Singhal, M. J. Cody, E. M. Rogers, & M. Sabido (Eds.), *Entertainment-education and social change: History, research, and practice* (pp. 97–116). Mahwah, NJ: Erlbaum.

Buller, D. B., Andersen, P. A., Walkosz, B. J., Scott, M. D., Cutter, G. C., Dignan, M. B., Kane, I. L., & Zhang, X. (2012). Enhancing industry-based dissemination of an occupational sun protection program with theory-based strategies employing personal contact. *American Journal of Health Promotion, 26,* 356–365.

Caplan, L. S., Erwin, K., Lense, E., & Hicks, J., Jr. (2008). The potential role of breast-feeding and other factors in helping to reduce early childhood caries. *Journal of Public Health Dentistry, 68,* 238–241.

CDC Study Finds Seat Belt Use Up to 85 Percent Nationally. (2011). Centers for Disease Control and Prevention. (4 January). Retrieved from http://www.cdc.gov/media/releases/2011/p0104_vitalsigns.html

Carpenter, C. J. (2010). A meta-analysis of the effectiveness of health belief model variables in predicting behavior. *Health Communication, 25,* 661–669.

Collins, R. L., Elliott, M. N., Berry, S. H., Kanouse, D. E., & Hunter, S. B. (2003). Entertainment television as a healthy sex educator: The impact of condom-efficacy information in an episode of *Friends. Pediatrics, 112,* 1115–1121.

Cram, P., Fendrick, A. M., Inadomi, J., Cowen, M. E., Carpenter, D., & Vijan, S. (2003). The impact of a celebrity promotional campaign on the use of colon cancer screening: The Katie Couric effect. *Archives of Internal Medicine, 163,* 1601–1605.

Davin, S. (2004). Healthy viewing: The reception of medical narratives. In C. Seale (Ed.), *Health and the media* (pp. 143–159). Malden, MA: Blackwell.

Dean, M. (2016). Celebrity health announcements and online health information seeking: An analysis of Angelina Jolie's preventative health decision. *Health Communication, 31,* 752–761.

DeSantis, A. D., & Morgan, S. E. (2003). Sometimes a cigar [magazine] is more than just a cigar [magazine]: Pro-smoking arguments in Cigar Aficionado, 1992–2000. *Health Communication, 15,* 457–480.

Diem, S. J., Lantos, J. D., & Tulsky, J. A. (1996). Cardiopulmonary resuscitation on television: Miracles and misinformation. *New England Journal of Medicine, 334,* 1578–1582.

Fewtrell, L., Kaufmann, R. B., Kay, D., Enanoria, W., Haller, L., & Colford, J. M. (2005). Water, sanitation, and hygiene interventions to reduce diarrhoea in less developed countries: a systematic review and meta-analysis. *The Lancet Infectious Diseases, 5,* 42–52.

Fishbein, M. (2000). The role of theory in HIV prevention. *AIDS Care, 12,* 273–278.

Fishbein, M., & Ajzen, I. (1975). *Belief, attitude, intention, and behavior: An introduction to theory and research.* Reading, MA: Addison-Wesley.

Fishbein, M., & Ajzen, I. (2011). *Predicting and changing behavior: The reasoned action approach.* New York, NY: Taylor & Francis.

Fishbein, M., & Cappella, J. N. (2006). The role of theory in developing effective health communications. *Journal of Communication, 56,* S1–S17.

Fishbein, M., & Yzer, M. C. (2003). Using theory to design effective health behavior interventions. *Communication Theory, 13,* 164–183.

Folb, K. (2000). "Don't touch that dial!" TV as a—what!?—positive influence. *SIECUS Report, 28*(5), 16–18.

Foss, K. A. (2013). "That's not a beer bong, it's a breast pump!" Representations of breastfeeding in prime-time fictional television. *Health Communication, 28,* 329–340.

Gantz, W., Fitzmaurice, M., & Yoo, E. (1990). Seat belt campaigns and buckling up: Do the media make a difference? *Health Communication, 2,* 1–12.

Gauthier, C. (1999). Television drama and popular film as medical narrative. *Journal of American Culture, 22,* 23–26.

Gebrian, B. (2014). Bottles to breastfeeding in rural Haiti. *Journal of Health Care for the Poor and Underserved, 25,* 1514–1519.

Gerbner, G., & Gross L. (1976). Living with television: The violence profile. *Journal of Communication, 26,* 173–199.

Gesser-Edelsburg, A., & Endevelt, R. (2011). An entertainment-education study of stereotypes and prejudice against fat women: An evaluation of *Fat Pig. Health Education Journal, 70,* 374–382.

Gillman, M. W., Rifas-Shiman, S. L., Camargo, C. A., Berkey, C. S., Frazier, A. L., . . . Rockett, R. H. (2001). Risk of overweight among adolescents who were breastfed as infants. *JAMA, 285,* 2461–2467.

Glik, D., Berkanovic, E., Stone, K., Ibarra, L., Jones, M. C., . . . Rosen, B. (1998). Health education goes Hollywood: Working with prime-time and daytime entertainment television for immunization promotion. *Journal of Health Communication, 3,* 263–282.

Glik, D., Nowak, G., Valente, T., Sapsis, K., & Martin, C. (2002). Youth performing arts entertainment-education for HIV/AIDS prevention and health promotion: Practice and research. *Journal of Health Communication, 7,* 39–57.

Grantham, S., Ahern, L., & Connolly-Ahern, C. (2011). Merck's *One Less* campaign: Using risk message frames to promote the use of Gardasil® in HPV prevention. *Communication Research Reports, 28,* 318-326.

Graves, K. N., Sentner, A., Workman, J., & Mackey, W. (2011). Building positive life skills the Smart Girls Way: Evaluation of a school-based sexual responsibility program for adolescent girls. *Health Promotion Practice, 12,* 463–471.

Greene, K., & Brinn, L. S. (2003). Messages influencing college women's tanning bed use: Statistical versus narrative evidence format and a self-assessment to increase perceived susceptibility. *Journal of Health Communication, 8,* 443–461.

Haroon, S., Das, J. K., Salam, R. A., Imdad, A., & Bhutta, Z. A. (2013). Breastfeeding promotion interventions and breastfeeding practices: a systematic review. *BMC Public Health, 13*(Suppl 3), S20.

Hicks, J. J. (2001). The strategy behind Florida's "truth" campaign. *Tobacco Control, 10,* 3–5.

Hornik, R. (2002). *Public health communication.* Mahwah, NJ: Erlbaum.

Horodynski, M. A., Calcatera, M., & Carpenter, A. (2012). Infant feeding practices: Perceptions of Native American mothers and health paraprofessionals. *Health Education Journal, 71,* 327–339.

Horton, D., & Wohl, R. R. (1956). Mass communication and para-social interaction: Observations on intimacy at a distance. *Psychiatry, 19,* 215–229.

Huffman, S. L., Zehner, E. R., & Victora, C. (2001). Can improvements in breast-feeding practices reduce neonatal mortality in developing countries? *Midwifery, 17,* 80–92.

Imdad, A., Yakoob, M. Y., & Bhutta, Z. A. (2011). Effect of breastfeeding promotion interventions on breastfeeding rates, with special focus on developing countries. *BMC Public Health, 11*(Suppl 3), S24.

Jacobson, S. W., Chiodo, L. M., & Jacobson, J. L. (1999). Breastfeeding effects on intelligence quotient in 4- and 11-year-old children. *Pediatrics, 103*(5), e71–e71.

Janz, N. K., & Becker, M. H. (1984). The health belief model: A decade later. *Health Education & Behavior, 11,* 1–47.

Kavanagh, K. F., Lou, Z., Nicklas, J. C., Habibi, M. F., & Murphy, L. T. (2012). Breastfeeding knowledge, attitudes, prior exposure, and intent among undergraduate students. *Journal of Human Lactation, 28,* 556–564.

Kearney, M. S., & Levine, P. B. (2014). *Media influences on social outcomes: The impact of MTV's* 16 and Pregnant *on teen childbearing* (No. w19795). National Bureau of Economic Research.

Kim, H. S., Ahn, J., & No, J. K. (2012). Applying the health belief model to college students' health behavior. *Nutrition Research and Practice, 6,* 551–558.

LaCroix, J. M., Snyder, L. B., Huedo-Medina, T. B., & Johnson, B. T. (2014). Effectiveness of mass media interventions for HIV prevention, 1986–2013: A meta-analysis. *JAIDS Journal of Acquired Immune Deficiency Syndromes, 66,* S329–S340.

Li, R., Hsia, J., Fridinger, F., Hussain, A., Benton-Davis, S., & Grummer-Strawn, L. (2004). Public beliefs about breastfeeding policies in various settings. *Journal of the American Dietetic Association, 104,* 1162–1168.

Madden, T. J., Ellen, P. S., & Ajzen, I. (1992). A comparison of the theory of planned behavior and the theory of reasoned action. *Personality and Social Psychology Bulletin, 18,* 3–9.

Maddock, J., Maglione, C., Barnett, J. D., Cabot, C., Jackson, S., & Reger-Nash, B. (2007). Statewide implementation of the 1% or less campaign. *Health Education & Behavior, 34,* 953–963.

Mahoney, L. M., & Bates, B. R. (2013). The impacts of an entertainment-education radio serial drama in Botswana on outcomes related to HIV prevention goals in the President's Emergency Plan for AIDS Relief. *Journal of African Media Studies, 5,* 353–367.

Martins, N., & Jensen, R. E. (2014). The relationship between "Teen Mom" reality programming and teenagers' beliefs about teen parenthood. *Mass Communication and Society, 17,* 830–852.

McCrory, C., & Layte, R. (2012). Breastfeeding and risk of overweight and obesity at nine-years of age. *Social Science & Medicine, 75,* 323–330.

McKinney, A. (2015). A lifestyle perspective on infertility and pregnancy outcome. *American Journal of Lifestyle Medicine, 9,* 368–377.

Montgomery, K. C. (1989). *Target: Prime time: Advocacy groups and the struggle over entertainment television.* New York, NY: Oxford University Press.

Moyer-Gusé, E. (2008). Toward a theory of entertainment persuasion: Explaining the persuasive effects of entertainment-education messages. *Communication Theory, 18,* 407–425.

Moyer-Gusé, E., Mahood, C., & Brookes, S. (2011). Entertainment-education in the context of humor: Effects on safer sex intentions and risk perceptions. *Health Communication, 26,* 765–774.

Moyer-Gusé, E., & Nabi, R. L. (2011). Explaining the effects of narrative in an entertainment television program: Overcoming resistance to persuasion. *Human Communication Research, 36,* 26–52.

Murray-Johnson, L., & Witte, K. (2003). Looking toward the future: Health message design strategies. In T. L. Thompson, A. Dorsey, K. I. Miller, & R. Parrott (Eds.), *Handbook of health communication* (pp. 473–495). Mahwah, NJ: Erlbaum.

Nattinger, A. B., Hoffmann, R. G., Howell-Pelz, A., & Goodwin, J. S. (1998). Effect of Nancy Reagan's mastectomy on choice of surgery for breast cancer by U.S. women. *JAMA, 279,* 762–767.

Oddy, W. H., Li, J., Whitehouse, A. J., Zubrick, S. R., & Malacova, E. (2011). Breastfeeding duration and academic achievement at 10 years. *Pediatrics, 127,* e137–e145.

Odijk, J. V., Kull, I., Borres, M. P., Brandtzaeg, P., Edberg, U., Hanson, L. Å., . . . Wille, S. (2003). Breastfeeding and allergic disease: A multidisciplinary review of the literature (1966–2001) on the mode of early feeding in infancy and its impact on later atopic manifestations. *Allergy, 58,* 833–843.

Østbye, T., Miller, B., & Keller, H. (1997). Throw that epidemiologist out of the emergency room: Using the television series *ER* as a vehicle for teaching methodologists about medical issues. *Journal of Clinical Epidemiology, 50,* 1183–1186.

Owen, C. G., Martin, R. M., Whincup, P. H., Smith, G. D., & Cook, D. G. (2006). Does breastfeeding influence risk of type 2 diabetes in later life? A quantitative analysis of published evidence. *The American Journal of Clinical Nutrition, 84,* 1043–1054.

Palmer, B. (1998). The influence of breastfeeding on the development of the oral cavity: A commentary. *Journal of Human Lactation, 14,* 93–98.

Pechmann, C. (2001). A comparison of health communication models: Risk learning versus stereotype priming. *Media Psychology, 3,* 189–210.

Pierce, J. P., Macaskill, P., & Hill, D. (2002). Long-term effectiveness of the early mass media led antismoking campaigns in Australia. In R. Hornik (Ed.), *Public health communication* (pp. 57–70). Mahwah, NJ: Erlbaum.

Piotrow, P. T., & de Fossard, E. (2004). Entertainment-education as a public health intervention. In A. Singhal, M. J. Cody, E. M. Rogers, & M. Sabido (Eds.), *Entertainment-education and social change: History, research, and practice* (pp. 39–60). Mahwah, NJ: Erlbaum.

Poindexter, D. O. (2004). A history of entertainment-education, 1958-2000. In A. Singhal, M. J. Cody, E. M. Rogers, & M. Sabido (Eds.), *Entertainment-education and social change: History, research, and practice* (pp. 21–38). Mahwah, NJ: Erlbaum.

Pratt, H. F. (1984). Breastfeeding and eczema. *Early Human Development, 9,* 283–290.

Quigley, M. A., Hockley, C., Carson, C., Kelly, Y., Renfrew, M. J., & Sacker, A. (2012). Breastfeeding is associated with improved child cognitive development: A population-based cohort study. *The Journal of Pediatrics, 160,* 25–32.

Reger, B., Wootan, M. G., Booth-Butterfield, S., & Smith, H. (1998). *1% or Less*: a community-based nutrition campaign. *Public Health Reports, 113,* 410.

Rice, R., & Foote, D. (2012). A systems-based evaluation planning model for health communication campaigns in developing countries. In R. Rice & C. Atkin (Eds.), *Public communication campaigns* (4th ed., pp. 53–68). Newbury Park, CA: Sage.

Rideout, V. J. (2008). Television as a health educator: A case study of *Grey's Anatomy*. Henry J. Kaiser Family Foundation.

Robinson, J. K., Rigel, D. S., & Amonette, R. A. (1997). Trends in sun exposure knowledge, attitudes, and behaviors: 1986 to 1996. *Journal of the American Academy of Dermatology, 37,* 179–186.

Roccella, E. J. (2002). The contributions of public health education toward the reduction of cardiovascular disease mortality: Experiences from the National High Blood Pressure Education Program. In R. Hornik (Ed.), *Public health communication* (pp. 73–83). Mahwah, NJ: Erlbaum.

Rogers, E. M., & Storey, J. D. (1987). Communication campaigns. In C. R. Berger & S. H. Chaffee (Eds.), *Handbook of communication science* (pp. 817–846). Newbury Park, CA: Sage.

Rothman, E. L. (1999). *White coat: Becoming a doctor at Harvard Medical School.* New York, NY: Morrow.

Sabido, M. (2004). The origins of entertainment-education. In A. Singhal, M. J. Cody, E. M. Rogers, & M. Sabido (Eds.), *Entertainment-education and social change: History, research, and practice* (pp. 61–74). Mahwah, NJ: Erlbaum.

Salmon, C. T., & Atkin, C. (2003). Using media campaigns for health promotion. In T. L. Thompson, A. Dorsey, K. I. Miller, & R. Parrott (Eds.), *Handbook of health communication* (pp. 449–472). Mahwah, NJ: Erlbaum.

Sharf, B. F., & Freimuth, V. S. (1993). The construction of illness on entertainment television: Coping with cancer on *thirtysomething*. *Health Communication, 5,* 141–160.

Sharf, B. F., Freimuth, V. S., Greenspon, P., & Plotnick, C. (1996). Confronting cancer on *thirtysomething:* Audience response to health content on entertainment television. *Journal of Health Communication, 1,* 157–172.

Sherry, J. L. (2002). Media saturation and entertainment—Education. *Communication Theory, 12,* 206–224.

Singhal, A. (2004). Entertainment-education through participatory theater: Freirean strategies for empowering the oppressed. In A. Singhal, M. J. Cody, E. M. Rogers, & M. Sabido (Eds.), *Entertainment-education and social change: History, research, and practice* (pp. 377–398). Mahwah, NJ: Erlbaum.

Singhal, A., & Rogers, E. M. (2004). The status of entertainment-education worldwide. In A. Singhal, M. J. Cody, E. M. Rogers, & M. Sabido (Eds.), *Entertainment-education and social change: History, research, and practice* (pp. 3–20). Mahwah, NJ: Erlbaum.

Singhal, A., & Rogers, E. M. (1999). *Entertainment-education: A communication strategy for social change.* Mahwah, NJ: Erlbaum.

Slater, M. D., & Rouner, D. (2002). Entertainment-education and elaboration likelihood: Understanding the processing of narrative persuasion. *Communication Theory, 12,* 173–191.

Snyder, L. B., & Hamilton, M. A. (2002). A meta-analysis of US health campaign effects on behavior: Emphasize enforcement, exposure, and new information, and beware the secular trend. In R. Hornik (Ed.), *Public health communication* (pp. 357–384). Mahwah, NJ: Erlbaum.

Sonnenschein-van der Voort, A. M., Jaddoe, V. W., Raat, H., Moll, H. A., Hofman, A., de Jongste, J. C., & Duijts, L. (2012). Fetal and infant growth and asthma symptoms in pre-school children: The Generation R Study. *American Journal of Respiratory and Critical Care Medicine, 185,* 731–737.

Sood, S. (2002). Audience involvement and entertainment-education. *Communication Theory, 12,* 153–172.

Sood, S., Shefner-Rogers, C. L., & Sengupta, M. (2006). The impact of a mass media campaign on HIV/AIDS knowledge and behavior change in North India: Results from a longitudinal study. *Asian Journal of Communication, 16,* 231–250.

Stanger-Hall, K. F., & Hall, D. W. (2011). Abstinence-only education and teen pregnancy rates: Why we need comprehensive sex education in the US. *PloS One, 6*(10), e24658.

Stuebe, A. M. (2014). Enabling women to achieve their breastfeeding goals. *Obstetrics & Gynecology, 123,* 643–652.

Stuebe, A. (2009). The risks of not breastfeeding for mothers and infants. *Reviews in Obstetrics and Gynecology, 2,* 222–231.

Sweat, M. D., Denison, J., Kennedy, C., Tedrow, V., & O'Reilly, K. (2012). Effects of condom social marketing on condom use in developing countries: A systematic review and meta-analysis, 1990-2010. *Bulletin of the World Health Organization, 90,* 613–622A.

Terlouw, D. J., Morgah, K., Wolkon, A., Dare, A., Dorkenoo, A., Eliades, M. J., . . . Hawley, W. A. (2010). Impact of mass distribution of free long-lasting insecticidal nets on childhood malaria morbidity: the Togo National Integrated Child Health Campaign. *Malaria Journal, 9,* 199–212.

U.S. Department of Health and Human Services. (2011). *The Surgeon General's call to action to support breastfeeding.* Washington, DC. Retrieved from http://www.surgeongeneral.gov/library/calls/breastfeeding/calltoactiontosupportbreastfeeding.pdf

Usdin, S., Singhal, A., Shongwe, T., Goldstein, S., & Shabalala, A. (2004). No short cuts in entertainment-education: Designing Soul City step-by-step. In A. Singhal, M. J. Cody, E. M. Rogers, & M. Sabido (Eds.), *Entertainment-education and social change: History, research, and practice* (pp. 153–176). Mahwah, NJ: Erlbaum.

Vaughan, W., Rogers, E. Singhal, A. & Swalehe, P. (2000). Entertainment-education and HIV/ AIDS prevention: A field experiment in Tanzania. *Journal of Health Communication, 5,* 81–100.

Verhasselt, V. (2010). Neonatal tolerance under breastfeeding influence. *Current Opinion in Immunology, 22,* 623-630.

Wakefield, M. A., Loken, B., & Hornik, R. C. (2010). Use of mass media campaigns to change health behaviour. *The Lancet, 376,* 1261–1271.

Walkosz, B. J., Buller, D. B., Andersen, P. A., Scott, M. D., Dignan, M. B., Cutter, G. R., & Maloy, J. A. (2008). Increasing sun protection in winter outdoor recreation: A theory-based health communication program. *American Journal of Preventive Medicine, 34,* 502–509.

Whittier, D. K., Kennedy, M. G., St. Lawrence, J. S., Seeley, S., & Beck, V. (2005). Embedding health messages into entertainment television: Effect on gay men's response to a syphilis outbreak. *Journal of Health Communication, 10,* 251–259.

Williams, A. F., Wells, J. K., & Reinfurt, D. W. (2002). Increasing seat belt use in North Carolina. In R. Hornik (Ed.), *Public health communication* (pp. 85–96). Mahwah, NJ: Erlbaum.

Winsten, J. A. (1993). Promoting designated drivers: The Harvard Alcohol Project. *American Journal of Preventive Medicine, 10*(3 Suppl), 11–14.

Witte, K. (1992). Putting the fear back into fear appeals: The extended parallel process model. *Communications Monographs, 59,* 329–349.

Worden, J. K., & Flynn, B. S. (2002). Using mass media to prevent cigarette smoking. In R. Hornik (Ed.), *Public health communication* (pp. 23–34). Mahwah, NJ: Erlbaum.

Wright, A. L., Bauer, M., Naylor, A., Sutcliffe, E., & Clark, L. (1998). Increasing breastfeeding rates to reduce infant illness at the community level. *Pediatrics, 101,* 837–844.

Wright, K. B., Sparks, L., & O'Hair, H. D. (2012). *Health communication in the 21st century* (2nd ed.). Malden, MA: John Wiley & Sons.

12

Communicating the Politics of Healthcare Systems

Heather Zoller & Shaunak Sastry

When you think about health and politics, what comes to mind? Medical care reform may be your first thought. However, consider the following issues raised in local and state ballots as well as national campaigns during the 2014 U.S. elections: The city of Berkeley, California, voted to tax soda distributors to raise funds to prevent diabetes; Denton, Texas, and two other communities voted to ban hydraulic fracturing gas drilling (fracking) based in part on health concerns; Massachusetts voted "Yes on 4," which allows workers to earn one hour of sick time for every 30 hours they work; Republican candidates continued to campaign against the Affordable Care Act (ACA or "Obamacare"); and governors debated whether and how to quarantine individuals who may have been exposed to Ebola. Across the world, in countries like Spain, Brazil, Greece, and Turkey, individuals, employees, and entire communities participated in mass protests against governmental "austerity" measures designed to shrink public investment in health.

This chapter describes the political complexities of health. What do we mean by politics? You are probably familiar with politics in terms of government policy making, public policy debates, and elections. Governmental policy has a profound influence on public health, including funding Medicaid and Medicare, crafting health and safety regulations, determining the legality of drugs such as marijuana, and mandating caregiver behavior in areas such as physician-assisted suicide. More broadly, governmental economic policy and even international trade agreements affect levels of employment, poverty, and public spending in ways that heavily influence public health outcomes. However, politics also encompasses "private" decision making that takes place in social institutions (e.g., corporations, workplaces, nonprofits, and voluntary associations) and in the negotiation of meaning in our everyday lives. Of course, citizens differ in the degree to which they actively engage in advocating for their own and others' health in medical and public health contexts (Rimal, Ratzan, Arntson, & Freimuth, 1997).

Communication is directly tied to political issues. Political communication is not just about the expression of political interests, although the ability to participate and have one's voice heard in public decision making is very important. Communication also involves the social construction of ideas and social agreements—often becoming taken-for-granted assumptions—that influence our experiences, our sense of self, and what we consider to count as knowledge. These taken-for-granted assumptions are formed and negotiated in a context of relations of power at governmental, institutional, and interpersonal levels.

In this chapter, we will describe (1) the political complexities of our taken-for-granted assumptions about health and illness causation, (2) the role of power in defining illness and establishing the scope of medical treatment, (3) the influence of economic decision making on health, and (4) the role of communication in medical care reform debates.

■ The Politics of Defining Health and Attributing Illness

Increasing numbers of employers are charging higher insurance rates or a monthly fee (a surcharge) for employees who smoke, have high cholesterol, have diabetes, or are deemed obese. Take the case of PepsiCo, which rolled out a wellness program that charges employees $50 a month if they smoke or have health issues such as diabetes, hypertension, and high blood pressure that are presumed to be avoidable or resolvable with changes in lifestyle or personal habits. Employees can avoid the surcharge if they attend classes to help them quit smoking or lose weight.

When we decide how to protect health, and how to distribute public health and medical resources, we draw from a set of beliefs about what it means to be healthy and what causes illness. Consider the workplace surcharges described above. When employers start these programs, they assume that (1) these conditions or activities cause illness and (2) these conditions or activities are controllable by individual employees. At first, these might seem like pretty straightforward assumptions, but many factors contribute to our health status. The way that we define health and illness has significant *political* implications.

These issues are political and not just scientific for several reasons. To start, *science is often uncertain* about the biological causes of illness. It is also important to remember that there is a difference between *agents* of disease and *causes* of disease, because multiple factors can lead to different biological vulnerabilities to the manifestation of disease. For example, two people may be exposed to a cold virus (an agent of disease) but only one may come down with the cold (a disease), due to a host of factors that influence the immune system, such as genetics, amount of sleep, adequate nutrition, and the existence of other illnesses. So when we explain what it takes to be healthy and what causes illness, we are selecting from multiple potential causes. When we attribute the cause of illness, we are also attributing *responsibility* for disease—a persuasive and rhetorical process rather than a solely scientific one (Kirkwood & Brown, 1995). These rhetorical choices influence how we treat people who are ill and how we distribute resources to prevent and treat disease. Thus, our theories about health and attributions of disease causation are linked to our beliefs about the proper organization of society (Tesh, 1994).

Thinking about the workplace surcharge, look at the list below of different theories of illness:

- The *lifestyle theory,* which holds that illness is caused by our personal choices, might be used to support employee surcharges for workers who are obese, have high cholesterol, or smoke. Proponents argue that higher costs will motivate workers to stop smoking and eat better.

- *Genetic theories,* on the other hand, might be used to question whether the policies discriminate against individuals who are genetically prone to high cholesterol or higher weight. (Generally, it is quite difficult to control cholesterol through behavior choices, and research is mixed about whether high cholesterol is bad for one's health.)

- *Environmental theories* might encourage us to consider the context of health choices: Does every person have equal access to safe and affordable ways to exercise and eat healthy food? Environmental theories also consider that our exposure to endocrine-disrupting chemicals such as bisphenol A and pthlalates may be contributing to obesity.

- Even *germ theories,* which attribute illness to microorganisms, play a role in this debate. Some researchers suggest that our "gut bacteria" might play an important role in our weight, seriously questioning the utility of common advice to just eat less as a way to lose weight (Wendelsdorf, 2013). This theory attributes weight gain to antibiotic use and sugar that may produce less diverse microbes.

- The *political/structural* perspective would point out that income level is the primary predictor of health status. Minority groups and low-income individuals are far more likely to live in places that are unsafe for exercise, have little access to healthy food, and have little time for healthy habits due to difficult work schedules and lack of childcare. Therefore, surcharges blame the individual for widespread social inequalities and further reduce income.

Table 12.1   Major Theories of Illness Causation

Theory	Attribution of Illness Causation	Primary Intervention
Lifestyle	Diet, exercise, and other choices	Individual choice-making
Genetic	Genetic make-up	Genetic therapy
Environmental	Factors in built and natural environments	Ecology, industry, political system
Germ	Microorganisms, viruses	Individual medical care
Political/Structural	Social and economic inequality	Structures supporting social, economic, and political marginalization

Considering these different theories, it becomes evident that questions about what causes illness are very complex. Perceptions about the causes of good health and illness are formed in everyday interactions, media accounts, and through institutional and governmental discourses. However, some people's definitions (such as PepsiCo) become policy because people support their theories of causation and they have power to implement changes (see Theorizing Practice 12.1).

As the surcharge example shows, debates about the causes of illness influence how we distribute resources such as insurance. It also influences how we design health interventions. For example, health communicators may address obesity by drawing from lifestyle theories to create health campaigns to encourage individuals to exercise, or draw from political/structural theories to advocate for safer neighborhoods. Further, by establishing responsibility for illness, these discourses direct blame and moral stigma. Indeed, when we attribute obesity to personal choices, we tend to blame and stigmatize overweight people more than if we emphasized genetic causes. Those who attribute obesity to political/structural factors tend to call out the food industry (such as PepsiCo) for aggressive marketing of cheap calorie-laden and sugary foods, and call for larger changes in our food system.

Heather, one of this chapter's authors, found that these theories of health played a big role during a community debate about a chemical plant that was releasing chemicals of concern in her neighborhood (Zoller, 2012). Some residents drew from envi-

HCIA 12.1

Does the U.S. Have a "Weight Problem"?

Lisa M. Tillmann

At Rollins College, I teach in a program of Critical Media and Cultural Studies (CMC). This major exposes students to pressing challenges like war, climate change, and economic inequality and to movements working for change. Through theory, library and original research, digital art, and social justice documentary filmmaking, CMC students become not only critical consumers of media and culture but critical *producers* as well. I try to model that through my own scholarship and creative work. Since the launch of our program in 2007, I have learned photo, sound, and video editing and have produced or coproduced three documentaries. Students have played important roles in all three films, from consulting on screenplays and music selections to contributing testimony and digital art.

Two of my three films began in sections of a course called The Political Economy of Body and Food. That class covers a lot of ground: from eating disorders and steroid abuse to food insecurity and farmworker justice. When I asked my 2011 student collaborators on what topic they wanted to center our work, they overwhelmingly chose cultural narratives of weight, fat, and "obesity." In other words: What stories circulate in our culture about fat, and how do those stories impact our bodies, lives, relationships, and public policy?

Following a practice encouraged by scholars in an interdisciplinary field known as Fat Studies, I put "obesity" in quotes to denote that this concept is a social construction that supports particular interests, such as those of the diet and drug industries. The quotes suggest that dominant narratives of "obesity" merit scrutiny, questioning, and critique.

The student testimony and digital art collected in 2011 provided the major building blocks for the film *Weight Problem: Cultural Narratives of Fat and "Obesity."* The U.S. indeed has a "weight problem," but in ways that differ from what we've been led to believe. *Weight Problem* addresses stereotypes and prejudices evident in our homes, with our peers, at primary and secondary schools, on college campuses, in the dating arena, and in mass media. The film directly challenges the rhetoric of the "obesity epidemic," which serves the $50–60 billion-per-year Diet Industrial Complex more than it improves public health.

Viewers hear from Tomas, who at age 15 undergoes a growth spurt in height and weight. He responds to criticism and teasing from his brother and schoolmates with dangerous patterns of self-starvation and weight cycling. Eric speaks of three years of weight-based harassment and bullying. We also meet Roxanne, who despite a hospitalization for anorexia, continues to experience stinging weight-based criticism from her mother.

Weight Problem offers several action items for viewers interested in helping redress the issues raised:

- Recognize that you have a stake in ending antifat prejudice—regardless of your current body shape or size. Exposure to cultural ideals for body shape and size lowers everyone's self-esteem, undermines our relationships with others, and drains energy and time from civic and community engagement.

- Eat a nutrient-dense diet and engage in regular physical activity for your own sake, not for weight loss.

- Vote with your wallet. Patronize companies and organizations that promote health for everyone, regardless of shape or size; withhold support from companies and organizations that sell products and services via antifat prejudice.

- Support antibullying policies inclusive of body shape and size, and interrupt harassment and bullying on these bases. Those classified as "overweight" and "obese" are more likely to be bullied than their so-called "normal"-weight peers, and people who have been bullied consider, attempt, and commit suicide at rates higher than those who have not.

- Lobby for antidiscrimination protections based on body shape and size. In the overwhelming majority of organizations, municipalities, and states, a person can be refused service in a shop or restaurant; denied a hotel room, house, or apartment; and even fired—on no other basis than body shape or size.

- Advocate for public policies, such as a living wage, that facilitate everyone's access to nutrient-dense food and to safe environments conducive to activity and play.

- Seek out sources of information independent of the Diet Industrial Complex.

Powerful forces wage the war on "obesity," and they have a lot to lose if we decide to pursue peace instead of war with our bodies. My student collaborators and I stand on the side of peace, health, equity, and justice. Learn more for yourself, then decide where you stand. For a full-length preview of *Weight Problem*, please email me at: lmtillmann@gmail.com. To learn more, please visit the website for *Weight Problem*'s production company, Cinema Serves Justice: http://cinemaservesjustice.com/index.html

(continued)

QUESTIONS TO PONDER

1. Have you ever lost and/or gained a significant amount of weight? If so, did that change in weight alter how you felt about yourself? If so, how? Did it alter how others (a dating partner, family member, friend, doctor, person on the street) treated you? How so?

2. When you hear the word "fat," what words or phrases come to mind first? How do those words and/or phrases reflect our culture's stereotypes about those labeled as "overweight" or "obese"?

3. About one third of people in the U.S. are classified as "overweight" and another one third as "obese." Given these statistics, what explains the fear and hatred of fat we find in mass media and public life?

Source: Tillmann, L. M. (Director, Producer, Writer). (2014). *Weight problem: Cultural narratives of fat and "obesity."* United States: Cinema Serves Justice. http://cinemaservesjustice.com/weight-problem.html

ronmental theories of health to call for reduced emissions from the company, EPA testing, and health department research into the effects of the chemicals. The company, and some residents, opposed such moves, using lifestyle theories of health to argue that research about company emissions was not needed because any increases in cancer and other illness were likely due to individual choices such as smoking and diet. Some residents also argued that cancer is caused by genetics, and nothing can be done about that.

Lifestyle theories of disease are becoming increasingly popular across the globe. During his research on HIV/AIDS risks faced by truck drivers in India, Shaunak, the second author of this chapter, found that most public health campaigns (as well as some truck drivers themselves) talked about AIDS as a "lifestyle" disease, emphasizing risky sexual behaviors and inadequate knowledge about contraception. However, very little attention was paid to the structural and economic context of truckers' lives: the fact that truckers were impoverished migrants forced to live away from their sexual partners for months at a time. Structural theories of health would point out the inequalities embedded in truck drivers' lives that compelled them to engage in risky behavior (Sastry, 2016).

A key issue in these debates is how much our health status is an *individual* and *private* versus *social* and *public* issue. Think about the debates over parents who refuse to vaccinate their children, arguing that it is their individual right to decide what risks their children take. These parents are concerned about their child's individual risk from vaccines. What these parents overlook is that not only are unvaccinated children at significant risk for disease, they are risking the lives of others, including infants who cannot yet get vaccinated and immuno-compromised individuals. Another example can be found in the media discussion of the Ebola Virus Disease (EVD) epidemic concentrated in the three West African nations of Guinea, Sierra Leone, and Liberia. While the spread of the virus may be a result of specific individual behaviors (like inadequate hygiene, or inappropriate disposal of patient waste), the disease is escalated to an epidemic status because of social factors: the lack of adequate public health infrastructure, medical facilities, hospitals, and so forth. In resource-poor countries like the ones mentioned above, the lack of adequate medical resources is a telling example of how health is determined through social causes. We will return to the Ebola example later in the chapter.

Although we may fall into the trap of thinking of individual and social causes as either-or, Levins and Lopez (1999) remind us to think about how these overlap:

> Consider the two propositions: (a) we are each responsible for our own health, and (b) health is socially determined. Both are claims about reality, and about the causes of disease. Both are also normative: each person should take responsibility for her or his own health, or our society should take collective responsibility for the health of all of us. Each proposition is separately false, but together they are jointly true. . . . When stated by policymakers, the first proposition blames the sick (or their parents) for being sick and justifies the denial of public resources for health improvement. The second, accepting social responsibility, would propose actions to improve healthcare, make it more available, or reduce environmental insults to our health such as pollution, but it leaves the individual out of the equation or as a passive onlooker. (p. 270)

We have described the political implications of defining health and naming responsibility for illness. In the next section, we describe how some conditions become "medicalized" and treated within the medical system.

HCIA 12.2

Learning to Talk about HPV "Like a Girl"

Jennifer A. Malkowski

When I was a teenager I tested positive for a high-risk strain of the human papillomavirus (HPV), a sexually transmitted disease known to cause cervical cancer. To care for the condition, I followed the doctor's orders and underwent some rigorous, painful treatments. At the time, I was not informed about the nature of HPV, nor how I might have been exposed to the virus in the first place. Most significantly, I left the doctor's office unclear about what an HPV-positive status meant for my future sexual health. WebMD and other e-health sites did not exist at the time. For the next two years, every three months I returned for an exam. Each report came back "clean." For the next decade, I remained uncertain about how to disclose my HPV status to sexual partners. What did a "clean" HPV-positive diagnosis mean for sexually responsible behavior?

Many years after my initial diagnosis, a public health awareness campaign was launched that urged me to "tell someone" about the link between HPV and cervical cancer, a link that I had not known about despite my HPV-positive status. The advertisements did not mention the sexual nature of transmission nor the male contribution to the problem. These omissions suggested some ground rules for discussion: I could talk about HPV in terms of cancer, but should I remain silent about its classification as a sexually acquired condition?

In June 2006, the approval of GARDASIL®, a vaccine that blocks infection by four strains of the HPV virus, became of interest to public health agencies, political institutions, and advocacy organizations that understood HPV to be the cause of 70% of all cases of cervical cancer and 90% of all cases of genital warts. The next wave of advertising, dubbed "One Less," promoted the vaccine as *the* method for ensuring that each vaccinated girl would become

(continued)

"one less" cancer victim. In this way, the new medical vaccination technology provided women with an opportunity to proactively intervene and protect themselves against a deadly condition, if they elected to get vaccinated. Moreover, the vaccination offered women a way to talk about HPV as a public health issue.

Once again, though, it appeared as if women were equipped and encouraged to talk about HPV only in terms of cancer prevention. Omission from public messaging of HPV's method of transmission and an overemphasis on cervical cancer as its health consequence (rather than focus on genital warts, a condition also caused by HPV that affects both women *and men*) implied an association between women, "responsible" behavior, and health "consequences." If individual women decided not to heed the advice of medical professionals to get vaccinated and share their HPV knowledge with others, then, at least in part, an HPV-positive status implied a connection between "irresponsible" behavior and "deserved consequences." As someone already carrying the virus, how was I to talk about HPV? More importantly, how could I ensure that I, too, would be "one less" cancer victim?

Since GARDASIL®'s introduction to market, understanding how women successfully communicate about HPV status has, thankfully, grown as an issue of concern among health scholars, professionals, and advocates alike. Indeed, many communication scholars, including myself, now study the ways public communication about health and medicine contributes to the adoption of individual health behaviors, the reputation of particular medical conditions, and the political and cultural responses to different types of disease prevention and treatment. Because my personal awareness about HPV was initiated by public health messaging about the condition, I have elected to focus on pharmaceutical advertisements as a mode of communication designed to inspire particular public responses to individual health conditions. Pharmaceutical giants, such as Merck, have raised much needed awareness about previously misunderstood or stigmatized health conditions, such as HPV. However, as communication critics, it is our job to think about the consequences of for-profit authorship of public health messages to ensure that the overall quality of individual lives—and especially those dealing with difficult health situations—are enhanced by public health communication.

Almost four years after its initial introduction to market, GARDASIL® launched the third installment of its national awareness campaign entitled "My Voice." Unlike the other waves of advertisements, this campaign claimed to represent the voices of people living with HPV. I decided to investigate the campaign materials from a rhetorical perspective to evaluate Merck's claims. Through close textual analysis, with attention to a history of women in medicine, I identified storytelling as a mode of persuasion used by Merck to gain the attention of female audiences more broadly and identified voice as the means by which Merck convinced female consumers to trust that GARDASIL® was the only way to resolve the HPV story. I concluded that Merck's use of contradiction and tension to tell that story appeared to encourage complacency, or inaction, among female health participants. As such, Merck's campaign may be functioning to keep women in a state of anxiety about HPV, a state that, perhaps intentionally, preserves problematic notions of both women and health. With this possibility in mind, how might we as communication scholars help to re-story health narratives in ways that empower women across health contexts and offset problematic patterns in public talk? Can we compete and/or partner with Big Pharma to improve everyday health experiences? As health communication specialists, I think we can and hope we do.

QUESTIONS TO PONDER

1. Based on your experiences, why do you think men and women experience health differently *even if the health condition is the same?*

2. Think about a pharmaceutical advertisement that you have recently seen either in print or on television. Describe what features of the ad make it persuasive. Is there anything that you find problematic about the advertisement? What and why?

3. In your opinion, whose responsibility is it to ensure that members of the general U.S. public know about contagious health conditions? Why this person, institution, or group in particular?

4. What makes talking about sexually transmitted infections and sexually transmitted diseases so difficult? Do you think public health advertisement campaigns help individuals to talk about these types of issues more easily? Why or why not?

Source: Malkowski, J. A. (2013). Confessions of a pharmaceutical company: Narrative, voice, and gendered dialectics in the case of Gardasil. *Health Communication, 29*, 81–92.

The Politics of Medicalization

How many absences are allowed in the course you are enrolled in right now? Does your instructor allow for "excused absences?" If you were too sick to work, would you be fired unless you had proof of illness? This is an important example of medicine as a site of social control: the unquestioned weight of a "sick note." Only a doctor has the power to decide whether one has a genuine reason for not participating in our social lives. Truancy, in school or at the workplace, must be reduced, and doctors have been vested the responsibility to make those judgments.

The Western medical establishment has come to dominate our thinking about health, illness, and our bodies. If asked to describe their bodies from the inside, chances are that most people would rely on anatomical descriptions. Think of the diagrams in school textbooks that reveal discrete, linear organs working in sequence like an assembly line. Are our bodies actually arranged like those diagrams? Or is it that our knowledge of our bodies has been completely formed by Western medical perspectives like anatomy? How did medicine develop this sort of legitimacy?

Michel Foucault (1975), a French philosopher, historian, and social theorist, investigated the development of professional control among the sciences, describing the confluence of knowledge and power. Professionals have gained the power to examine, classify, and create categories of health and illness, which is sometimes referred to as the "medical gaze." The medical gaze defines normality and abnormality, and extends through the growth in professional surveillance of the public and its health habits, bodily routines, social interactions, and mental status. Communicating expertise deepens the reach of their professional control. Western biomedical professionals often have a monopoly over diagnosis based on perceptions of objectivity and technical expertise. Medical sociologists like Deborah Lupton (2012) have argued that Western medicine has emerged as a site for the control and distribution of social ideologies, wherein it propagates ideas that justify the status quo and seeks to rectify dissonant ideas. For instance, until the early 1970s, the medical establishment's views on homosexuality mirrored the general social attitudes, and it was considered to be a form of mental illness. As a matter of fact, the Diagnostic and Statistical Manual (DSM), which categories the different kinds of mental illnesses, had an entry for homosexuality, which included a set of diagnostic criteria, prognoses, and treatment options.

Medicalization is a contested process by which social, health, or behavior issues come to be defined and treated as medical problems. Processes that were once thought of as natural such as childbirth, breastfeeding, and aging are now treated as medical events. Foucault argues that medicalization was a historical process that accompanied (and continues today) the development and professionalization of allopathic medicine in society. Broad-based changes in the economic, political and social organization of 19th-century European society were central to the development of professional medicine. In the backdrop of the industrial revolution and the great demand for industrial labor, social institutions began to differentiate between the sick and the poor (which up to this point were jointly regarded as "destitute"). Medicalization helped demarcate bodies that could be productively used as labor. Foucault notes that the process of medicalization, the regular surveillance of bodies and the maintenance of hygiene, was made possible by the development of the nuclear family, which subsequently emerged as the locus of responsibility for an individual's health.

Medicalization defines normality and deviance, for instance, in deciding whether a child is "rambunctious" or has attention deficit/hyperactivity disorder (ADHD). Gays and lesbians organized for many years to contest the American Psychiatric Association's classification of homosexuality as a mental illness, as mentioned above. Medicalization brings important benefits such as the legitimation of a diagnosis, reduction in personal blame, access to care, insurance benefits, social support, and other resources, as well as allowances from school, work, and social burdens (think about how medicalization has helped people with post-traumatic stress disorder (PTSD). On the other hand, medicalization may also increase stigmatization, and brings behavior into the purview of the medical care system. It may promote unneeded treatments that can lead to *iatrogenic disease* (illness caused by medical treatment). Furthermore, the process of medicalization may act politically to adapt individuals to currently dysfunctional social arrangements rather than changing those social circumstances. For example, giving children ADD medication allows them to fit into existing school structure rather than adapt those structures to the children (e.g., smaller class sizes, more time for exercise). Lynn Payer (1992) described attempts to make well people feel sick as *disease mongering*. Health professionals and marketers may invoke very broad definitions of illness to include more people in diagnoses, or inflate the risk of relatively minor disorders. Pharmaceutical marketing has worked with the American Psychiatric Association to develop new disorders in its Diagnostic and Statistical Manual and then marketed those disorders to promote drug sales such as Sarafem for "premenstrual dysphoric disorder" (Frances, 2013; Koerner, 2002). Medicalization is apparent through the constant creation of new medical conditions and categories, like "restless leg syndrome" and "chronic fatigue syndrome," among others, that make increasing sections of the population dependent on pharmaceutical drugs.

These issues show how deeply personal the politics of medicine can be. The discussion also points out how business concerns such as pharmaceutical marketing influence health. Next, we describe linkages between public health and the economy. But first, consider theories of policy making in Theorizing Practice 12.2.

Theorizing Practice 12.2
Theories of Policy Making

In democratic countries, citizens elect officials to represent their interests when creating public policies (the U.S. Congress, for example) and executing laws by appointing heads of government (the U.S. president, for example) and enforcing laws through federal and enforcement agencies and police. Among political scientists, sociologists, and communication researchers there are long-standing, competing theories about how our political system operates and whose interests it serves. Read and consider the following positions on how public policies occur:

- **Elite theories** (Mills, 1956; Schattschneider, 1960) argue that political elites (wealthy, well-connected people, often with big business interests) have the information, political skills, and influence to dominate policy processes. Because these groups can influence elected officials and other policy makers, they prefer to keep debates private, that is, off the public agenda, in order to maintain their control. This theory suggests that policy makers tend to make policies such as tax breaks that benefit the interests of powerful, wealthy, politically connected groups.

- **Pluralist theories** (Dahl, 1958) suggest that because different social and political interests can organize to represent their interests, and may work together in coalitions to gain strength, no single interest group dominates the process. Rather than a political process controlled by a few, this theory suggests that our political system represents a wide variety of public interests and concerns. (This theory would suggest that college students, for instance, could organize to pressure state governments to offer financial aid and reduce tuition.)

- **The Punctuated Equilibria Model** (Baumgartner & Jones, 1993; Conrad & McIntush, 2003) suggests that long periods of policy consensus (that is, times when policy does not change) are punctuated by sudden social change (for example, problems of lack of access to medical care mounted for years until anyone proposed significant changes in how we offer health insurance). The model argues that elite individuals and groups, often from large business interests, are tightly organized and have more money and prestige, which allows them to influence the political process better than fragmented non-elite groups such as students or consumers. However, non-elite publics can play a role in the political process. Nonelites are likely to participate at moments when they believe their interests are affected and they feel they have a voice. (For example, as we mentioned, public concern about water quality has led some communities to fight larger energy companies by passing local bans on fracking.)

- **From a communication perspective**, Conrad (2004) reminds us that in order for an issue to be addressed in the policy process, long-standing issues must be defined as problems important enough to require action, apparent solutions must be made available, and political pressure from the public must be adequate to overcome policy elites' desire for keeping debates behind closed doors. Groups must frame benefits and costs through their rhetorical skills. Conrad reminds us that politics is emotionally contentious rather than a rational process as different groups mobilize support for their positions (Conrad & McIntush, 2003). Which theory best describes the U.S. political system? Is our political system dominated by wealthy elites or is it open to public participation by everyday people? Whose interests are reflected in government policies?

HCIA 12.3

Gender Stereotypes, Media Portrayals, and the Prophylactic Mastectomy Narrative

Tasha Dubriwny

Narratives about health in the media offer us information not only about the health issue at hand but also about who we are, and who we can be, in relation to a given health issue. In one recent project, I analyzed how women's health issues are represented in popular media texts (news, films, and bestselling books), and I suggested that these representations coalesce into dominant narratives that construct a specific identity for women: the "vulnerable empowered woman." This identity positions women both as *vulnerable* to the female body's supposed frailty and as *empowered* to make choices about their medical care. However, it is important to think critically about the health information we receive in the media, especially in terms of how such information may be reproducing harmful gender stereotypes. For example, in the media narrative about prophylactic mastectomies, the representation of the vulnerable empowered woman as empowered to choose prophylactic surgery is concerning because the narrative positions all women as mothers and frames prophylactic mastectomies as a cosmetic procedure that can give women perfect breasts.

By "prophylactic mastectomies," I am referring to the procedure of removing healthy breasts as a way to reduce one's risk for eventually developing breast cancer. In the media coverage I explored, most women that elected the procedure had also received positive results from a genetic test for the breast cancer gene mutations BRCA1 and BRCA2. Women with these gene mutations have up to an 85% chance of developing breast cancer in their lifetime.

The narrative that develops in media coverage about prophylactic mastectomies emphasizes the high risk that women with the BRCA1 and BRCA2 gene mutations face, to the extent that the risk of cancer is often equated with actually having cancer. For example, in *Gossip Girl*, writer/producer Jessica Queller's memoir about her experience with prophylactic mastectomies, she describes finding herself literally in the position of a breast cancer patient; she is sitting in the waiting room in an oncology office, filling out forms with women who had lost their hair from chemotherapy treatments. The difference between testing positive for a gene mutation and having cancer disappears, and breast cancer is depicted not as a possibility but as her destiny. The media narrative also routinely emphasizes the horrors of breast cancer. Coverage of actress and mother of six Angelina Jolie's decision to remove both breasts after receiving a positive result from a genetic test, for example, included information on Jolie's mother Marcheline Bertrand whose eight-year battle with breast and ovarian cancer resulted in her death. Stories of the pain caused by cancer and its treatments combined with a sense of "cancer as destiny" propel the vulnerable empowered woman of the prophylactic mastectomy narrative to remove her breasts in an effort to remain cancer-free.

Such a choice is understandable given the fear and uncertainty of a breast cancer diagnosis, but I critique the narrative that develops in the media for positioning the choice as compulsory. What makes the choice compulsory is the connection between the vulnerable empowered woman's pursuit of a cancer-free life and her position as a mother (or, as often, a potential mother). Women, according to this narrative, must do all they can to rid themselves of the risk of cancer for the sake of their children. Moreover, the promise of a *future* family works as well to support the framing of the choice as compulsory; in Jessica Queller's case, her memoir ends with details about her plans to become pregnant. Reducing women to the position of mothers is problematic, as not all women are or will be mothers. Positioning women's health decisions as driven by motherhood reproduces stereotypes about what it means to be a woman in contemporary society (women are first and foremost seen as nurturers of *others*, with care for the self coming in a distant second place).

If the narrative about prophylactic mastectomies in the media is problematic because it reduces women to their status as mothers, it is also problematic because in the end the narrative reproduces cultural standards about what women's bodies should look like. For example, Queller's memoir details how her "new" breasts are better and more suited to her than her old breasts. Coverage of Jolie has unabashedly examined her bust line, using words such as "fuller" and "perkier" to describe her new appearance. Prophylactic mastectomies and the often grueling procedures of reconstructive surgery are thus aligned with the growing culture of body modification through cosmetic surgery. In this narrative, interest in women's long-term health is displaced by a focus on the vulnerable empowered woman maintaining an appropriately feminine appearance.

Health narratives can be thought of as tools for helping us work through life situations. However, as I have suggested here, some narratives are problematic because they reduce the complexity of health events and propel medical choices that depend on gender stereotypes.

QUESTIONS TO PONDER

1. Can you think of other examples of media narratives about health issues that rely on gender stereotypes about women and/or men?

2. How do you see health narratives as influencing your own health decisions? Can you think of an example of (for instance) a celebrity's story that has influenced your approach to health?

3. Thinking critically about health narratives means being aware that narratives often offer only one perspective on a given health issue. Outside of mainstream media sources, where can we find alternative health narratives that may not reinforce gender stereotypes?

Source: Dubriwny, T. N. (2013). *The vulnerable empowered woman: Feminism, postfeminism, and women's health.* New Brunswick, NJ: Rutgers University Press.

Health and the Economy

Although we may not always realize it, economic decisions are an important part of the politics of healthcare. Economic development is important to public health. Advances in nutrition and sanitation that resulted from improved standards of living played a larger role in improving the health of the public in Europe and the U.S. than developments in medicine (McKeown & Brown, 1976). Unfortunately, there are also long-standing conflicts between business interests and public health. Early conflicts included business resistance to quarantining ships to prevent the spread of contagious disease in the 1800s (Tesh, 1994). Today, some of the most significant influences on health are corporate policies. Corporations are responsible for resource depletion and environmental pollution, as well as occupational injury and disease in Western countries and are compounded in "sweatshop" conditions in the Global South. The production, sales, and marketing of harmful products such as tobacco, fast food, and dangerous chemicals puts corporate interests in conflict with public health (Freudenberg, 2014).

For example, concentration among food companies means that a handful of very large corporations determine what we eat. Popular author and journalist Michael Pollan, in the film *Food Inc.* (Kenner, 2008), argues that the grocery store gives only the appearance of variety. Because of massive government spending on corn subsidies for large agricultural businesses, we have made junk food appear to be very inexpensive. Companies can buy this corn for an artificially low price. As a result, it is difficult to find products without high fructose corn syrup. Hidden sweeteners in our food contribute to obesity, diabetes, and other costly health problems. Cattle eat inexpensive corn instead of grass, which makes the price of meat cheaper at the store but raises the risk of E. coli contamination and antibiotic resistance. Livestock raised in concentrated animal feeding operations produce millions of gallons of liquid manure that run off into neighboring wells and cause gastrointestinal illness, fatal respiratory illness in babies, and is associated with miscarriage and developmental defects (Pojda, 2010). Workers are exposed to pesticides and face high rates of occupational injury in agricultural work and in meatpacking plants. These practices increase profits for the companies, but they do so by "externalizing" the costs and risks, which means shifting them to the public—taxpayers, workers, consumers, and neighbors.

Corporate public relations and issue management are central to this system. Food companies lobby elected officials to maintain government subsidies (that is, government payments for commodities like corn) (Nestle, 2013). "Veggie libel laws" (food disparagement laws) passed in several states are a good example of this corporate influence. These laws allow food manufacturers to sue members of the public for making disparaging comments about their food. Oprah Winfrey was famously sued by a Texas beef company for suggesting that she would no longer eat hamburgers because of the Mad Cow Scare, resulting in lower beef sales. Although the company lost the suit, the high cost of her defense had a chilling effect on other advocates (Kenner, 2008). Food companies avoid stricter regulations and enforcement through the *revolving door,* in which corporate leaders move from their positions with food companies to head the agencies such as the USDA and FDA that are supposed to regulate those companies. This system can lead to *regulatory capture,* wherein the agencies that are supposed to police an industry actually come to advocate for the profitability of those companies instead.

It is also important to remember that by failing to educate ourselves about what is in our food, and allowing the price we see on the fast-food menus and store shelves to guide our choices, we *consent* to the hidden costs of tax subsidies to corporations, increased disease, obesity, animal cruelty, low wages, and environmental damage.

Despite the power and influence of the food industry, there are signs of public *resistance* as groups advocate for regulating and reforming the industry, and develop alternatives to factory farming. Movies such as *Food, Inc.* and *Fed Up* shine a light on the government policies and corporate practices hidden behind the packaging. Many communities are supporting local food by hosting farmers' markets, and allowing urban residents to raise chickens and goats. More people are learning to garden and grow their own food. The Slow Food movement (versus "fast food") is a global network that seeks justice in the food system by advocating for better food policies, as well as by encouraging changes in the way we eat. As Slow Food USA website (https://www.slowfoodusa.org/) describes, "A better, cleaner and fairer world begins with what we put on our plates—and our daily choices determine the future of the environment, economy and society." They add, "If you care about local farmers, ranchers, fishers; animal welfare; the joy of a shared meal; preserving food culture; protecting the environment or avoiding GMOs, we have a place for you at our table." The Equitable Food Initiative (EFI) is a partnership of nonprofits such as Oxfam, agricultural unions, large produce farming operations, and grocery chains such as Costco to create a certification system that guarantees the produce was harvested and packed by workers who have been trained to identify and address potential food safety threats, that workers and consumers are exposed to fewer pesticides, and that workers receive fair wages. The project demonstrates that workers, consumers, and food companies can all benefit from safer food practices that reduce food-borne illness and recalls, and reduce environmental impact.

Earlier in this chapter, we mentioned the Ebola Virus Disease (EVD) epidemic that was declared as a "health emergency of international concern" by the World Health Organization in August 2014. Concentrated in the three West African countries of Sierra Leone, Guinea, and Liberia, the disease has resulted in more than 11,300 deaths (Centers for Disease Control and Prevention, 2016). It is known that bats are carriers of the virus, and at some point, bats entered the food chain in one of the three countries, leading to the human spread of the virus.

While media reporting on the epidemic has focused on the dangers of eating bats and other "bush meat" (a term that technically only means meat that is not recognized as food in mainstream Western cultures), we encourage you to think about the economic aspects of Ebola. Until recently, why were these three countries, despite significant international efforts, unable to effectively prevent, manage, and treat the cases of Ebola? Another way to ask this question is to ask why these particular countries reached epidemic status while neighboring countries like Ivory Coast, Benin, and Mali did not. The lack of adequate public health infrastructure to deal with an epidemic may lie in the economic arrangements in the affected countries. It is common knowledge that underdeveloped countries in Africa receive aid and financial support from the United Nations (UN) and the World Bank (WB). Why, then, were these countries unable to effectively apply quarantine and prevention measures to isolate the virus, as was done in the United States, Spain, and other countries?

Resource-poor countries like those in West Africa have historically depended on loans and financial support from Western countries and international organizations like the World Bank, the World Trade Organization (WTO), the International Monetary Fund (IMF), as well as influential governmental organizations like the United States Agency for International Development (USAID). These organizations provided huge loans to impoverished nations, in the name of "developing" their economies. However, these loans come at a high cost, often accompanied by the condition that they be used to develop markets, private enterprise, and free trade at the cost of public infrastructure like hospitals, clinics, and schools. Recipient countries are required to reduce spending on public infrastructure in favor of repayment of interest on the loan, often with devastating consequences on health. These *neoliberal* economic policies promoting deregulation, austerity (minimal government spending on public goods), and privatization (the transfer of public functions to private industry) have had negative effects on public health in many countries, particularly impoverished nations.

Medical anthropologist and physician Paul Farmer described how neoliberal economic policies in Haiti exacerbated the economic deprivation of poor Haitians, making them more vulnerable to contracting HIV/AIDS (Farmer, 2006). The construction of large hydroelectric dams in central Haiti flooded several villages there and displaced hundreds of indigenous Haitians. In Haiti, as in many underdeveloped countries, basic infrastructure like continuous electricity is not guaranteed. Hydroelectric energy (tapped by damming major waterways) has commonly been used by international agencies in the developing world. As it turns out, the lucrative contracts for these dams were awarded to private Western construction companies who then instituted local offices and branches in Haiti, hiring engineers, laborers, and other local employees. Hydroelectric dams require large reservoirs of stored water, which, in Haiti, were created over existing agricultural villages.

Forced out of their lands, which were now inundated by the reservoir, many rural Haitians had to leave and go to urban centers to survive. But jobs were not easy to come by, and some Haitians had no recourse but to take to sex work in order to sustain themselves and their families, putting them at higher risk for HIV/AIDS. Here, an infrastructural project purportedly undertaken for the development of Haiti ended up ravaging the health of large sections of its population. Activists seek to put these development policy issues on the public health agenda and question whose voices are heard in the formation of these policies and whose definition of development is applied.

We now turn to the role of health politics closer to home: the much-debated history of medical care reform in the United States.

■ Politics and Communicating Medical Care Reform

Since Congress passed the Affordable Care Act (ACA) or "Obamacare" into law in 2011, it has become the focus of attention of all health policy-related discussions in the United States. Its proponents have endorsed it, given that the U.S. is the only developed country without universal health coverage, whereas opponents have consistently tried to repeal it. A political commercial paid for by a group called "Generation Opportunity" urges young college-age students to "opt out of Obamacare." The commercial opens with a typical scene: a young woman going in for a regular check-up at an obstetric/gynecologic (Ob/Gyn) clinic. The nurse notices that she has "signed up for Obamacare" and asks her to change into a gown and wait for the doctor. The doctor asks a few routine questions and then prepares the patient for a vaginal exam, saying, "Okay, let's take a look." However, instead of proceeding to examine the patient, the doctor leaves the room. The patient is confused by this turn of events, when suddenly, she sees an oversized, caricatured Uncle Sam emerge from under the stirrups. As the patient screams in shock, the commercial cuts to text that reads: "Don't let the government play doctor." The commercial ends with cutting back to Uncle Sam, complete with eerie grin and speculum in hand, followed by the message, "Opt out of Obamacare."

Critics of Obamacare have propagated the idea that medicine is a "private" transaction between doctor and patient, and this commercial suggests that the government is now literally interested in the citizen's private parts. This sort of childish (and rather patriarchal) depiction of the government's role in health has been the most prominent mode of public debate around health. How has the discussion drifted this far?

Americans often tout our reputation for having "the best healthcare in the world." The U.S. does provide innovative, life-saving interventions. However, high costs, uneven access, and medical mistakes contribute to the U.S. ranking poorly compared with the healthcare systems of other nations. The "healthcare trilemma" (Conrad & McIntush, 2003) involves managing trade-offs among cost, access, and quality. From a communication perspective, arguments about reform tend to emphasize different parts of that equation.

The U.S. Healthcare System

The Affordable Care Act (ACA) requires that individuals have health insurance coverage. Thus the U.S. medical care system is a mix of private (nongovernmental) and public (governmental) options. Private insurance may be self-financed but is often offered through the workplace. Congress offers employers tax breaks (public money) to offer health insurance to employees (Morone & Ehlke, 2013). Public financing includes Medicaid for a percentage of low-income people, Medicare for the elderly, and state-by-state Child Health Insurance Programs. The U.S. also has a patchwork of public hospitals and clinics that provide some treatment for low-income and uninsured individuals.

Data generally show that although the U.S. has the highest per capita spending on healthcare, it has poor health outcomes compared with other economically developed countries. In 2014, we spent roughly 17% of our Gross Domestic Product (GDP), or about $8,895 per person on healthcare, and our life expectancy was 78.7 years. Hong Kong, by contrast, spent 5.3% of its GDP ($1,944 per person), and its life expectancy was 83.5 years. Japan spent 10.2% of its GDP or $4,752 and had an 83-year life expectancy and universal health coverage (Bloomberg Best [and Worst], n.d.a).

In 2010, prior to the ACA, 48.2 million adult Americans were uninsured, or roughly 18% of the adult population (Ward, Clarke, Freeman, & Schiller, 2015). Lack of insurance was most common among young adults. Over the last two decades, employers have been reducing benefits and employing part-time and temporary workers who do not qualify for employer-based insurance (Kaiser Commission on Medicaid and the Uninsured, 2010 in Weitz, 2013). Prior to the ACA, insurance companies could deny coverage to people with preexisting illnesses or other conditions. Estimates suggest that roughly 25 million Americans were underinsured, not having enough coverage to pay for their medical expenses (Weitz, 2013).

A lack of health insurance leads to a lack of preventive care, which creates increased costs for more advanced problems in emergency care. Approximately 18,000 deaths each year can be attributed to insufficient or no care due to lack of insurance (Morone, Litman, & Robins, 2008). Lacking insurance also leads to loss of work days and jobs, bankruptcy, and homelessness. In 2005, researchers found that at least 46% of bankruptcy filings were triggered by healthcare bills (about 2 million medical bankruptcies each year) (Himmelstein, Warren, Thorne, & Woolhandler, 2005). Of those who filed for bankruptcy, 56% were classified as middle class. In a process called *rescission,* many people diagnosed with illness found their insurance company cancelled their coverage or refused to pay for treatment based on minor discrepancies in paperwork or because prior illnesses were determined to be a "preexisting condition." For example:

The day before she was scheduled to undergo a double mastectomy for invasive breast cancer, Robin Beaton's health insurance company informed her that she was "red flagged," and they wouldn't pay for her surgery. The hospital wanted a $30,000 deposit before they would move forward. Beaton had no choice but to forgo the life-saving surgery. She had never missed a payment, but that didn't matter. Blue Cross cited two earlier, unrelated conditions that she hadn't reported to them when signing up—acne and a fast beating heart—and rescinded her policy. (Potter, 2009a)

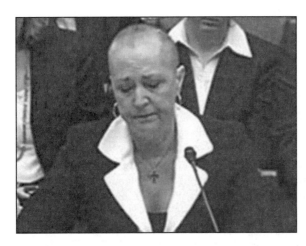

Ms. Robin Beaton at a press conference after her surgery and insurance cancellations. (Image source: https://flic.kr/p/6Mttf3)

In addition to access and cost, quality is another important piece of the healthcare trilemma. The Institute of Medicine estimated that 44,000 to 98,000 people die annually from medical errors (cited on "How Common Are," 2016), although others put the number much higher at 225,000 deaths per year (Starfield, 2000). Hospital infection rates may be as high as 2 million cases per year. Prescription drugs save lives, but they can also be dangerous. Between 1969 and 2002, 75 drugs were removed from market for safety reasons (Egilman & Ardolino, 2010). Research techniques frequently underreport side effects and overreport potential benefits (Egilman & Ardolino). These numbers remind us that *more* care is not always *better* care. As we will discuss, these statistics are important when we consider how different healthcare reform proposals address the "trilemma" of cost, access, and quality healthcare. Next, we discuss some of these healthcare reform debates.

History of U.S. Reform Attempts

There have been many attempts to reform U.S. healthcare. Each attempt shows us how different interest groups have framed the debates and negotiated the policy process.

- In 1912, presidential candidate Theodore Roosevelt proposed national health insurance.
- In 1942, President Franklin Roosevelt supported national health insurance through Social Security (to ward off calls for socialism) (Weitz, 2013). Fearing

that health insurance would jeopardize social security, he did not strongly endorse the proposal (Marmor, 2000).

- In 1943, the Murray-Wagner-Dingell bill proposed a comprehensive insurance system. Congress refused to hold hearings on the bill. President Truman shifted his attention to coverage for the aged population (Medicare).

The American Medical Association played a major role in defeating these proposals, due to concerns that national programs would reduce incomes or autonomy for its physician members (Weitz, 2013). Some labor unions such as the American Federation of Labor also opposed national health insurance because offering insurance was a major benefit of joining a union. Conservatives equated national insurance with socialism (and later communism), and the growth in access to Blue Cross and Blue Shield insurance in the 1930s meant middle-class people who were covered were not motivated to create a national plan.

- In 1964, President Lyndon Johnson campaigned on health issues. Medicare (elderly) and Medicaid (percentage of the poor) legislation passed in 1965, accompanied by massive Democratic victories in Congress, despite the efforts of hospital and physician groups.

- In 1993, President Bill Clinton proposed the Health Care Security Act. The proposal maintained private insurance and private medical care but created purchasing options for lower-cost insurance. The insurance and pharmaceutical industries along with many large employers lobbied hard against the program, fearing it would affect their profits. The groups outspent supporters four to one (Weitz, 2013) and used growing fears of "big government" to defeat the plan.

You can see from this discussion that a number of different groups play a role in healthcare reform debates. Figure 12.1 lists some of these groups. As we describe the policy process, consider the stake that these groups have in different proposals.

The following organizations represent groups with a significant stake in healthcare reform policies and often seek to influence debates about the issue:

- The American Medical Association represents physicians.

- The American Hospital Association, Federation of American Hospitals, and other groups represent hospital interests.

- The Pharmaceutical Research and Manufacturers of America (PhRMA) is the lobbying arm for the pharmaceutical industry.

- American Health Insurance Providers (AHIP) is a lobbying and advocacy group for the health insurance industry.

- Big business has a number of associations that participate in healthcare debates, such as the Chamber of Commerce, Business Roundtable, and the American Legislative Exchange Council.

- Patients and healthcare consumers are represented through smaller, often fragmented organizations, such as American Association for Retired Persons, Families USA, Public Citizen, and other advocacy groups.

Figure 12.1   Interest Groups

Communication and the U.S. Policy Process

Morone and Ehlke (2013) describe four stages of the governmental policy process: (1) agenda setting, (2) policy formation, (3) policy adoption, and (4) policy implementation. Strategic and everyday discourses interact at each stage to influence the possibilities for medical care reform.

Agenda setting involves gaining enough attention for an issue to create policy debates. Agenda setting determines which issues are debated and brought into the realm of policy making and which go unaddressed. For example, medical care reform often receives more attention than public health spending unless the public is concerned about the spread of a high-profile contagious disease.

From a communication perspective, agenda setting is not only about which issues get discussed, but also *how* they are talked about. *Framing*, or providing interpretive "structures that render events and occurrences subjectively meaningful, and thereby function to organize experience and guide action" (Snow & Lessor, 2010, p. 285), is powerful because it influences how discourses are understood. For example, opponents of universal healthcare coverage often framed the U.S. system as "the best medical care system in the world," which obscured problems in an effort to persuade the public that no reform was needed. Opponents also framed healthcare reform as expensive, something that we cannot afford given our rising deficit. Prior to the passage of Obamacare, *proponents* of healthcare reform framed the need for healthcare reform by comparing the amount of money the U.S. was spending on the Iraq war ($12 billion per month in 2008 according to the *Huffington Post*; see Hanley, 2008) versus what it would spend insuring all Americans. They also framed healthcare reform as "deficit-reducing" because it would control healthcare costs and increase preventive care.

Problem definition is a key means of influencing the policy agenda. Often, problems are defined and communicated in ways that fit the solutions interest groups already want to promote (Conrad & McIntush, 2003). For example, you've probably heard of Health Maintenance Organizations (HMOs). Advocates first promoted the use of "gatekeeper" physicians in HMOs to solve the problem of overseeing medical quality, and then as public priorities shifted to concerns about healthcare costs, they promoted HMOs to solve the problem of medical cost overruns. Other examples:

- Insurance companies discuss the problem of high costs from medical providers, but rarely address the problem of access to health insurance.

- Physicians groups tend to promote the problem of access to care rather than cost. When physicians do address the problem of medical costs, they blame them on the rising price of malpractice insurance. The American Medical Association's (AMA) solution proposes limiting consumers' ability to sue caregivers (tort reform).

- Groups who advocate for universal healthcare coverage often define wasteful duplication and bureaucracy of our mixed public and private system as the problem, and propose government negotiation of healthcare costs (sometimes called a Single Payer system) in order to reduce overhead costs and create universal access to care.

Groups often use *narratives* to influence the policy agenda. Proponents of reform share stories about people without healthcare, or who have been denied coverage or services. During the debates over the ACA, commercials by those opposed to reform highlighted problems in the Canadian medical system. Stories are powerful because they give us a personal and emotional connection to the issue (Sharf, Harter, Yamasaki, & Haidet, 2011).

Policy formation is the process through which solutions are defined and policies written and introduced into the legislative process. Although elected officials introduce legislation in Congress and in state legislatures, policies are formed through a process of negotiation among political parties and interest groups.

When different plans are introduced, proponents and opponents seek to frame the legislation for the public. Groups who successfully frame policies in ways that resonate with dominant social values have an advantage in policy debates. For example, the ACA requires that everyone be covered by health insurance or pay a fine. (The plan requires that businesses with more than 50 employees offer insurance, creates health exchanges to buy private insurance at more affordable prices, and expands access to Medicaid for low-income citizens.) The *mandate* requiring insurance coverage was (and remains) a hot political topic during debates. Republicans and other opponents framed the mandate as government intrusion into the public's lives. Interestingly, when Republicans proposed an individual healthcare mandate in 1993, it was framed in terms of the need to require individuals to take personal responsibility to get coverage (Roy, 2012).

Naming and word choice are central to policy formation debates. Proponents of comprehensive medical care reform such as Physicians for a National Health Plan describe their Canadian-style proposal, in which the government sets prices as the single purchaser of healthcare, as "single payer" whereas critics use the label "socialized medicine." (A single-payer system does have a significant government role, but it is not socialized medicine. Although healthcare payments come from the government, healthcare is delivered through the private sector.) Indeed, the term "socialized medicine" is now used for almost any attempt to reform healthcare.

These buzzwords are an example of what Richard Weaver called *ultimate terms,* which include *god terms*—those terms that merit the highest cultural respect and often go unquestioned—and *devil terms*—those terms that merit cultural revulsion. "Choice" is a god term often used to ensure that any plan must promote consumer choice of physicians. Other god terms may include "efficiency" and "free market." The name of President Obama's plan—"The Patient Protection and Affordable Care Act"—includes god terms like "protection" and "affordable." It is difficult to argue against affordability, for example.

Devil terms like "socialism" and "communism" have long plagued attempts to provide national health insurance in the U.S. "Government-run" healthcare was often used as a devil term in debates about the Affordable Care Act. Wendell Potter, the former vice president of communication at Cigna Insurance, shared a memo with journalist Bill Moyer:

> I have a memo written by Frank Luntz who we discovered, in the spring, has written the script for opponents of healthcare reform. "First," he says, "you have to pretend to support it. Then use phrases like, 'government takeover,' 'delayed care is denied care,' 'consequences of rationing,' 'bureaucrats, not doctors prescribing medicine.'" (Potter, 2009a)

These terms are designed to short-circuit thoughtful debate and create negative impressions for the public. For example, the devil term "rationing" sounds like a threat to our access to care. This is a fallacy, however, because all care is rationed in some way (in the U.S., we ration care by ability to pay).

Although it was played for laughs, late night television host Jimmy Kimmel highlighted the importance of terminology when he interviewed people on the street, many of whom said they supported the Affordable Care Act but not Obamacare. Some people knew they were the same thing, but many people shown had a preference for one or the other.

Policy adoption entails Congressional lawmaking. Public debate may influence this process, as does interest group lobbying and other strategies. *Corporate lobbying, political donations,* and *advertising* play a significant role in which legislation is passed, particularly in the wake of the Citizens United vs. the Federal Election Commission decision that allows for unlimited corporate donations to political candidates. CNN estimated that groups spent $600 million on lobbying, campaign contributions, and television ads in 2008, with $400 million of that coming from the healthcare industry (Liberto, 2009). In addition, AHIP, the health insurance lobby, gave the U.S. Chamber of Commerce more than $86 million in 2009 to oppose the legislation on their behalf without disclosing the source (Armstrong, 2010). Among Democrats, those individuals that opposed the public option in the Patient Protection and Affordable Care Act received the largest political donations from insurance companies (Renick Mayer, 2009).

Many well-funded industry groups know that the public will mistrust information they provide because it appears biased. So instead, they promote their viewpoints using *front groups*: apparently neutral research or advocacy groups that actually serve some other interest, whose sponsorship is hidden.

- Wendell Potter (former vice president of communications for Cigna Insurance) described the Healthcare Leadership Council as a front group for the insurance industry that sought to defeat reform (Potter, 2009b). The group lobbied members of Congress, providing talking points to elected officials and conservative talk show hosts and editorial page editors.
- The Center for Medicine in the Public Interest also sought to prevent healthcare reform. Although it sounds like a consumer group, it is a project of the Pacific Research Institution, itself a front group that Philip Morris used to create academic support for the tobacco industry (Fang, 2009).
- The National Federation of Independent Business (NFIB) appears to represent small business. However, it lobbies for issues that serve the interests of larger corporations, and it receives millions in contributions from large corporate interests without revealing these sources (Center for Media and Democracy, n.d.b).

Astroturf is paid corporate PR that appears to be grassroots organizing. In other words, groups are funded and formed by corporate interests but appear to be everyday citizens who care enough to express their views through protest. For example, many advertisements during the most recent healthcare debate were aired in the name of groups like "Patients United Now," which sounds like a patient advocacy group but was actually funded by Americans for Prosperity, an organization led by the heads of Koch Industries. In fact, the initial protests against the ACA were organized and paid for by Americans for Prosperity. But they appeared to be just angry citizens who chose to protest at representatives' town hall meetings (Center for Media and Democracy, n.d.c).

Protestors against the ACA sometimes held signs reading "Hands Off My Healthcare." These signs framed healthcare reform as unnecessary government intervention. Notice what this draws our attention to, and what it draws our attention away from. For example, "our healthcare" assumes that viewers have health insurance coverage and would continue to do so, despite rising costs. It also draws our attention away from the control of our healthcare by health insurance companies and medical providers.

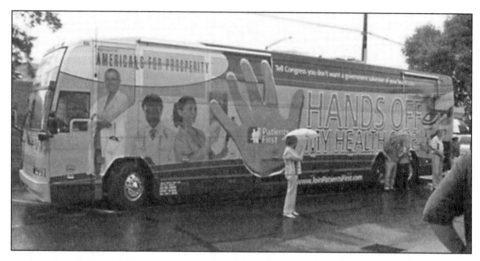

A "Hands Off My Healthcare" rally.

The *implementation* step often receives less attention, but it is a key phase where governmental departments write and enforce rules. For example, in the United States, the AMA fought against the creation of Medicaid in 1965 by labeling it socialized medicine. During implementation, however, the AMA negotiated highly lucrative "standard fees" for physicians (http://kff.org/health-reform/issue-brief/national-health-insurance-a-brief-history-of/), meaning that healthcare providers themselves set the prices with little oversight, and were paid by public dollars. The Hill Burton Hospital Survey and Construction Act in 1946 provided $12 billion to fund hospital construction. Although liberals in Congress included a requirement that these hospitals treat people who could not afford to pay, this requirement was never enforced (Morone & Ehlke, 2013).

The New York Times reported that after the passage of the Affordable Care Act in 2010, health insurance companies shifted from trying to defeat the legislation to lobbying federal and state officials over how it would be implemented. In particular, they wanted to avoid regulation of premium costs and profits (Pear, 2010). The rules that federal agencies write to enforce the law are central to its impact. More than 40 provisions require rules of enforcement; for example, one provision bars insurance companies from unreasonable premium increases without justifications to regulators, but does not define unreasonable.

This is the stage where laws are put into practice. Implementation for the ACA has been uneven. The rollout of healthcare.gov, the website used to enroll in a health insurance exchange, was stymied by major technical problems so that the deadline for enrolling had to be pushed back. However, the required number of people did eventually enroll. At the time of this writing, 17 states have refused federal money to expand access to Medicaid, barring affordable healthcare coverage for thousands of qualified citizens ("Where States Stand," 2016). In 2014, Freedomworks and Americans for Prosperity ran ads persuading the public not to get covered by highlighting citizens who claimed to have increased costs or lost coverage under the ACA (fact-checkers showed that most people telling their stories actually saved money under the ACA). Generational Opportunity, also funded by the Koch brothers, launched a campaign to discourage college students from gaining insurance through the exchanges. In addition to the Uncle Sam ad described earlier, they rolled out parties on campus with games, pizza, and free giveaways, where organizers asked college students to sign a pledge that they would not enroll in insurance through "Obamacare" (Moody, 2013).

Debate during ACA passage has led to a great deal of confusion about the law. In 2015, a significant number of people opposed Obamacare and were unaware that they were enrolled in the program through their state exchange, and were happy with their insurance. State governors who created the exchanges through which insurance is purchased have sought to hide the connection and take credit for the insurance program. These debates are so heavily influenced by interest groups that they often distract us from some very basic questions: How should we distribute healthcare? Should healthcare be distributed by the ability to pay? Is it a public right? Is it a public good that we should promote? See how well you know the ACA in Theorizing Practice 12.3.

Theorizing Practice 12.3
How Well Do YOU Know the Affordable Care Act (ACA)?

Take the following quiz, using items adapted from the Henry J. Kaiser Family Foundation (http://kff.org/quiz/health-reform-quiz/):

1. Does the health reform law require nearly all Americans to have health insurance or else pay a fine?

2. Does the health reform law establish a government panel to make decisions about end-of-life care for people on Medicare?

3. Does the health reform law give states the option of expanding their existing Medicaid program to cover more low-income, uninsured adults?

4. Does the health reform law allow undocumented immigrants to receive financial help from the government to buy health insurance?

5. Does the health reform law increase the Medicare payroll tax on earnings for upper income Americans?

6. Does the health reform law require employers with 50 or more employees to pay a fine if they don't offer health insurance?

7. Does the health reform law provide financial help to low- and moderate-income Americans who don't get insurance through their jobs to help them purchase coverage?

8. Has the health reform law created a government-run insurance plan to be offered along with private plans?

9. Does the health reform law create health insurance exchanges or marketplaces where small businesses and people who don't get coverage through their employers can shop for insurance and compare prices and benefits?

Answers: 1. Yes, 2. No, 3. Yes, 4. No, 5. Yes, 6. Yes, 7. Yes, 8. No, 9. Yes
The Kaiser Family Foundation also has a helpful video that explains the law: http://kff.org/health-reform/video/youtoons-obamacare-video/

■ Conclusion

The political complexities of public health and medical encounters also include many other issues, including the rise of the AMA and the regulation of competition among caregivers, patients' rights issues such as right-to-die controversies, and debates about technology and wrongful birth. Medical research has been marked by a history of racism, sexism, and nationalism, and there are ongoing concerns that these biases may influence debates about how to manage genetic testing and interventions. As this chapter has demonstrated, in everyday interactions, institutional settings, and policy making, communication constitutes public perceptions of health, illness, and ideal social relations in ways that profoundly influence how we organize and address health issues. The politics of health play out through the communicative construction of knowledge regarding how to achieve health and manage illness, access decision making, and have a voice in the policy process.

Discussion Questions

1. Are you concerned about environmental sources of illness? If so, how does that affect your behavior? If you found that an organization was polluting your neighborhood with potential carcinogens, what would you do? Do you believe the government does too much, too little, or about the right amount to regulate polluters? Should companies adopt more environmentally sustainable practices voluntarily?

2. Consider a diagnosis such as attention deficit disorder. Do you think we are diagnosing too many children with this label? Or, do children benefit from the diagnosis? Should we address problems by making changes, such as reducing class sizes allowing more time for physical activity at school, or by using medication?

3. Should soda companies and others who sell highly sugary foods have responsibility to pay for medical care costs due to obesity, diabetes, and other resulting health problems?

4. We discussed the political-economic basis of the Ebola epidemic. Can you describe the political economic context of another major global epidemic, like HIV/AIDS?

5. Is some level of healthcare a basic right of all humans? Is providing healthcare to all citizens a sign of a strong nation or an intrusive government? Or, do you believe that healthcare should be distributed by the ability to pay? Do you think that insurance companies, hospitals, and other healthcare providers should operate as for-profit or not-for-profit institutions?

6. Do you find it difficult to talk with people who have different positions from yours regarding healthcare? How have your own experiences with healthcare (for example, whether you have always had insurance coverage, whether your family experienced any major illnesses or injuries, whether your family is middle-class or working two jobs to get by?) influenced your position on healthcare reform? Consider talking with someone who has had very different healthcare experiences. How have those experiences shaped his/her political positions?

REFERENCES

Armstrong, D. (2010, November 17). Health insurers gave $86 million to fight health law. *BloombergBusiness*. Retrieved from http://www.bloomberg.com/news/articles/2010-11-17/insurers-gave-u-s-chamber-86-million-used-to-oppose-obama-s-health-law

Baumgartner, F., & Jones, B. D. (1993). *Agendas and instability in American politics*. Chicago, IL: University of Chicago Press.

Bloomberg Best (and Worst). (n.d.a) Most efficient health care 2014: Countries. Retrieved from http://www.bloomberg.com/visual-data/best-and-worst/most-efficient-health-care-2014-countries

Center for Media and Democracy. (n.d.b). National Federation for Independent Business. Retrieved from http://sourcewatch.org/index.php?title=National_Federation_of_Independent_Business

Center for Media and Democracy. (n.d.c) Americans for prosperity. Retrieved from http://www.sourcewatch.org/index.php?title=Americans_for_Prosperity

Centers for Disease Control and Prevention. (2016, February 14). 2014 Ebola outbreak in West Africa—case counts. Retrieved from http://www.cdc.gov/vhf/ebola/outbreaks/2014-west-africa/case-counts.html

Conrad, C. (2004). The illusion of reform: Corporate discourse and agenda denial in the 2002 "corporate meltdown." *Rhetoric & Public Affairs, 7*, 311–338.

Conrad, C., & McIntush, H. G. (2003). Organizational rhetoric and healthcare policymaking. In T. L. Thompson, A. M. Dorsey, K. I. Miller, & R. Parrott (Eds.), *Handbook of health communication* (pp. 403–422). Mahwah, NJ: Erlbaum.

Dahl, R. (1958). A critique of the ruling elite model. *American Political Science Review, 52*, 463–469.

Egilman, D., & Ardolino, E. (2010). The pharmaceutical industry, disease industry: A prescription for illness and death. In W. H. Wiist (Ed.), *The bottom line or public health* (pp. 193–224). New York, NY: Oxford University Press.

Fang, L. (2009, November 18). Exclusive: Attacks on health reform orchestrated by yet another shadowy corporate front groun—"CMPI." *THINKPROGRESS*. Retrieved from http://thinkprogress.org/economy/2009/11/18/69874/cmpi-front-group/

Farmer, P. (2006). *AIDS and accusation: Haiti and the geography of blame*. Berkeley: University of California Press.

Foucault, M. (1975). *The birth of the clinic: An archaeology of medical perception* (A. Sheridan, Trans.). New York, NY: Vintage.

Frances, A. (2013). *Saving normal: An insider's revolt against out-of-control psychiatric diagnosis, DSM-5, Big Pharma, and the medicalization of ordinary life*. New York, NY: HarperCollins.

Freudenberg, N. (2014). *Lethal but legal: Corporations, consumption and protecting public health.* New York, NY: Oxford University Press.

Hanley, C. J. (2008, March 28). Studies: Iraq costs US $12B per month. *Huff Post Politics.* Retrieved from http://www.huffingtonpost.com/2008/03/10/studies-iraq-costs-us-12b_n_90694.html

Himmelstein, D. U., Warren, E., Thorne, D., & Woolhandler, S. (2005). Illness and injury as contributors to bankruptcy. *Health Affairs, (Web Exclusive),* W5-63–W5-73.

How common are medical mistakes? (2016, March 1). *CureResearch.com.* Retrieved from http://www.cureresearch.com/mistakes/common.htm

Kenner, R. (Writer). (2008). *Food, Inc.* [Los Angeles, CA]: Magnolia Home Entertainment.

Kirkwood, W. G., & Brown, D. (1995). Public communication about the causes of disease: The rhetoric of responsibility. *Journal of Communication, 45,* 55–76.

Koerner, B. (2002, July/August). Disorders made to order. *Mother Jones,* 222–227.

Levins, R., & Lopez, C. (1999). Toward an ecosocial view of health. *International Journal of Health Services, 29,* 261–293.

Liberto, J. (2009). $600 million spent to influence health care debate. *CNN.* Retrieved from http://money.cnn.com/2009/11/18/news/economy/health_care_lobbying/

Lupton, D. (2012). *Medicine as culture: Illness, disease and the body in Western societies* (3rd ed.). Thousand Oaks, CA: Sage.

Marmor, T. R. (2000). *The politics of Medicare* (2nd ed.). Hawthorne, NY: Aldine de Gruyter.

McKeown, T., & Brown, R. G. (1976). *The modern rise of population.* New York, NY: Academic Press.

Mills, C. W. (1956). *The power elite.* New York, NY: Oxford University Press.

Moody, C. (2013, September 19). Creepy Obamacare ad hits college campuses and your nightmares. *Yahoo! News.* Retrieved from http://news.yahoo.com/obamacare-battle-moves-to-college-campuses-200027191.html

Morone, J. A., & Ehlke, D. (2013). *Health politics and policy* (5th ed.). Stamford, CT: Cengage Learning.

Morone, J. A., Litman, T. J., & Robins, L. S. (2008). *Health politics and policy* (4th ed.). Clifton Park, NY: Delmar.

Nestle, M. (2013). *Food politics: How the food industry influences nutrition and health* (rev. ed.). Los Angeles: University of California Press.

Payer, L. (1992). *Disease mongers: How doctors, drug companies, and insurers are making you feel sick.* Hoboken, NJ: John Wiley.

Pear, R. (2010). Health insurance companies try to shape rules. *The New York Times.* Retrieved from http://www.nytimes.com/2010/05/16/health/policy/16health.html

Pojda, J. A. (2010). Food and agriculture industry. In W. H. Wiist (Ed.), *The bottom line or public health* (pp. 281–298). New York, NY: Oxford University Press.

Potter, W. (2009a, July 10). Wendell Potter on profits before patients. *Bill Moyers Journal.* Retrieved from http://www.pbs.org/moyers/journal/07102009/profile.html

Potter, W. (2009b, September 15). Wendell Potter: How corporate PR works to kill health care reform. *PR Watch.* Retrieved from http://www.prwatch.org/news/2009/09/8552/wendell-potter-how-corporate-pr-works-kill-health-care-reform.

Renick Mayer, L. (2009). Key Senate Democrats opposing public option get more cash from insurers and pharmaceutical companies. *OpenSecrets.org.* Retrieved from http://www.opensecrets.org/news/2009/09/committee-members-opposed-to-p/

Rimal, R. N., Ratzan, S., Arntson, P., & Freimuth, V. S. (1997). Reconceptualizing the "patient:" Health care promotion as increasing citizens' decision-making competencies. *Health Communication, 9,* 61–74.

Roy, A. (2012, February 7). The tortuous history of conservatives and the individual mandate. *Forbes.* Retrieved from http://www.forbes.com/sites/theapothecary/2012/02/07/the-tortuous-conservative-history-of-the-individual-mandate/#12bc6435597a

Sastry, S. (2016). Long-distance truck drivers and the structural context of health: A culture-centered investigation of Indian truckers' health narratives. *Health Communication, 31,* 230–241.

Schattschneider, E. E. (1960). *The semi-sovereign people: A realist's view of democracy in America.* New York, NY: Holt.

Sharf, B., Harter, L., Yamasaki, J., & Haidet, P. (2011). Narrative turns epic: Continuing developments in health narrative scholarship. In T. L. Thompson, R. Parrott, & J. F. Nussbaum (Eds.), *The Routledge handbook of health communication* (2nd ed., pp. 36–51). New York, NY: Routledge.

Snow, D. A., & Lessor, R. G. (2010) The cases of obesity, work-related illnesses, and human egg donation. In J. C. Banaszak-Holl, S. R. Levitsky, & M.N. Zeld (Eds.), *Social movements and the transformation of American health care* (pp. 284–299). New York, NY: Oxford University Press.

Starfield, B. (2000). Is US health really the best in the world? *Journal of the American Medical Association, 284,* 483–484.

Tesh, S. (1994). *Hidden arguments: Politics, ideology and disease prevention policy.* New Brunswick, NJ: Rutgers University Press.

Ward, B. W., Clarke, T. C., Freeman, G., & Schiller, J. S. (2015, June). Early release of selected estimates based on data from the 2014 National Health Interview Survey. Retrieved from http://www.cdc.gov/nchs/nhis.htm

Weitz, R. (2013). *The sociology of health, illness & health care.* Boston, MA: Wadsworth.

Wendelsdorf, K. (2013). Gut microbes and diet interact to affect obesity. *National Institutes of Health, IH Research Matters.* Retrieved from http://www.nih.gov/researchmatters/september2013/09162013obesity.htm

Where states stand on Medicaid expansion. (2016, January 13). *The Advisory Board Company.* Retrieved from https://www.advisory.com/daily-briefing/resources/primers/medicaidmap

Zoller, H. M. (2012). Communicating health: Political risk narratives in an environmental health campaign. *Journal of Applied Communication Research, 40,* 20–43.

13

Communicating the Culture-Centered Approach to Health Disparities

Mohan J. Dutta & Satveer Kaur

Maria[1] came to work in Singapore when she was 26, hoping to make enough money to send back to her children in the Philippines for school. Maria's husband worked on the family farm, but the produce did not yield enough money for education or emergency expenses. And when her father-in-law became ill, the family sold the land to pay for the medical bills. Taking a job in Singapore as a domestic worker seemed to be a viable way for Maria to support her family back home.

■ Globalization, Neoliberalism, and Health Disparities

Stories like Maria's depict the flows of capital and labor across international spaces. Maria's struggles with not having enough money to take care of the education and health of her family in the Philippines pushed her to look for domestic work in Singapore. Her story suggests how health vulnerabilities (for example, not having enough money to afford healthcare in the Philippines) traverse across nations, from extreme areas of poverty and the effects of natural disasters in the Philippines to commercial affluence in Singapore. Singapore, a global financial hub that is consistently ranked as the "easiest place to do business" (http://www.doingbusiness.org/data/exploreeconomies/singapore) and as the "city with the second best investment potential" (http://www.usnews.com/news/best-countries/invest-in-full-list), serves as a destination of economic migration from poorer nations in the region. Existing research suggests that globalization—the flow of jobs, capital investments, products, services, and labor across countries—results in worldwide inequalities of access to a variety of resources including income, education, food, and health (Dutta, 2008, 2015). These global inequalities of access to employment and resources, in turn, result in inequalities in morbidity and mortality (Dutta & Kreps, 2013; Harvey, 2005).

At the crux of globalization are neoliberal reforms; that is, there are political and economic reforms across countries based on the principle of the free market. The narrative of the free market says that an open global exchange of products and services across national boundaries is designed to take care of people and their health needs by creating conditions for the economy to grow and by generating profits that will trickle down to the poor. Free market reforms call for minimized government policies of regulation so the market can operate freely, as well as minimized welfare policies and state-supported programs.

There are great discrepancies when the larger narrative of free markets that will improve the health conditions of everyone is compared with the reality of the lived experiences of the poor (Dutta, 2011, 2015). The worldwide hegemony or domination of neoliberalism is founded on stories celebrating individual freedom, liberty, capitalist democracy, and consumption as the tools of progress, positioning the free market as the solution to human health and well-being (Dutta, 2011; Dutta & Kreps, 2013). However, neoliberal policies have contributed to large-scale global inequalities by leading to rising unemployment rates, international movement of jobs from one country to another, weakening of worker unions, displacement of the poor from rural sources of livelihood, corporatization of agriculture, and privatization of public health resources. The economic impoverishment of large segments of global populations is linked to the heavier burdens of health risks and illnesses borne by these segments as compared to the health of the well-off (Dutta, 2015). People with low incomes, many of whom are then forced to become migrants in order to find work, live in substandard conditions with inadequate nutrition, a lack of jobs that pay a living wage, and an increased exposure to toxicities and infections. Such conditions result in much higher incidence of physical diseases and psychological problems, without access to proper healthcare. These are the dynamics of what we are calling *health disparities* since the risk of many health problems is much higher for people living in these conditions compared to the rest of the surrounding population.

In this chapter, we discuss the culture-centered approach as a framework for evaluating how free market health narratives contribute to global health inequalities, such as those experienced by Maria and other foreign domestic workers. We also examine the ways in which local stories expose and challenge these global health inequalities. To do so, we describe the Respect Our Rights campaign created in partnership with our university-based research team, the nongovernmental organization Humanitarian Organization for Migrant Economics (HOME) that serves foreign domestic workers in Singapore, and an advisory board of foreign domestic workers. This campaign creates an opportunity for disenfranchised communities to share personal stories and create messaging strategies targeting policy makers and employers in the mainstream.

■ The Culture-Centered Approach

The *culture-centered approach (CCA)*, a framework for listening to voices of subaltern[2] communities, privileges accounts of lived experiences of health from the margins (Dutta, 2004, 2008, 2015). Narratives grounded in the experiences of the poor across the world interrupt the continually recycled stories of growth, progress, and modernity that are sold as features of the free market, thus creating spaces for the unheard voices of people who experience poverty and health inequality. Health disparities are addressed by drawing attention to the adverse health effects produced by neoliberal policies (Dutta, 2015; Dutta & Kreps, 2013). For instance, culturally centered stories from members of the Philippine farming communities highlight the economic disenfranchisement, lower health, and diminished well-being of the rural poor that resulted from free market reforms in the Philippines (Borras, 2001, 2007; Borras, Carranza, & Franco, 2007).

Foreign domestic workers like Maria migrate to Singapore because they are unable to provide adequate resources for their families in their countries of origin (Rodriguez, 2010). Foreign domestic workers experience a range of poor physical and mental health outcomes. In the absence of unions representing domestic workers, including enforcement of health regulations, foreign domestic workers often lack adequate labor protections, health insurance coverage, access to preventive health services, and access to food and spaces for exercising.

Listening to the voices of domestic workers from the Philippines through the framework of the CCA offers a map for comparing the stories of disenfranchisement with the dominant stories of neoliberalism. Maria's "story" (a compilation of several domestic workers' stories) challenges unhealthy policies by showing that economic growth does not translate into better health outcomes for the poor. The rhetoric of trickle-down economics is juxtaposed against stories of migrant workers such as Maria who live at the margins of global economic centers (mostly large cities) of production and exchange and struggle to access affordable or quality healthcare. As in the story of Maria, not having enough to pay for healthcare is a reality that does not correspond with the narrative that growth will trickle down to benefit the poor. This experience is represented in the voice of Maria, recalling her hard life in the Philippines: "It was always hard. Never easy. Struggled to meet even the basic needs, and worked many jobs together. Still we could not afford the treatment when my father-in-law became ill. Had to sell everything. That's why I came to work here."

Maria migrated because the economic reforms in the Philippines that were sold as tools for improving her life resulted in further marginalizing her family. Stories like Maria's offer insight into avenues for change in regional, national, and global policies. Through stories narrated by cultural members, new interpretations, rituals, meanings, and opportunities for change are introduced into the cultural context, offering templates for new imaginations and alternative rationalities for addressing health disparities.

▪ The Culture-Centered Approach and Narratives

Narratives frame health experiences (Mattingly, 1998). As you've read throughout this book, the literature on narratives in health communication emphasizes their storied nature. According to the CCA, community members participate in their everyday negotiations through the stories circulated within their culture about health and healing. Stories express the lived experiences of community members with health, resources of health, social and contextual constraints on health, and the broader cultural expectations regarding the interpretation of health, wellness, illness, prevention, treatment, and healing. Stories are the expressions of cultures and cultural norms, and are sites of cultural change.

Consider, for instance, the following story shared by Maria: "I felt very sad when I started my work. Felt light headed and dizzy, it was all the sadness that got into my body. Always stress in my body. Never thought how I could be treated like this, like I am not a human being. My employer slapped me, scold me, it is never good work, what I do." Maria's expectations of being treated with dignity as a domestic worker in Singapore sharply contrast with the treatment she experienced. Referring to her health as being intertwined with the treatment she experienced, she co-constructs dignity as central to her understanding of well-being. Her voice, emerging through conversations among foreign domestic workers, fosters an entry point for cultural change, depicting ill-treatment by employers as health threatening and therefore as a site for a communication intervention.

Along similar lines, Maria experiences stress after not having been paid her salary for eight months: "I worked for all these months, for what? No money. The employer didn't pay me the salary. Always kept saying, 'We'll pay you the next month,' and after eight months, still no salary." Her story of not getting paid her salary after having worked hard for eight months disrupts the cultural narrative of neoliberalism that frames migration as a strategy for pulling individuals and households out of poverty. Her story also disrupts the discursive constructions of contracts as papers that ensure that migrant workers are paid their due. A health communication program rooted in Maria's story would include envisioning strategies for ensuring that foreign domestic workers in Singapore are paid in full and on time as stipulated by the contracts they sign.

■ The Intersections of Culture, Structure, and Agency

The three concepts of culture, structure, and agency form the guiding posts in the CCA (Dutta, 2008, 2015). Culture reflects the shifting and dynamic values, beliefs, norms, rituals, and everyday health practices that form the fabric of the community. Cultures offer the interpretive frameworks and cues to action, rendering meaningful a wide range of templates for action. Cultures, as represented in the stories shared by community members, are integral to the generational transfer of values and meanings, and to the creation of transformative spaces. For example, investigating how domestic workers like Maria are treated is a culturally constituted value, tied to notions of hierarchy, class power, and communicative expectations.

Structures, referring to systems of organizing that enable and/or constrain access to resources of health, are rooted in material conditions. Economic access to resources forms the bases of structures and at the same time is shaped by these structures. Opportunities for health, housing, and access to spaces of living, education, adequate and healthy food, spaces for exercising, and quality healthcare are all elements of structures. For Maria, the home in Singapore where she worked, the rules and regulations imposed on her, and the treatment meted out to her by her employers are all structures to which she must adapt. According to Maria, "The employer can treat me like an animal because she has the money and she pays me. She took away my hand phone the day I came. My passport and ID are also with her. How can I talk to my family? I can't contact anyone."

Maria's isolation and her separation from her family are structured into the realm of domestic work and the power that is tied to the economic position of her employer. She feels that she can be meted out inhumane treatment because of her position as a domestic worker.

Agency depicts the community, family, and individual-level participation in ordinary processes of sensemaking, in everyday acts of negotiation, in adapting to structures, and in collective participation in processes of structural transformation. For instance, in responding to their lack of access to health structures such as health insurance, preventive care, and hospitals, domestic workers narrate a variety of strategies that they negotiate in order to secure healthcare. They suggest following multiple pathways of healing, making health decisions, while being keenly aware of the constraints imposed by the structures. Maria shares, "I know that stress is no good. I tell myself, keep calm. All this will someday be gone. I talk to myself."

Another avenue for sensemaking and negotiation occurs as Maria and other domestic workers collaborate with our research team to put together the Respect Our Rights campaign, which seeks to create awareness about the dignity of domestic work and the basic rights of domestic workers. Thus domestic workers' agency is reflective of both local sensemaking processes as well as fields of action in which community members participate. Through their expressions of agency reflecting everyday practices embedded within cultures, as well as through their participation in processes that seek change in policies, community members imagine alternative stories.

These stories thus are situated at these intersections of culture, structure, and agency, as reflections of the interplay between these three elements in dynamic contexts. Theorizing Practice 13.1 asks you to consider how your own personal stories might work at these intersections.

Theorizing Practice 13.1
Relating the CCA to Your Family's Storied Health

As we have described, 26-year-old Maria, a foreign domestic worker in Singapore, struggles amid very limited resources to make sure that she can send home to the Philippines enough money for the care of her own children. Her identity as a parent wanting to educate her children is the primary motivation that drives her hard work. Now, consider your own background, including stories of health in your family:

• What are the most salient features of your health identity?

• Juxtapose these family health stories with the culture-centered approach that has been described. How do your stories work at the intersections of culture, structure, and agency?

HCIA 13.1

Silence, Stigma, and Sexual Risk

Patrick J. Dillon

In the United States, estimates suggest that more than half of the nearly 1 million people living with HIV/AIDS are men who were infected through sex with other men. Studies also indicate that, within the general population of men who have sex with men (MSM), the risk of HIV infection is significantly higher among African Americans and Latinos. In order to address this disturbing trend, researchers and practitioners have, in recent years, called for efforts to understand how social, cultural, and structural factors influence racial/ethnic disparities in HIV-infection rates. Ultimately, such information can be used to inform health campaigns/interventions seeking to lessen HIV-infection risk within minority MSM populations.

Despite the urgent need to address HIV/AIDS disparities, this issue has received limited consideration from health communication scholars. As a starting point for future communication research on this topic, we synthesized qualitative research (i.e., 12 interview and focus group studies) conducted by scholars from other disciplines. Our analysis identified several factors that contribute to increased HIV-infection risk within these populations. Although African American and Latino MSM do not constitute a homogenous group, we observed a great deal of commonality across participants' experiences.

A primary contributor to HIV-infection risk among both African American and Latino MSM is the social stigma attached to same-sex relationships within their cultural communities. Study participants explained that cultural definitions of masculinity, such as notions of the "strong Black man" in African American communities and the concept of "machismo" for Latinos, created perceptions that engaging in same-sex relationships made one less of a man. Furthermore, African American and Latino MSM noted that associations between their cultures and Christian churches that consider sex between men to be morally wrong also contribute to the stigma. In either case, the stigma compelled some participants to feel guilty about their same-sex relationships; for others, it led them to experience and/or fear rejection by their loved ones and faith communities. One Latino male, for example, explained that upon disclosing to his mother that he had been infected with HIV through sexual contact with another man, "she just shook her head and said it was because of [his] evil choice to be that way."

The threat of rejection by their loved ones and the stigma associated with sex between men led African American and Latino MSM to engage in sexual behaviors that put them at risk for HIV. These behaviors included: (1) inconsistent condom use, and (2) consuming alcohol and/or drugs before sexual encounters. Although most study participants were aware that condom use reduced the risk of HIV infection, they noted that the desire to hide their same-sex relationships often led them to engage in spontaneous, often anonymous, sexual encounters. The spontaneous nature of such encounters diminished the likelihood of participants using condoms. Participants further stated that these anonymous, spontaneous encounters frequently took place in locations, such as bars and bathhouses, where alcohol and drug use are common practices. Consuming these substances lowered men's inhibitions and increased their likelihood of forgoing condom use during sexual contact.

The desire to avoid being "found out" also led many African American and Latino MSM to simultaneously maintain romantic and/or sexual relationships with women. In many of these relationships, the men chose to avoid condom use with their female partners in order to avert suspicion about their other sexual behaviors. For example, one African American man stated, "You go in the house and got Trojans in your pocket, you're getting accused of something."

Concurrent with social stigma and risky sexual practices, many participants also experienced limited access to health resources and had inadequate knowledge about HIV/AIDS. African American and Latino MSM are minorities within minority groups, and the marginalizing impacts of racism and heterosexism restricted their access to gainful employment, housing, education, and health insurance. For some men, economic insecurity, in particular, meant that purchasing condoms was beyond their means; for others, it led them to exchange sexual favors (often without condoms) for money and/or other resources. Economic insecurity also limited participants' ability to access general medical care and HIV/AIDS prevention and testing services. Our study indicated that, even when free HIV/AIDS services were available, MSM of color were often unwilling to access them because they mistrusted the healthcare system and/or were afraid of sacrificing their anonymity. Participants' inability and/or reluctance to access these services meant that many of them lacked important information about HIV/AIDS. Several participants, for example, believed that the HIV virus could not be transmitted through oral sex.

As evidenced by our study, HIV-infection risk for African American and Latino MSM is influenced by a number of social, cultural, and structural factors. Through enhanced understanding of these factors, health communication scholars and practitioners are more prepared to address these populations' needs and work to eliminate racial/ethnic HIV/AIDS disparities.

QUESTIONS TO PONDER

1. Why is it important for health communication scholars to understand how social, cultural, and structural factors influence racial/ethnic health disparities in HIV-infection risk?

2. How did stigma influence study participants' HIV-infection risk? Can you think of other examples where stigma might influence people's health behaviors?

3. If you were asked to design a communication program (e.g., a public communication campaign or community-based health intervention) to address HIV-infection risk among African American and Latino MSM, what might that look like? How might you integrate some of the findings described above?

Source: Dillon, P. J., & Basu, A. (2014). HIV/AIDS and minority men who have sex with men: A meta-ethnographic synthesis of qualitative research. *Health Communication, 29,* 182–192.

■ The Role of Community Participation in the CCA

The CCA recognizes the absence of subaltern voices from dominant spheres, noting that structural oppressions contribute to these erasures. For instance, the erasure of Maria's voice from spaces of policy making in both the Philippines and in Singapore are tied to her experiences of poor health as a foreign domestic worker in Singapore. Through dialogues with subaltern communities and the stories voiced by community members, CCA seeks to offer entry points for knowledge creation and action steps. Thus the community is viewed as a space for challenging the structures that constrain members and result in poor health outcomes through poor labor regulations, poor access to health insurance, and poor access to food (Dutta, 2008, 2015; Nelson & Wright, 1995).

Culture, as a fluid and dynamic web of meanings constituted in the interactions and co-constructions of cultural members, is voiced in participants' stories (Dutta,

2008, 2015). By centering the voices of cultural actors in the context of health structures, strategies for addressing health inequities may be developed (Dutta, 2007; Dutta
& Pal, 2010). For instance, in our conversations with Maria, we learn about her meanings of health as intertwined with her limited access to basic food resources. She
describes her life in our conversations, sharing how she wakes up at 5:00 A.M. and
goes to bed at 11:30 P.M. She begins her day with half a piece of toast, eats half a bowl
of rice at lunch, and for dinner, only consumes any leftovers brought home by her
employers. She describes how she feels weak from having to work those long hours
with very little food in her stomach. One day, she felt so weak that she fell from a lad-
der while cleaning one of the ceiling fans in the house.

From Maria's story, we learn how she has been surviving without receiving her
salary to financially support her. She is not allowed to go outside of the house and,
therefore, has no way of securing more food. She describes how her employers asked
her why she needed to eat more, given that she was spending all day in the home.
Tears flowing down her cheeks as she recounts this experience, Maria shares with us
stories of growing up in the Philippines when she had enough rice to eat, and how she
migrated to Singapore feeling she would now be able to eat and send money home for
her children to be able to eat. Maria's story, depicted in the context of Singaporean
domestic work, draws attention to the need for change in attitudes of employers
toward foreign domestic workers. Culture, narrated in Maria's recollection of growing
up in the Philippines with enough rice to eat, is placed in conversation with Maria's
understanding of the culture of a household of employers in Singapore who offer her
little food and bring her their leftovers to eat at night. These stories of not having
enough food to eat become sites of intended change in a culturally centered health
communication intervention developed by foreign domestic workers.

HCIA 13.2

"Peeled Off the Mold . . . , Because It's What I Had to Eat"

Vandhana Ramadurai

Food insecurity is one of the nation's leading public health problems, especially in inner-
city neighborhoods isolated by poverty and crime and, less obviously, in rural communities
isolated by distance and scarce resources. It is defined by the unavailability within a reasonable distance of nutritionally adequate and safe foods and the inability to access such foods
in socially acceptable ways, without resorting to stealing or scavenging. This formal definition was aptly illustrated by Maya, one of our participants:

> [B]efore I got pregnant I would go two or three days without eating. Just try and
> conserve on the food. Now being pregnant . . . I go [a] whole day, I might eat one honey
> bun, and I mean that's it for the day. [I] wait till the next day and try and eat [a] little,
> 'cause, you know I am trying to feed myself, my husband, [and] my mom. It is a 15-, 16-
> mile trip just one way [to the regional food program]; it is hard to do. I don't have a cell
> phone that works. You know if something happens, like the other day. I had a severe
> blow out and no way of getting [in] touch with anyone. What am I going to do if it is
> dark outside and I am driving and something happens?

Despite its prevalence and importance, this problem has not received sufficient consideration from health communication scholars. In an effort to help remedy that lack of attention, we conducted a series of 12 focus groups (N = 86) in nine central Texas rural communities. Though we initially sought to find disparities by race and ethnicity, such differences in our diverse sample seemed minor compared with commonalities due to rural location.

The food-related problems experienced by rural residents were due to structural problems associated with community institutions such as groceries, churches, and governmental and nongovernmental agencies, as well as everyday personal obstacles faced by individuals and families. For instance, at the structural level, grocery stores were frequently criticized for selling expensive products of substandard quality, lack of food variety, and relative unavailability of stores in rural locations. In order to avoid hunger, participants ate foods that had expired and were nutritionally compromised. Additionally, many voiced concerns about how the cost of food hindered their management of health conditions such as diabetes.

Both governmental and nongovernmental organization (NGO) programs had been established to aid in alleviating food insecurity. However, timing was problematic. Often assistance was provided by these organizations early in the month when participants had some personal resources to procure food. But when household money ran short, so did food items provided by the assistance programs, so some residents, if they had a means of transportation, had to travel to multiple regional food banks to acquire enough food to last a month. Additionally, eligibility for NGO programs was dependent on where rural residents lived. Hence, it was common for participants to be turned down by multiple programs due to the location of their residence. Residents attended church gatherings as a means not only to observe spiritual practices and to socialize but also to obtain food. Unfortunately, the traditional menus at church gatherings were typically unhealthy, featuring fried and fatty foods.

At a personal level, traveling distances for employment, long work hours, and easy access to fast food all affected how our participants and their families ate. Spouses exerted considerable influence on food choices; many residents expressed frustration with their partners for being resistant to their positive suggestions. Also, the amount of money people spent and the chances of food insecurity were increased by significant others' differing dietary preferences or their need for medications.

Concurrent with the problems associated with food insecurity, our participants also spoke about creative coping, both individually and at a community level. Though poor in conventional material resources, our rural participants described forms of social capital, expressed as feelings of responsibility for the well-being of their communities and enacted through social networks and interpersonal support. Examples included sharing information about health and nutrition, cooked meals and garden surplus, and transportation. Church plays an important role in rural life, providing not only a religious space, but also representing a place for residents to connect and build social relationships.

By taking the time and effort to understand contextual nuances of specific communities, health communication scholars are better prepared to engage in collaborative problem solving with community members and to help develop health campaigns that both address local problems and make use of available social capital.

QUESTIONS TO PONDER

1. Why is food security an important issue to discuss in relation to health communication?
2. If you were asked to design a communication program (public communication campaign or community-based empowerment training) to address food insecurity in a rural area of

(continued)

your own state, what might that look like? What kinds of information about those communities do you think you would need to learn about before designing a program?

3. Think of a public health problem in your own community. If not food insecurity, it might be obesity, drug abuse, refusal to vaccinate, or any number of other issues. What are some structural obstacles that make the problems worse? What forms of social capital could be employed to help remedy the problems?

Source: Ramadurai, V., Sharf, B. F., & Sharkey, J. R. (2012). Rural food insecurity in the United States as an overlooked site of struggle in health communication. *Health Communication, 27*, 794–805.

■ The Respect Our Rights Campaign

The Respect Our Rights campaign (http://respectfdwrights.com), a national-level campaign directed at all Singaporeans, and especially those who hire foreign domestic workers, began with the question, "What does health mean to you?" An advisory group of foreign domestic workers like Maria who reside at a shelter supported by the nongovernmental organization (NGO), Humanitarian Organization for Migrant Economics (HOME), developed the campaign. The advisory board meetings were organized jointly by our research team and HOME. The campaign seeks to raise awareness about the rights of domestic workers and the dignity of domestic work, and to target attitude and behavior change in how employers treat domestic workers.

As depicted by Maria's story, paying close attention to the narratives shared by subaltern communities provides insights about the shared cultural meanings of health and the ways in which these shared meanings are located in relationship to broader structures (Dutta, 2008). For instance, in listening to multiple stories voiced by disenfranchised foreign domestic workers in Singapore, we make sense of their health needs as being in conflict with the larger structures that determine their recruitment into the country, the wage policies governing domestic work, and the broader policy environment around domestic work. Domestic workers articulate their health rights as being able to secure basic resources such as access to clean and fresh food, access to medical resources, receiving a weekly day off, being paid on time every month, working in a safe environment, and not having to pay hefty agency fees to come to Singapore for work.

Moreover, by focusing on health rights, culturally centered stories told by domestic workers suggest their health needs will not be met if they are not covered under the employment act (a state level policy) in Singapore that would offer these basic provisions of healthy working conditions to domestic workers. The domestic workers tell us that the unregulated market forces in the informal domestic work economy leave them vulnerable to health risks. Their narratives point to the minimal protection they receive during their employment; they indicate that the invisible nature of domestic work in the private spaces of homes leaves them vulnerable to oppression and health risks. The absence of labor protection serves the interests of employers and agents who recruit migrant workers, with the absence of guarantees for basic health needs of domestic workers. Maria asks, "Who is going to care for us domestic workers? We don't have the money or the connections or the power." Narratives voiced from the margins in the form of the Respect Our Rights campaign thus offer entry points for changing attitudes and behaviors of employers, public opinion, and public policies governing domestic work.

Inverting Narrative Structures and Expectations

The participation of foreign domestic workers in our culture-centered project inverts how stories of health are told and who gets to tell these stories (Dutta, 2008; Nelson & Wright, 1995; Peterson, 2010). Through their participation as advisory board members, domestic workers take charge of defining their health problems and developing corresponding health solutions. The power of expertise as the producer of knowledge is placed in the voices of domestic workers who come together to produce stories directed at powerful stakeholders such as policy makers, recruitment agencies, and employers.

A Subaltern Studies reading of these narrative structures interrogates the assumptions underlying the accounts circulated in public spheres, questioning our narrative expectations and assumptions in the mainstream. Foreign domestic workers identifying health problems, developing communication strategies, and sharing their experiences of health and well-being through photographic images and video storytelling disrupt dominant expectations that target domestic workers as subjects of one-way interventions designed by experts (Dutta, 2008). Accounts of health narrated from the margins question the narratives of trickle-down economics that circulate polished stories in the mainstream discourse of domestic work as a means for poor families to work their way out of poverty.

Subaltern accounts of domestic work narrated in the form of print and television advertisements directed at the Singapore public and policy makers in the Respect Our Rights campaign foreground the lack of fundamental access to food as a narrative entry point to understanding the health consequences for foreign domestic workers in Singapore. The narrative structure of a television advertisement co-created by foreign domestic workers disrupts the dominant narrative structure of communication in which advertising and public relations campaigns are designed by experts hired by advertising agencies, public relations firms, and transnational corporations, targeted to migrant workers as tools for educating them. Specific forms of storytelling such as songs, poetry, street theatre, and performance emerge from the subaltern contexts as openings for disrupting taken-for-granted stories told by the status quo (Beverley, 2001, 2004a, 2004b). Theorizing Practice 13.2 on the following page now asks you to consider the experiences of subalterns in your own community.

Culture and Communicative Inversions

One of the strategies employed by dominant power structures is the strategy of *communicative inversion* (Dutta, 2015). Communicative inversion refers to the strategic use of stories to articulate reflections of events, processes, and instances that are diametrically different from the material roots (i.e., verifiable circumstances) of these events, processes, and instances. Communicative inversions represent the opposite of the materially grounded experiences and relationships of everyday life in subaltern contexts, deploying the power of communication to circulate misrepresentations of subaltern communities.

Theorizing Practice 13.2
Recognizing Subalterns in Your Own Community

While subalterns may not be a term with which you are familiar, the phenomenon of people who are socially marginalized is all too familiar no matter where we live. Consider your own communities (e.g., cities with which you've been associated, neighborhoods in which you grew up, or people on your campus) to answer the following questions:

- Who are the people within those communities who "have been systematically erased from dominant discourse due to social status" and for what reasons specifically?

- What are the aspects of culture and/or structural elements that function to erase these group(s) from the dominant discourses that characterize power, privilege, and opportunity?

- What efforts are being made, that you are aware of, for individuals within these group(s) to increase their sense of agency and acquire voice that will be heard and respected within the larger community?

Stories are integral to the processes of communicative inversions, forming the basis for public relations and propaganda. For instance, the stories about neoliberal reforms in the Philippines narrate the trickle-down effects of privatization and minimization of trade barriers, inverting the material realities of large-scale displacement, inequalities, and threats to health posed by these reforms (Borras, 2001, 2007; Borras et al., 2007). The glossy stories of foreign domestic workers working in Singapore and earning high incomes in economies of scale that dig them and their families in the Philippines out of poverty are disrupted by the stories of foreign domestic workers that reveal they are earning only $20 a month because of hefty salary deductions and do not have enough money to buy the food, let alone send money home.

For example, the foregrounding of stories of foreign domestic workers like Maria reveals the health threats and vulnerabilities brought about by policies solely predicated on growth-driven change. Maria laments the harsh economic conditions in the Philippines that force her to be separated from her children. She shares: "I cry for my children every night. What mother leaves her children behind to come work someplace else? I miss them very much. My daughter was only a few months old when I came to work here." Maria's story inverts the story of growth-driven migration to economic centers as the solution to poverty, depicting the vulnerabilities and disruptions that are produced by global movements of labor. The stories of trickle-down and growth-driven development are interrupted by stories of struggles and entrapment in the poverty cycle in spite of backbreaking hard work. In this next section, we will explore specific methods of storytelling within the framework of the CCA, attending to the contributions of the CCA to the narrative method in health communication.

■ Stories for Method and Theory

The CCA addresses health disparities through its emphasis on listening to subaltern voices. Especially in the context of health risks experienced by subaltern communities, these stories navigate the dual issues of developing an effective strategy for addressing the problems voiced by subaltern communities and guarding some stories as stories not to be shared to protect the identities and struggles of the participants. Communities of activists, subaltern members, and academics question and negotiate which stories to share and which stories to keep hidden.

There is a dialectical tension between safekeeping some stories and sharing other stories for purposes of bringing about change, guided by co-conversations among academics, practitioners, and community members. For Maria and her friends, strategies of resisting employer harassment are stories to be kept secret in order to protect domestic workers from the possibilities of employer and agent retaliation and also in light of the many instances of ongoing legal cases. The participation of domestic workers in the Respect Our Rights campaign actively negotiates the possibilities of employer retaliation and legal ramifications by not sharing certain stories, changing Maria's name, making Maria a composite character in this chapter, disguising identities in the documentary, and not revealing people or specific identifying features in photos, among other strategies. Deciding which stories to share is also guided by the objective of the sharing and the effect sought determined by the advisory board of domestic workers. Consider one of our field notes:

> Are all stories "stories?" Are all stories to be written up for consumption by the academic audience in the Western metropole? This question I struggle with often when working with foreign domestic workers in Singapore. Many of the stories of loss and pain emerge as sites of activism and advocacy. The stories call for action, shaped by the urgency of the context. Sitting down to write down these stories at these moments is both a luxury and a distraction. For many of these other stories, there is something inherently violent about writing down the stories, about personally benefiting from the suffering of the subaltern. Who ultimately benefits from the telling of the story also perhaps has a lot to do with the very power structures we inhabit as bourgeoisie academics. The stories we write (or do not write) and the stories we tell (or do not tell) tread this delicate balance of ethical considerations, power relationships, and questions of impact.

For instance, Maria and her domestic worker friends sheltered at HOME discuss the importance of stories to foreground their dignity as human beings and as workers. For Maria, being respected as a worker is tied to the capability of foreign domestic workers to secure the dignity of work and to address structural injustices, thus contributing to better health and well-being. The ethics of the stories we share as a collaborative project then needs to be grounded in the power of the stories to address the dignity of domestic work as a fundamental right, an objective for the change effort decided on by the advisory board of domestic workers.

The CCA points toward reflexivity as an opening for interrogating the stories circulated in dominant structures and for examining closely our own value positions and privileges as academics. Academic cultures may construct stories about subaltern communities, often participating in the political economy of profiteering that operates by commoditizing subaltern knowledge (Dutta, 2008). The meaningfulness of the action of sharing Maria's story then needs to be evaluated by the criterion of the capability of the story to offer a framework of change.

The stories we tell from our own fieldwork are constituted in this complex terrain of power, commoditization, and profits and need to be interpreted and negotiated with the disenfranchised communities with whom we work. These stories in the CCA need to be evaluated on the basis of their capability in addressing health disparities and in transforming unhealthy structures, placed within a broader ethical framework that continually questions the purpose of storytelling. Moreover, the accountability for these stories is anchored in the subaltern communities at the margins rather than in the dominant structures of knowledge production, policy development, and practice. Whether a project addressing health disparities in a specific subaltern community works or not depends upon the metrics through which the community members evaluate success.

Performing Stories and Reflexivity

Stories embody lived experiences, constituted amid the social contexts that frame the realms of possibilities and impossibilities. Therefore, as health citizens, we perform stories through our own bodies and the positioning of our bodies amid relationships of power. Our own vulnerabilities are intertwined with the vulnerabilities that we witness when listening to stories. We co-create our stories as we listen to and share the stories of the disenfranchised communities with whom we work. These stories become reflections of our own privileges and the ways in which these privileges may foreclose possibilities for listening. By understanding our own stories and our own situatedness within the broader structures of relationships, we come to understand the oppressions and communicative processes that produce silences (Basu & Dutta, 2010).

The treatment of stories as performance brings health communication researchers, practitioners, and community members into shared spaces. Reflexivity as method therefore teaches us that our own subject positions as students and scholars of health communication are deeply intertwined with the subjects we study. We can't disentangle these relationships and we can't extricate ourselves from the complexities of these storytelling relationships. Thus, when I (Mohan) listen to Maria's story, I have to negotiate my own stories of privilege, having lived with domestic workers in my own home. I recall my childhood and think of Lalmadidi, who works in my own home now in Singapore. She cares for our children, supports us in our everyday household chores, and frees up the time for my academic-activist labor. Reflecting on Maria's story, I, on one hand, feel good about the relationship of care my family has with Lalmadidi and the ways in which we care for her through our relationship. On the other hand, I become cognizant of the need for continued vigilance in our familial relationship with Lalmadidi, working to ensure that we treat her as a professional (this is a key theme of the Respect our Rights campaign).

There are imaginative openings for new narratives through these individual stories and accounts of marginalization, connected in solidarity with other stories of marginalization across global sites of exploitation. Maria's story of everyday struggles with poverty in the Philippines and her struggles with access to basic food in Singapore as a domestic worker disrupts the public relations imageries of neoliberal development. Maria understands her health as compromised by her lack of access to food in spite of her hard work. Her story calls for alternative frameworks for distributing health resources and addressing the needs of the global poor.

The role of the researcher in engaging reflexively with stories on the ground becomes one of listening critically to these stories. The very act of listening transforms the inequities that constitute marginalization at local, national, and global levels. The stories of foreign domestic workers in Singapore shared through the Respect Our Rights campaign reflexively seek to create a cultural environment that respects the rights of foreign domestic workers. Consider, for instance, our experience with an academic reviewer asking us "how is Maria's story anything about health?" Maria's story disrupts the privilege of the reviewer by constructing a plot that stands in resisting, conveying the moral that the struggle to secure access to food within the confines of foreign domestic work is a fundamental struggle of/for health.

Moreover, note how Maria makes sense of her lack of food by referring us to a broader social system of capitalism and wealth accumulation with very little room for empathy: "Everyone is busy making money in this city, but there is no heart," she shares. "My employer does not care, as long as her family is making the money, it does not matter whether I eat or not. She thinks, even if I eat a little food, that will take away from how much money she can make. My health is declining every day. I lost so much weight, but no one in the family notices. The money and the busy life that make you without a heart."

For Maria, it is the deep-rooted individualism, extreme capitalism, and search for wealth that renders employers without compassion. Also, she points to the problems of a free market framework for managing domestic work, noting, "How can I say anything when laws are not there or even when they are there, either I am not aware or I am going to have a very difficult time getting justice?" She seeks to resist and invert the free market structuring of domestic work by co-opting the individualistic narrative of neoliberalism in voicing a narrative of "right" rooted in the collective experiences and solidarity of domestic workers. The framing of rights of domestic workers as worker rights disrupts the "unregulated free market" framework for domestic work and suggests the need for policies to ensure that domestic workers have their fundamental rights be respected.

Thus, in listening to Maria's story, we are able to co-create a plot that not only questions the policy space but also questions privileges of academic theorizing. Too often this theorizing is situated within the global structures of neoliberalism and rife with the individualistic and false assumptions about human identity, human relationships, and human communication. According to Maria, "Each and every domestic worker has the right to be treated with respect. I am a worker, and all domestic workers are workers. We are not your slave. So give us the respect that you want for yourself when you go to work. Treat us like you want to be treated when you work. We are not slaves in your home."

Note here how Maria juxtaposes her narrative against a backdrop of a collective story of domestic work, anchoring the experiences of domestic workers in solidarity and weaving them together in possibilities of change. The solution to threats to health is present in fundamental cultural shifts in beliefs, attitudes, and values around domestic work, thus inverting the structures that constitute domestic work.

Maria's story constructs health in relationship to the vulnerabilities and risks that are tied to the nature of domestic work. The mainstream individual-level narrative of health that frames health in the realm of behavior (such as eating healthily and exercising) and as a product of individual choice is disrupted by a collective narrative that situates health of foreign domestic workers amid the structures of domestic work. That the health of Maria is structured in the attitudes and behaviors of her employers and is intertwined with the broader structure of policies is an articulation that resists the individualism in the free market narrative. Maria says that people coming to Singapore and seeing how good the infrastructure is would probably have no idea of the experiences of foreign domestic workers within the four walls of homes; thus her story and the stories of other domestic workers narrate the plot of another Singapore as experienced through the everyday lived experiences and struggles of foreign domestic workers. This sharing of "other" stories becomes the basis for the Respect Our Rights campaign.

Solidarity, the connection among multiple sites of storytelling, is an important tool in changing local, national, and global policies around health. A key element of solidarity in the CCA is the relationship between the researchers and subaltern communities. As researchers working on addressing health inequalities through communication, our methodological engagements within the framework of the CCA work in solidarity with communities at the margins that are at the receiving end of the unequal neoliberal policies. Solidarity, understood as friendships of support and sustenance between academics and subaltern communities, works through localized collaborations on processes of social change. The erasure of subaltern communities from spaces of recognition and representation is the site for structural transformation based on the argument that listening to participants' stories from their own contexts opens up avenues for disrupting structures by introducing alternative theories of health, grounded in subaltern understandings and lived experiences.

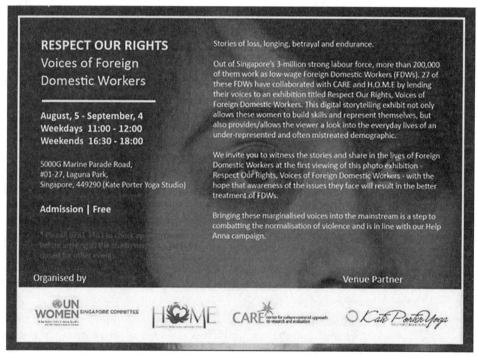

A promotional advertisement for the Respect Our Rights photovoice exhibit (Solidarities for Social Change).

Solidarity thus is the recognition of subaltern agency and the simultaneous recognition of the politics of the scholar's own participation in processes of social change. In our collaborations with foreign domestic workers in Singapore, we partner in the creation of scripts, in the production processes, camera work, editing work, and developing an implementation strategy of a campaign addressing the rights of foreign domestic workers. The campaign, depicting images and story lines crafted by the domestic workers, draws attention to the everyday struggles, physical, emotional, and sexual abuse, and challenges to health experienced by foreign domestic workers. Solidarity between researchers and subaltern communities thus turns into an active process of collaboration in an actual project of social change, developing story structures and story forms for a campaign on the health rights of foreign domestic workers. Discussing solidarity as "concrete friendship with poor," Beverley (1999) notes:

> The desire for solidarity must begin, however, with a relation of what Gutierrez calls "concrete friendship with the poor": it cannot be simply a matter of taking thought or "conversation," or for that matter of romanticizing or idealizing the subaltern . . . in making the shift from "objectivity" to "solidarity," we cannot simply disavow representation under the pretext that we are allowing the subaltern to "speak for itself." . . . And there is a way in which the (necessarily?) liberal political slant Rorty gives the idea of solidarity may also be, as the 1960s slogan has it, part of the problem rather than part of the solution, because it assumes that "conversation" is possible across power/exploitation divides that radically differentiate the participants. (p. 39)

Solidarity is first and foremost recognition of the power one occupies as a scholar in her/his relationship with subaltern communities and the ways in which this power forecloses the possibilities of participation. The lens thus is turned on the very nature of scholarship, interrogating the hierarchies in scholarly projects of social change that engage with subaltern communities, as well as exploring the privileges that shape narratives, the structures of these narratives, the framing of the various actors within these narratives, and the plots of the narratives. Getting into dialogic moments of concrete friendships with subaltern communities calls for an openness to storytelling that emerges from within community spaces. For instance, in the Respect Our Rights campaign, Maria's story takes center stage, narrated in a form that is meaningful to her (but as a documentary, the script has been written by an advisory board of foreign domestic workers).

Structural transformation, primarily reflected in policy changes and the creation of programs and infrastructures, is achieved through the spaces of storytelling grounded in subaltern rationalities and imaginations. Maria discusses her interpretation of solidarity in the work that she carried out in collaboration with the other domestic workers and the research team in coming up with the idea of the Respect Our Rights campaign and in carrying out the campaign. She shares: "We came up with all this. We decided together what we would like to achieve and what are the goals of our campaign. Hopefully all this work we did will change the lives of other domestic workers. We will all be treated well because of what this campaign achieved." Maria's celebration of the campaign's success is the recognition of the creativity and agency of her collective of advisory board members who mapped out the problems, devised the solutions, came up with the strategies and tactics, and collaborated with the research team in the implementation and evaluation processes.

HCIA 13.3

Let's Talk About Sex:
Digital Storytelling for Puerto Rican Youth

Aline Gubrium ■ Jeffery Chaichana Peterson

As part of a project called *Let's Talk About Sex*, we ran three, 4-day digital storytelling (DST) workshops, each with 10 Puerto Rican Latinas aged 15–19. During the workshops, participants produced short, first-person stories that synthesized digital images, audio recordings, music, and text. The workshops were facilitated by the Center for Digital Storytelling (now called StoryCenter: www.storycenter.org) and were held at a local partner agency that works to improve sexual health education policy and provides access to sexual health programming for youth.

The city where our project is located contains a large Puerto Rican community, where teens give birth to children at a rate much higher than their peers around the country. Teens also report higher rates of HIV and other sexually transmitted infections. Research tells us that there are many potential reasons for this disparity, including those related to education, economics, and other social and cultural factors. However, popular explanations are often influenced by fears related to stereotypes. For instance, despite evidence to the contrary, Latinas are perceived to begin sexual activity at relatively earlier ages, reproduce at abnormally high rates, and overuse medical and other social services. These perceptions lead to anxieties that the U.S. is soon to be overwhelmed by immigration pressures, which will displace "legitimate" Americans. Historically, solutions to the "population problem" have focused on family planning and birth control, instead of critically investigating why disparities in teen birth rates exist. This history shapes the ways sexuality currently is or is not discussed within and among families, communities, schools, and between individuals and healthcare providers.

We designed our project to encourage conversations around sexuality that often are silenced for young women, especially in a community where sexuality tends to be stigmatized. Public health research projects often create one-size-fits-all interventions that are ineffective because they ignore the historical contexts and the environmental and social realities of communities and do little to promote self-determination or self-sufficiency, much less change the system. Or they fail because they understand culture at a superficial level and treat it as something that is stagnant and fixed instead of dynamic and vibrant.

Some health communication research asks individuals to tell stories that address health promotion from their unique, cultural point of view. This research shows that culturally "tailored" *messages* are persuasive in shaping *audiences'* health attitudes, beliefs, and behaviors. However, we believe that these projects often miss the point that the *process* of telling stories also has a positive effect on the *storytellers*. In digital storytelling workshops, we promote a collaborative process that encourages participants to reflect as deeply as they can about themselves and their lives so they can express their own meanings of sexuality and well-being, instead of parroting ideas they may have learned from messages created by outside experts who tell them what they should think and do to be healthy.

First, we encouraged participants to write about one of the following "moments": when they learned about sex, experienced pleasure and desire, understood what love is all about, felt really strong or really helpless in a relationship, learned about contraception or tried to get or use it, were afraid that they had an STD, found out they were pregnant, were scared to ask about reproductive or sexual health care, or knew they were in a good or bad relationship. We used similar prompts in previous workshops and found they help to provide a guide for storytellers who are struggling to pinpoint a story topic. Providing a focus to the content supports storytellers to identify a meaningful moment to share out loud. Participants received feedback, from peers during group work and from workshop facilitators in one-on-one contexts.

Our team observed and assisted with the DST workshop process during story brainstorming and scripting, image collection, and video-editing activities. We also wrote field notes, conducted participant observation, and conducted an interview with participants after they completed a DST workshop. The final activity during each DST workshop was a screening and sharing of all of the stories created throughout the process.

We believe that if we can get people together to talk about and reflect on difficult issues and support each other through an increased sense of solidarity that develops over the course of the workshop, we can begin to address issues in a way that meets the individual or community "where they are." However, it is notoriously difficult to get teenagers to talk about anything, much less such an intimate topic! According to one of our participants, DST can be helpful:

> Um, it was actually a really good experience. Because . . . there was a lot of girls there, who at first, to me I am more of a(n) observer, so they didn't look as comfortable. And then once they started to getting to work with everyone and talking about their stories and hearing other people's stories . . . I feel like, everybody got connected and everybody just . . . expressed themselves. They weren't scared or anything.

The original focus of the *Let's Talk About Sex* project came from a community-based agenda to address sexuality in relation to high rates of teen pregnancy and birth among Puerto Rican Latina youth in the local area. However, through the process, we saw the young women instead wanting to speak about the need to attend to past traumas and address mental health issues, which wrack their community and their own well-being. This is an area that has been underprioritized and overshadowed in the local area by top-down prevention efforts that have misunderstood the priorities and needs that might be characterized by the community. We are committed to conducting research that meets people on their own terms. As this project demonstrates, sometimes that means being willing to change the discussion entirely.

QUESTIONS TO PONDER

1. What stereotypes do you know of that are communicated about culture, ethnicity, or race and sexuality? How do they affect how we feel about health issues that these communities face?

2. How do we put priority on valuing the opinions of the community members, while still taking into account what might be learned from experts outside of the community?

3. What can be communicated, if anything, via digital stories that cannot be expressed in other ways?

Sources: Gubrium, A. (2009). Digital storytelling: An emergent method for health promotion research and practice. *Health Promotion Practice, 10,* 186–191. Gubrium, A., Krause, E. L., & Jernigan, K. (2014). Strategic authenticity and voice: New ways of seeing and being seen as young mothers through digital storytelling. *Sexuality Research & Social Policy, 11,* 337–347. Peterson, J. C., Antony, M. G., & Thomas, R. (2012). "This right here is all about living": Communicating the "common sense" about home stability through CBPR and Photovoice. *Journal of Applied Communication Research, 40,* 1–24.

Resisting Communicative Inversions/Erasures

In listening to stories from the subaltern margins, we collaborate on inverting the dominant structures of knowledge production, policy making, and practice. Here is a reflection from one of our journal notes:

> The story of Maria is a central story of our culture-centered campaign Respect Our Rights, conceptualized, co-created, and co-implemented by foreign domestic workers in Singapore and foregrounding Maria's experiences with abuse in the hands of her employers. The narratives of foreign domestic workers constituted at the intersections of feminization of labor, oppressive labor practices carried out by employers in the global metropole, and the North-South boundaries of labor, bear witness to the violence and threat to health structured within everyday practices of neoliberal organizing of the metropole. Maria narrates the story of her abuse in the hands of an employer who had taken away her passport from her, who gave her [the equivalent of] only one meal a day, and who did not pay her what she was promised in her contract.

The voice of Maria in our culture-centered campaign disrupts mainstream narrative expectations, in which the mainstream academic/expert/producer creates and imposes a story on Maria's lived experiences. Instead, with us witnessing her lived experiences with abuse and exploitation and in co-creating the narrative structure of a communication campaign, Maria provides the story, which disrupts the communicative expectations of mainstream civil society, policy makers, and academics, where the subaltern is a passive target audience.

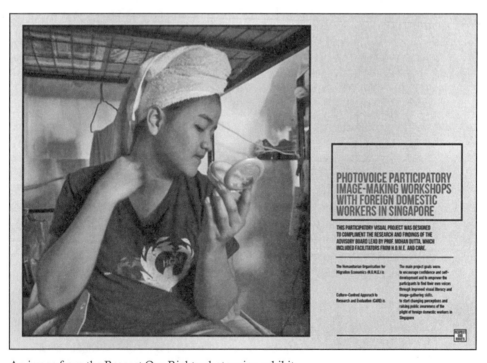

An image from the Respect Our Rights photovoice exhibit.

The communicative structure of the video in the Respect Our Rights documentary emerges as a tool for narrating her account of exploitation in the realm of domestic work. The narrative structure of images and videos are designed by the foreign domestic workers, situating the narratives in relationship to opportunities for structural transformations, grounded in the aspirations of the foreign domestic workers and the objectives they have collaboratively established. For Maria, inequalities in domestic work are addressed in the television advertisements and documentary film designed by her team of advisory board members.

In their struggles to be heard, subaltern communities share their stories of being at the margins—stories that are constituted in relationship to dominant structures of social, political, and economic organizing. In the CCA, the role of the researcher is redefined along the ambits of participating in the politics of structural transformation through journeys of solidarity with subaltern communities (Dutta, 2004, 2008). When projects are embedded in the narrative sensibilities of communities that have been erased, the narrative structures and expectations of research processes, research objectives, and accountability in research are fundamentally shifted to the hands of the community. These shifts in the power of storytelling in the hands of subaltern communities foster openings for new imaginations of communication solutions addressing health disparities. Research takes up new meaning in its relationship to communities at the margins, with its structures of accountability, casting of characters, narrative plots, and narrative functions being driven by local community interpretations of problems and corresponding solutions. Amid large-scale global inequalities, the CCA offers unprecedented openings for inviting new stories that reimagine and transform unequal, underlying structures. Theorizing Practice 13.3 invites you to further consider global health inequalities.

Theorizing Practice 13.3
Communicating to Address Health Inequality

Health inequalities are on the rise across the globe. Consider the patterns of inequalities in the U.S., as well as the various demographic characteristics that you might draw upon to study health inequalities. You can, for instance, draw upon gender to examine the unequal health outcomes for men and women. Or consider the disparate health outcomes experienced by African Americans as compared to Caucasians. You can similarly draw upon social class to examine the unequal health outcomes between the rich and the poor. Choose one characteristic that would serve as a meaningful marker for examining health inequalities.

- Based on the characteristic (gender, for instance), describe the health inequalities and the pathways through which these health inequalities are produced.
- What is the role of communication in these pathways of health inequalities? How does communication produce health inequalities?
- What communication strategies would you suggest for addressing the underlying factors that produce health inequalities?

■ Epilogue

Maria dreams that she will someday go back to her family in the Philippines. Yet for Maria and many women like her, having the money to return home to the Philippines is a distant dream. So Maria continues working year after year, chasing the dream that she will someday have enough money to feed her children, send them to school, and care for the health of her family. Until then, Maria's hope lies in telling stories that she considers as openings for change. The policy changes and implementation she suggests are two key mechanisms for ensuring her health and well-being. Maria believes that as more foreign domestic workers share their stories, these changes will come.

■ Conclusion

The CCA puts forth the argument that stories lie at the heart of global health inequalities, producing scripts of individual freedom and liberty that work as justifications for neoliberal policies, which in turn reproduce poverty, inequality, and disenfranchisement of subaltern communities from their sources of livelihood. The narratives of everyday life thus are connected to the narratives shaped within broader structures. Powerful political, economic, and social actors frame stories that threaten the health of people living in subaltern communities. Constructed at the intersections of culture and structure, these stories reproduce health disparities through communicative erasures and communicative inversions. Academic narratives, framed within the dominant structures of knowledge production that uphold and reproduce neoliberalism, carry out the project of individualism by constructing stories that solely focus on the individual.

Narratives voiced in the subaltern sectors of the globe, bring together voices that have hitherto been erased and offer entry points for addressing health disparities. In the CCA, the unheard voices of subaltern communities find entry points into the dominant platforms of knowledge production and practice. These unheard voices disrupt the dominant logics of neoliberalism, depicting the gaps and the inversions in the often circulated narratives of the free market. Performance, reflexivity, solidarity, and resistance are the key methodological tools of the CCA when engaging in academic–community partnerships in addressing health disparities. Through these tools, the assumptions in the narratives constructed by academics in the mainstream are brought to question.

By listening to stories voiced by subaltern communities in the Global South, opportunities are fostered for organizing politics of social change and structural transformations. Stories of the dignity of domestic work from subaltern contexts offer alternative frameworks for participating globally in processes that seek to contribute to human health. For the foreign domestic workers who participate in our co-constructive journey, respecting domestic work as "work" and respecting the dignity of domestic work are integral to the creation of policies and practices that uphold the health of domestic workers. Listening to Maria's story of how she does not have enough food to eat on an everyday basis is a reminder of how a fundamental threat to health is situated within a broader cluster of beliefs, attitudes, and values in a capitalist society.

The everyday interactions, relationships, and experiences of subaltern communities are shaped by the broader structures that organize a society. However, new narrative structures and communicative inversions—like the Respect Our Rights campaign—can change these structures. Maria's and the other participants' stories create entry points for addressing the health disparities experienced by subaltern communities at the global margins.

Discussion Questions

1. What is the relationship between communication and health inequality? Specify the pathways through which communication influences health inequality.

2. What stories can you tell that relate to the importance of building global spaces with more equitable health outcomes? How would you tell these stories to influence equitable health policies?

3. What role do you think solidarity plays in communication about health? Please suggest three strategies for building solidarity when working as a health communicator with a subaltern community.

4. How would you apply the concept of communicative inversion to understand the ongoing U.S. debate of "black lives matter" vs. "all lives matter"? How would you apply the concept toward creating communication solutions for addressing disparate proportions of health burdens borne by African Americans in the U.S.?

5. What are the overarching health concerns of migrant and refugee communities across the globe? How can communicators work toward addressing these health concerns?

NOTES

[1] Maria's story as depicted in this chapter is a composite, woven together as a collective narrative of the many foreign domestic workers who participated in our Respect Our Rights project.

[2] Subaltern refers to the condition of being systematically erased (i.e., rendered without agency or voice) from dominant discourse due to social status. The term stems from postcolonial and Marxist theories (see, for example, Guha, 1981, 1983, 2001; Landry & MacLean, 1996; Spivak, 1988, 1996, 1999).

REFERENCES

Basu, A., & Dutta, M. (2010). *Born into Brothels*: Neocolonial moves and unheard voices. *Feminist Media Studies, 10,* 101–105.

Beverley, J. (1999). *Subalternity and representation: Arguments in critical theory.* Durham, NC: Duke University Press.

Beverley, J. (2001). The impossibility of politics: Subalternity, modernity, hegemony. In I. Rodríguez (Ed.), *The Latin American subaltern studies reader* (pp. 47–63). Durham, NC: Duke University Press.

Beverley, J. (2004a). *Subalternity and representation: Arguments in cultural theory.* Durham, NC: Duke University Press.

Beverley, J. (2004b). *Testimonio: On the politics of truth.* Minneapolis: University of Minnesota Press.

Borras, S. M., Jr. (2001). State-society relations in land reform implementation in the Philippines. *Development and Change, 32,* 545–575.

Borras, S. M., Jr. (2007). "Free market," export-led development strategy and its impact on rural livelihoods, poverty and inequality: The Philippine experience seen from a Southeast Asian perspective. *Review of International Political Economy, 14,* 143–175.

Borras, S. M., Jr., Carranza, D., & Franco, J. C. (2007). Anti-poverty or anti-poor? The World Bank's market-led agrarian reform experiment in the Philippines. *Third World Quarterly, 28,* 1557–1576.

Dutta, M. J. (2004). The unheard voices of Santalis: Communicating about health from the margins of India. *Communication Theory, 14,* 237–263.

Dutta, M. J. (2007). Communicating about culture and health: Theorizing culture-centered and cultural sensitivity approaches. *Communication Theory, 17,* 304–328.

Dutta, M. J. (2008). *Communicating health: A culture-centered approach.* Cambridge, UK: Polity Press.

Dutta, M. J. (2011). *Communicating social change: Structure, culture, and agency.* New York, NY: Routledge.

Dutta, M. J. (2015). *Neoliberal health organizing.* Walden, CA: Left Coast Press.

Dutta, M. J., & Kreps, G. L. (2013). *Reducing health disparities: Communication interventions.* New York, NY: Peter Lang.

Dutta, M., & Pal, M. (2010). Dialog theory in marginalized settings: A subaltern studies approach. *Communication Theory, 20,* 363–386.

Guha, R. (1981). *Subaltern studies I: Writings on South Asian history and society.* Delhi, India: Oxford University Press.

Guha, R. (1983). *Subaltern studies II: Writings on South Asian history and society.* Delhi, India: Oxford University Press.

Guha, R. (2001). Subaltern studies: Projects for our time and their convergence. In I. Rodríguez (Ed.), *The Latin American subaltern studies reader* (pp. 35–46). Durham, NC: Duke University Press.

Harvey, D. (2005). *A brief history of neoliberalism.* Oxford, UK: Oxford University Press.

Landry, D., & MacLean, G. (1996). *The Spivak reader: Selected works of Gayatri Chakravorty Spivak.* New York, NY: Routledge.

Mattingly, C. (1998). *Healing dramas and clinical plots: The narrative structure of experience.* Cambridge, UK: Cambridge University Press.

Nelson, N., & Wright, S. (1995). *Power and participatory development: Theory and practice.* London, UK: Intermediate Technology Publications.

Peterson, J. C. (2010). CBPR in Indian Country: Tensions and implications for health communication. *Health Communication, 25,* 50–60.

Rodriguez, R. M. (2010). *Migrants for export: How the Philippine state brokers labor to the world.* Minneapolis: University of Minnesota Press.

Spivak, G. C. (1988). Can the subaltern speak? In G. Nelson & L. Grossberg (Eds.), *Marxism and the interpretation of culture* (pp. 120–130). Champaign: University of Illinois Press.

Spivak, G. C. (1996). Bonding in difference: Interview with Alfred Arteaga. In D. Landry & G. MacLean (Eds.), *The Spivak reader: Selected works of Gayatri Chakravorty Spivak* (pp. 15–28). New York, NY: Routledge.

Spivak, G. C. (1999). *A critique of postcolonial reason: Toward a history of the vanishing present.* Cambridge, MA: Harvard University Press.

14

The Story Unfolds
Linking Complexities

Patricia Geist-Martin

International investment banker Azim Khamisa (1998) tells the story of the life-changing night in his life that fueled his commitment to establish and continue to serve in a nonprofit foundation devoted to stopping youth violence:

> On the night of January 21, 1995, an emotional nuclear bomb dropped on my life. . . . I had no way of knowing that January 21, 1995 marked the end of the life I had known, and that January 22 would usher in a terrifying new era. I had no way of knowing that my . . . only son, Tariq—a 20-year-old student at San Diego State University—was shot and killed while delivering pizza for an Italian restaurant in San Diego. . . . The last words Tariq uttered in this life were, "Help me! No! No!" The shot, through a rolled–up window, into a moving car, from the hand of an inexperienced gunman, could have gone anywhere. It could have missed completely. It could have inflicted an insignificant wound. But it didn't. It penetrated Tariq's shoulder, and continued through his left lung, then his heart, then his right lung. The car shuddered to a stop. The Black Mob ran down the street and disappeared. . . . In the Volkswagen, the pizzas and my son's body grew cold in the January night air. In his pocket, the delivery slip showed the amount due for the order: $27.24. (Khamisa, 1998, pp. 1, 2, 34–35)

The gunman, 14-year-old Tony Hicks, remains in prison as the youngest person to face criminal charges in California history at the time of his sentencing in 1995. Gang violence is an enduring epidemic in cities across the nation with serious consequences, and the epidemic of youth violence continues today. The most recent statistics on youths' deaths due to gun violence are offered by the Centers for Disease Control and Prevention (2012):

- In 2010, 4,828 young people ages 10 to 24 were victims of homicide—an average of 13 each day.

- Homicide is the 2nd leading cause of death for young people ages 15 to 24 years old.

- Among homicide victims 10 to 24 years old in 2010, 86% (4,171) were male and 14% (657) were female.
- Among homicide victims ages 10 to 24 years old in 2010, 82.8% were killed with a firearm.
- Each year, youth homicides and assault-related injuries result in an estimated $16 billion in combined medical and work loss costs.

However, gangs and violence against youths are not the only threats that citizens face in staying healthy and alive. Today, we live in a world where school shootings, community shootings, and police shootings are front-page news. December 14, 2015 marked the third anniversary of the tragedy at Sandy Hook Elementary School in Newtown, Connecticut, where 20-year-old shooter Adam Lanza killed 20 schoolchildren, six school staffers, his mother, and himself (Sandoval & Pearson, 2015). Unfortunately, this tragedy is one of many where young people have been murdered in school shootings.

The startling realities concerning guns and deaths in the United States include: (1) the U.S. leads the world in guns per capita, (2) U.S. gun violence kills significantly more people than terrorism, (3) mass shootings in the U.S. have tripled in the last three years, and (4) firearm deaths are one of the leading causes of death in the U.S. (behind heart disease and auto accidents) (Sanchez, 2015). A recent article suggests that more young Americans die from guns than cars:

> The United States is one of the greatest nations in the world. But compared to our peers, we're one of the worst when it comes to gun violence. In America, you can be shot at an elementary school. You can be murdered at a church or movie theatre. You can even be executed on live TV—and yet there's no real expectation of gun reform. Gun-related violence and death is a real public health problem in America. (Diamond, 2015a)

Diamond (2015b) indicates that while more than 32,000 people are killed each year by guns, and there is growing consensus that gun violence is a public health problem, not enough is being accomplished to address this health issue.

In one interview, U.S. Surgeon General Dr. Vivek Murthy highlights five crucial health issues facing Americans: gun violence, walkable neighborhoods, mental health, diet, and sleep (Gebreyes, 2015). The first one Dr. Murthy mentions is gun violence:

> Whenever you have large numbers of people who are dying for preventable reasons, that constitutes a public health issue. . . . In the past I've said that gun violence is a public health issue. That's not news to anybody that's worked in a hospital or visited a hospital. And I stand by that statement. (Gebreyes, 2015)

What does all of this mean for you? We have asked you to consider the ways you can better equip yourself to be a more effective health citizen and we have offered a wide range of stories to help you become more aware of the complexities, contexts, and competencies that communicating health and illness entail. If you listen *with* these stories, as Chapter 1 suggests, you can begin to equip yourselves with the competencies to enact your own health citizenry.

Throughout this book, we have invited our readers to consider the personal, cultural, and political complexities across lives and contexts (e.g., families, groups, clinics, organizations, and the public arena). We know that an expansive array of experiences and messages have formed, shaped, and molded who we are and what we believe about health. Each chapter in this book has asked you to consider just a few of the contexts or circumstances surrounding health or illness that may be communicated throughout your lifetime. We gain insight from the stories that everyday people tell others about their experience as patients, providers, or family members. We learn what people know or have learned about health and illness, their thoughts and feelings, and the ways communication has validated, invalidated, included, or excluded their views. We learn that our health and illness identities are powerfully and subtly embedded in ideas of how the world is and the way we are "supposed" to live our lives. But as well, we learn what it means to actively engage in health citizenry, including our conceptions of health status and medical care.

Think back, to all the changes you have experienced from childhood until now. Consider how communication with friends, parents, siblings, and even yourself (through journaling, art, music, or other forms of expression) figured prominently in your efforts to make sense of your changing identity. Take a moment to write the story asked for in Theorizing Practice 14.1.

Theorizing Practice 14.1
A Formative Life Passage

People go through an array of formative health-related life passages that they know in their heart have a tremendous impact on who they are, what they know and believe, and who they have become. Take a moment to write a story about just one of these formative life passages, featuring the communication that occurred as you moved through this life passage and how this one experience has impacted who you have become.

In this final chapter, I describe the Tariq Khamisa Foundation as an exemplar of the storied nature of health communication and how we can use these stories as currency for raising awareness about an important public health issue—in this case, gun violence. Next, I return to some of the *key themes* woven throughout each chapter. After that, I review some of the *competencies* that the chapters recommend in communicating health. Finally, I close with an invitation for you to consider your own *health citizenry* and the ways that you may communicate to become an advocate or activist for health—your own, your family's, or a community of strangers that you want to support. The story of the Tariq Khamisa Foundation (TKF), which began this chapter, offers an exemplar of *health activism*—a challenge to the existing prevalence of a health issue (i.e., gang violence) and the mission to change the status quo (reduce the number of deaths due to gang violence) (Zoller, 2005). As one form of health activism, taking action on a public health issue such as gun violence, focuses our attention on barriers to good health (Nathanson, 1999; Zoller, 2005).

■ TKF as Activist for the Public Health Issue of Gun Violence

The Tariq Khamisa Foundation (TKF), founded more than 20 years ago, has engaged in health activism by serving more than 500,000 youth in San Diego County, ages 10–15, through educational, mentoring, and community programs ("TKF celebrates," 2015). TKF believes that no one is born violent, and their programs are designed to empower children to make the right choices through communication competencies of nonviolence, empathy, compassion, forgiveness, and peacemaking.

To accomplish their mission, TKF has focused its effort on violence-prone communities and schools by developing a Safe School Model, Violence Impact Assemblies, community service programs promoting good citizenship, and mentorship programs. The practical results of this public health initiative are very real and tangible.

> TKF has consistently measured its programs and services to gauge results and adjust its methods to improve its outcomes. The positive impact over two decades tells the story. Among the students participating in TKF's mentoring programs, behavioral misconduct incidents were reduced 67 percent, and truancy by 72 percent. Ninety percent of the youth attending TKF's assemblies learn significant and lasting lessons about the consequences of violence. ("TKF celebrates," 2015)

The competencies of forgiveness and nonviolence are at the center of these lessons. The unique feature of all of TKF's efforts is the way in which it focuses on the stories that youth tell about the prevalence of violence in their families and the struggles they face in comprehending and living through and beyond the violence.

In a year-long investigation of PeaceWorks, one of TKF's semester-long middle school programs, researchers indicate that:

> Public health initiatives, such as TKF's PeaceWorks, promote healthy choices and nonviolent behaviors among our most vulnerable youth (e.g., youth who live and go to school in neighborhoods that have a record of violence or whose family situations may not provide healthy role models). We see, too, how the stories that the students tell each other become strategic resources for change. This is especially true when the teachers listen and learn from the stories, revisioning the role they can play in mobilizing each and every story students tell as a resource for moral reflection. (Miller, Geist-Martin, & Beatty, 2005, p. 313)

The research, focusing on classroom interaction in PeaceWorks, and the stories, poems, and letters that students wrote about their experience with violence, revealed that the narratives functioned in three ways:

> (1) as *deliberation* where teachers and students communicate in ways to invent new ways of thinking about and responding to violent episodes, (2) as *recognition* where teachers and students appreciate as valid and worthy the stories of violence that each has to tell, and (3) as *reclamation* where students and teachers communicate in ways to cultivate peace and forgiveness. (Miller et al., 2005, p. 316)

Clearly, the narratives that these youth write and speak through their participation in TKF's programs become an opportunity to negotiate the demanding moments and changing identities in their personal lives (Hanne, 1994) and to become activists for their own and others' health and well-being.

As I move to discuss some of the key themes in the book, I hope you will consider the complexities, contexts, and competencies that are part of your own stories of health and illness. And I hope that by the close of this chapter you have envisioned some bright spots and lessons in terms of your own health, important public health issues, and the need for change in health policy.

■ Reflecting on the Key Themes in the Book

The main premise of our book is that health and illness are storied experiences that necessarily entail personal, cultural, and political complexities. For all of us, communicating health and illness necessitates a continuous negotiation of these complexities and a delicate balance between what we learn from healthcare providers about the biology of illness and our own very personal, subjective experience of being ill.

One prominent theme woven throughout the book is the idea that now, more than ever, we are recognizing that our physical and psychological states of being are imbued with and complicated by social and cultural meanings that are communicated in our families, in our communities, and in public health information. Harrington (2008) emphasizes the need to move from a focus primarily on the symptoms of the body to an appreciation and understanding of the ways that the stories people tell offer an understanding of the complexities of health and illness. For example, in Chapter 4 we learn how interdisciplinary dialysis healthcare providers overcome barriers to communication by engaging in role blurring (i.e., flexible disciplinary boundaries) to offer patients encouragement and emotional support. Chapter 5, as another example, reveals how technology complicates communication between providers and patients, but at the same time offers them an opportunity to dialogue together about what they have learned in the digitized health environment.

A second and related theme presented in our book is that personal stories can raise social awareness, destigmatize disease, inspire or affect policy decisions, and highlight the many identities and roles that we can play as we embrace our role as health citizens. We use the term *citizen* throughout the book to convey this sense of universality among all members of a society, as well as the rights, responsibilities, and privileges that accompany such participation. One example of this theme can be found in Chapter 13, which describes the culture-centered approach (CCA) as an opportunity to learn from people who may be disenfranchised by poverty, health inequality, or health policies. In this way, the complexities of their lived experience offer insight into their perceptions of constraints on their health and the meanings they have for health, illness, treatment, and healing. A second example of this theme occurs in Chapter 8, which focuses our attention on the stigma and marginalization of people who are obese. The dialogue between Kelli, Cris, and Maggie helps to raise our awareness of how the language of the biomedical model of medicine marginalizes and stigmatizes people with different-sized bodies. We learn, too, that by communicating about healthy eating and physical fitness, rather than body size, we engage in health citizenry that may help to minimize the stigmatization and medicalization of fat.

A third theme woven into each chapter of the book is the necessity of thinking with the stories of health and illness that we and others tell. As Frank (1995) suggests: "To think about a story is to reduce it to content and then analyze that content. . . . To

HCIA 14.1

Is Breast Really Best?

Joan B. Wolf

When it comes to feeding your baby, the overwhelming message from doctors, researchers, and public health officials is that breast is best. Breastfeeding, we're told, protects against ear and respiratory infections, leukemia, heart disease, diabetes, and obesity, among other health problems. As they grow older, children who were breastfed are less likely to wet the bed. They are smarter and more socially mobile. They even make more money as adults.

The trouble is, the science behind breastfeeding's health benefits is dubious. Why, despite this weak evidence, have we become so convinced that breastfeeding is the greatest gift a mother can give her baby? In *Is Breast Best? Taking on the Breastfeeding Experts and the New High Stakes of Motherhood* (2011) I argue that we misunderstand breastfeeding (and so many other health issues) because we ignore three critical questions we should ask every time someone tells us how to be healthy.

What's causing what? Correlation, as the saying goes, does not equal causation. Here is the primary problem with breastfeeding research: Studies compare breastfed and formula-fed babies, but they don't explain sufficiently whether the environments in which these babies are raised are also different. For example, researchers know that women who are middle class or educated are more likely to breastfeed. So they try to figure out whether the health benefits that are linked with breastfeeding have more to do with economic or educational status than breast milk. And it turns out that the more researchers control for confounding variables—that is, the more they examine the environments in which feeding takes place—the less breastfeeding seems to make much of a difference.

Specifically, breastfeeding studies do not address whether breastfeeding mothers (and/or those with whom they share care) behave in other ways that might produce healthier children. If teenagers and adults who were breastfed are, on average, less obese, is it because they were breastfed or because their parents fed them less junk food and encouraged them to exercise? If they are more intelligent, is it because they were breastfed or because their parents talked and read with them and otherwise stimulated their intellectual development? If they have fewer respiratory infections, is it because they were breastfed? Or is it because their parents kept sick people from their homes, made sure that anyone who handled the baby had washed their hands, and avoided taking their baby grocery shopping when stores are packed with people?

In the developed world, most of the benefits linked to breastfeeding are small and could be explained by social environment. In fact, a careful reading of the evidence suggests that breastfeeding or bottle feeding makes little difference to the overwhelming majority of children in industrialized societies.

What are the trade-offs? Every choice has costs and benefits. Trade-offs are unavoidable, and behavior that reduces costs or risks in one domain is virtually always accompanied by increased costs or risks in another. This is no less true for health decisions. For example, extensive evidence demonstrates that many women feel guilted into breastfeeding and that the process often entails profound physical, emotional, and economic costs. Mothers who breastfeed when they'd rather not are more likely to be depressed, which is not healthy for them, their babies and families, or an economy that depends on functional workers. Mothers and fathers both complain that breastfeeding establishes a routine of "mommy first" that is difficult to overcome even after weaning. Research also indicates that women who breastfeed suffer significant reduction in their short- and long-term income and that mothers who are marginalized in the workforce because they care for babies and small children are at greater risk for economic hardship when they are older. If they divorce, both they and their children suffer.

Breast milk is packed with environmental pollutants. In fact, milk is such a good conduit for these pollutants that toxicologists often use it as a barometer of environmental contamination. But our current research tools do not enable us to determine the existence or extent of any long-term effects. In truth, we just don't know. Critics who argue that bottle-feeding mothers needlessly put their children in danger ignore that breastfeeding also comes with risks.

Who pays? Culturally, we tend to concern ourselves with risks to children that mothers can alleviate, and we pay little attention to the costs involved. We embrace a philosophy of "total motherhood" in which mothers are expected to prevent virtually *any* risk to their children, regardless of how unlikely or poorly understood that risk is or what it will cost them in the process. This is why so many people say that breastfeeding is free: because costs to mothers don't register.

Imagine if men had functioning mammary glands. Would breastfeeding seem as urgent? Or would we concede that its benefits are marginal, at best, and do not warrant the kind of disruption breastfeeding would bring to fathers' lives? Would we say that breastfeeding is free, or would we worry that it is too expensive?

There is no cost- or risk-free way to feed babies, or to be healthy. As consumers of health information, we would be wise to let go of the idea that we can make perfect health choices and instead figure out which unhealthy consequences we can accept.

QUESTIONS TO PONDER

1. Can you identify trade-offs in the choices you've made that you thought were completely healthy? How do you go about assessing risks and benefits of advice you're offered about health?

2. Whom or what do you consult to obtain credible information about health issues that are important to you? How willing are you to question these informational sources?

3. The research summarized for you in this feature is likely to contradict information you've heard or received from other authoritative sources. What are your responses and why? What happens when you hear contradictory health information and how do you try to make sense of the contradictions?

Source: Wolf, J. B. (2011). *Is breast best? Taking on the breastfeeding experts and the new high stakes of motherhood*. New York: New York University Press.

think with a story is to experience its affecting one's own life and to find in that effect a certain truth of one's life" (p. 23). In our book, we have invited you to think with the stories of individuals living with the inherent challenges and unexpected opportunities of other health-related situations, including addiction/mental illness (Chapter 1), aging (Chapter 2), cancer (Chapters 3 and 5), dialysis (Chapter 4), developmental disabilities (Chapter 6), sexual harassment (Chapter 7), obesity (Chapter 8), miscarriage (Chapter 9), alopecia (Chapter 10), breastfeeding (Chapter 11), politics of medical care reform (Chapter 12), health threats to immigrant workers (Chapter 13), and youth violence (Chapter 14). The stories offered in each chapter demonstrate that "storytelling is one of the most potent medicines at our disposal" (Bettencourt, 2015, preface).

So, the question is how do you make sense of the essential themes offered in our book and put these themes into practice? As Susan Sontag (1978) suggested, we all hold passports in the world of the well. In her words:

> Illness is the night-side of life, a more onerous citizenship. Everyone who is born holds dual citizenship, in the kingdom of the well and in the kingdom of the sick. Although we all prefer to use only the good passport, sooner or later each of us is obliged, at least for a spell, to identify ourselves as citizens of that other place. (p. 3)

Throughout our lifetimes we move back and forth between these worlds. Many of us find ourselves in a liminal, in-between state, when communication about our health or illness is disorienting, confusing, ambiguous, or even contradictory. Liminality can be experienced as a continual disruption when we have difficulty reconciling all the stories told—by providers, healers, family members, and ourselves (Honkasalo, 2001; Jackson, 2005). We move along this continuum of liminality, being ill and communicating toward wellness, or being well and communicating to maintain that state, or in some cases, fearing or perceiving illness or the onset of illness.

The Tibetan Buddhist religion has a concept known as *bardo,* which "literally means 'in between.' It indicates a number of transitional or liminal conditions" (Goss & Klass, 1997, p. 380). Elaborated in another source, *bardo* is a transition or gap between the completion of one situation and the onset of another that are occurring continuously and "are junctures when the possibility of liberation, or enlightenment is heightened" (Rinpoche, 1993, p. 99). Interestingly, bardo in the context of life and death, "helps the living to resolve their grief by focusing on their providing spiritual assistance to the deceased" (Goss & Klass, 1997, p. 393). In our day-to-day lives, embracing the meaning of bardo encourages people to take action, to engage in a citizenry that moves them from a focus on the grief that they may find disabling or paralyzing to a focus on the present moment and moving forward to the future.

If we consider bardo as something that happens to all of us, all the time—in health and illness, not just after the death of someone, then bardo "can be applied to every moment of existence. The present moment, the now, is a continual bardo, always suspended between the past and the future" (Fremantle, 2001, p. 54). Enacting our own health citizenry on a daily basis, we encounter moments of bardo—not feeling well physically, mentally, socially, spiritually, or ecologically—and in this suspension between illness and wellness, we communicate to move forward to well-being. We may not always resolve this liminality, but we can enact a citizenry that allows us to engage with supportive communities to construct a story of health and well-being, as Charlie and his family did in Chapter 10, drawing support from the gymnastic community to advocate for him. As well, in Chapter 9, Elissa and Jay moved through a bardo as they navigated communication with providers, family, and friends in the challenges of pregnancy, miscarriage, and transitions. Health citizenry therefore necessarily invokes not only the personal complexities but as well the political and cultural complexities that surround and propel or paralyze us.

Our book is designed to offer a wealth of information about health communication so that you can make healthy choices for yourself, your family and friends, and your communities. Chapter 1 introduced you to the concept of *communication competencies*—the combinations of knowledge and skills that are aimed at helping you to become a dynamic health citizen in a number of different contexts. These skills could include focusing on the *process* of communicating about health and illness with providers and family, as well as developing a self-efficacy in negotiating what you need or want in your health and illness care (Parrott, 2004). We hope our book offers you strategies for strengthening these competencies in the face of the personal, cultural, and political complexities that may impede your efforts to enact your own health citizenry.

■ Developing Competencies in Communicating Health

The complexities we face throughout our lives in communicating through health and illness demand a wide range of communication competencies. First, competencies can be something that people construct individually. For example, a by-product of health activism is the perception of *self-empowerment*, which is a feeling of being more powerful and in control of our own lives because we have chosen to devote time, energy, and resources to bettering the health-related problems that impact us. Conversely, *disempowerment* is the feeling of having little or no control, that our lives are being determined by other people or circumstances beyond our influence. So we define competencies as something you construct and practice individually in your communication about health and illness with others. As well, we see competencies in the ways we communicate collaboratively with others to translate competencies to activism. Zoller (2005) suggests that health activism can be constructed in three illness-focused categories: "(a) medical care access and improvement, (b) illness and disability activism, and (c) public health promotion and disease prevention activism" (p. 348).

Consider for a moment the health communication competencies you have developed and learned about through this text. What are they? Have you practiced these competencies in ways that inspired you to take action? What competencies do you want to develop? In the next sections, I offer a review of the competencies presented in this text, the ways that practicing these competencies can inspire others to practice them, and a discussion of competencies in action as they are collaboratively constructed in communities.

Health Communication Competencies Presented in this Text

Throughout this text, we have highlighted a wide range of *competencies* aimed at enabling you to better navigate the healthcare system and to become an effective health citizen. Through Elizabeth's story in Chapter 1 we learn the importance of *honoring* people's stories and resisting the temptation to stigmatize or silence their voices. Hilda and Gene's story in Chapter 2 reveals the intricate and compelling difficulties of aging, but as well, we learn the competency of *appreciating* life, in spite of health limitations, and *resisting* the stereotype of aging as decline. In Chapter 3, we learn from Hannah's story the competency of *persisting* in gathering health information and searching for a physician that meets her needs. The collaboration of the dialysis team in Chapter 4 highlights the competency of *listening* and being open to new ideas. Joe and Jane's story in Chapter 5 opens our eyes to the competency of *realizing* the value of digital and personal support on the wellness trail. The story of the participants in Collaborative Art International (CAI) in Chapter 6 shows the competency of *connecting* with others through artistic expression. Allyson's story in Chapter 7 reveals the ways that work environments can become toxic and unhealthy and the competency of *organizing* sources of information and support. The conversation between Kelli, Cris, and Maggie in Chapter 8 uncovers the competency of *incorporating* diverse meanings for health represented in biodiversity and *resisting* the stereotypes that often accompany different body sizes. Elissa and Jay's story, in Chapter 9, of the challenges of coping with loss and grief reveals the competency of *supporting* in their relationship with one another and in the community of providers, friends, and family. Charlie's story in Chapter 10 indicates the importance of *assembling* community support in resisting stigma and *finding empowerment* in a personal definition of health. Chapter 11 presents information about health campaigns and develops the competency of *evaluating* that information in making decisions about our health behaviors. Chapter 12 offers the story of *deliberating* the political complexities of our taken-for granted assumptions about health and illness, including the role of communication in medical care reform. Maria's story in Chapter 13 engages us in the competencies of *resistance, solidarity, and reflexivity* when addressing health disparities and disenfranchised communities through a culture-centered approach.

In this final chapter, we ask you to consider this collection of competencies that may improve your own sense of empowerment and activism across health contexts. While each chapter in this text offers a unique set of competencies, the underlying theme is empowering individuals to move in some way along a path to health and healing, in some cases against all odds. We also learn that individual empowerment ripples out to others in powerful ways, as individuals and organizations inspire others to practice health competencies.

Inspiring Others as a Health Competency

One of the missions of TKF is to inspire others to practice nonviolence and forgiveness. The competencies that TKF teaches in schools whose neighborhoods have a history of violence include enhancing communication skills, teaching problem-solving skills, discussing consequences, promoting healthy decision making, encouraging civic engagement, and providing adult role models (www.tkf.org). The founder of TKF, Azim Khamisa, has a powerful impact wherever he speaks, and he has met with leaders throughout the world to share his message of forgiveness and peace, including the Pope, the Dalai Lama, and President Obama. Every semester that Azim comes to San Diego State University to share his message of forgiveness to the students (100–170 in number) enrolled in Introduction to Health Communication, he inspires students to take action and practice new competencies, as the three stories from students reveal:

> When I was listening to him, I was thinking about an old friend. We had a falling out a few years ago and neither of us were ready to forgive one another. In hearing Mr. Khamisa's story, it really encouraged me to reach out to my friend and forget the petty thing we had been holding grudges over. I came to the realization that life is too short and it truly is not worth it to stress over small things. If Mr. Khamisa could forgive and love someone who did something terrible to him, then I can certainly forgive an old friend. (Kyra)

> Azim Khamisa is one of the most inspiring people I have ever had the pleasure of meeting. He lost his son, yet he stands in front of us and tells us that this was his

spiritual purpose. I had not given substantial thought to violence in our society, but after hearing him speak, I was enlightened. I will never be violent to another human being, because if Azim could avoid violence after his son was shot, then anyone can. His story is heartbreaking, but his work is inspiring. I aspire to be like him, and his words have touched me deeply. (Cole)

My favorite part of Mr. Khamisa's presentation was his gentle spirit. The entire class felt like a wave of peacefulness washed over us when he was in the room. I liked that he brought to our awareness that violence is very much a learned behavior so nonviolence can also be learned; we just have to teach it. I liked that I felt like I could go out and help change the world—and I can, just starting with myself. I can practice nonviolence and self-forgiveness and show people, as Mr. Khamisa did, that once you do it for yourself you will experience a more satisfying life. The line that stuck with me the most from his presentation was "spirit is mightier than intellect and emotion." I do agree with him, everything starts from what's within you. You, yourself have to make changes in your life to be happy and at peace. (Samantha)

These are just a few of the powerful stories that students tell of competencies they are developing and how they are inspired to action by Azim's message. Interestingly, it was Azim Khamisa's story that inspired Megan Bettencourt (2015) to write the book *Triumph of the Heart: Forgiveness in an Unforgiving World.* Here's how she told the story of her curiosity and her inspiration:

In early 2012, I found myself writing a magazine story about a remarkable man. Seventeen years earlier, Azim Khamisa was working as an international investment banker based in San Diego when his only son, a college student working a pizza delivery job, was shot to death by an aspiring teenaged gang member. . . . I wanted to know why he forgave. I wanted to know how. And I wanted to know what it meant—for him, for me, for all of us. I was intrigued, if more than a little unsettled, for reasons I couldn't quite identify. Forgiveness had never been my forte, nor my aspiration. If I thought of forgiveness at all, I did so with distain, as something weak and almost pathetic. . . . Sometimes it takes a powerful story to take you out of your own and set you on a new, better path. . . . Over the past twenty years, multiple studies have shown that forgiveness can indeed improve physical and emotional well-being, and that it may even be a crucial survival skill developed throughout human evolution. Wanting to learn more, I embarked on an inward and outward adventure. (Bettencourt, 2015, pp. xi, xxi)

And the result of that adventure was her book. In the end, she tells us that "through developing our innate ability to seek and grant forgiveness, we can bolster our health and happiness, improve our relationships, and maybe even make the world a more peaceful place" (Bettencourt, 2015, p. xxii). Extensive research has provided evidence of a link between practicing forgiveness and improving health status (Rey & Extremera, 2015; Row, 2008; Svalina, 2012; Toussaint, Owen, & Cheadle, 2011; Webb, 2013; Webb, Toussaint, & Conway-Williams, 2012; Worthington, 2007; Worthington, Van Oyen Witvliet, Pietrini, & Miller, 2007).

Embracing a similar communication competency of forgiveness, for a much longer period of time is Eva Mozes Kor, who, along with her twin Miriam, at the age of 10 were taken to Auschwitz and subjected to the horror of medical experimentation by Dr. Josef Mengele. Both survived, but Miriam died in 1993 of bladder cancer, as a consequence of the experiments. Eva contributed her story to The Forgiveness Project (www.theforgivenessproject.com), a nonprofit founded in 2004 as an opportunity for people to tell their stories of their quest for restoration and healing in response to being harmed. In the words of the founder Marina Cantacuzino, who has since published a book about forgiveness (Cantacuzino, 2015), "The stories reflect the complex, intriguing and deeply personal nature of forgiveness, occupying a space of inquiry and authenticity rather than dogma or the need to fix it." The story that Eva Kor has told throughout the world since her speech in 1995, at the anniversary of the liberation of Auschwitz, is one that focuses on the healing power of forgiveness. In Eva's words:

> Forgiveness is really nothing more than an act of self-healing and self-empowerment. I call it a miracle medicine. It is free, it works, and has no side effects. I believe with every fiber of my being that every human being has the right to live without the pain of the past. For most people there is a big obstacle to forgiveness because society expects revenge. It seems we need to honor our victims but I always wonder if my dead loved ones would want me to live with pain and anger until the end of my life. Some survivors do not want to let go of the pain. They call me a traitor and accuse me of talking in their name. I have never done this. Forgiveness is as personal as chemotherapy—I do it for myself. (Cantacuzino, 2015, pp. 37–38)

Consider for a moment your own competency of communicating empowerment by answering the questions in Theorizing Practice 14.2.

Theorizing Practice 14.2
Empowerment as Medicine

Describe a situation in which you have felt disempowered. What happened to make you feel this way? Is there anything you would have chosen to say or do differently that might change the situation for the better?

Now, describe a health-related situation in which you have felt empowered. What factors helped you to feel this way? What actions did you choose to take? What impact did the feeling of empowerment have on your health? Do you continue to feel empowered? If not, why?

Azim, Megan, and Eva inspire others to practice forgiveness. Nonprofits throughout the nation do the same, inspiring communities to engage and practice a wide range of health competencies, as the next section reveals.

■ Competencies in Action: Collaboratively Constructed Health in Communities

Health communication competencies may extend beyond the individual to become something that individuals create in community with others. As a result of a complex combination of social, political, and economic factors that include the

The Meaning of Active Health Participation

Barbara F. Sharf

I want you to put me in the grave with all my limbs.

That is the personal objective that Gina, a 34-year-old woman from Louisiana, shared with Dr. Winner, an endocrinologist she was seeing for the first time. Gina, who had recently moved to Houston for work, comes from a large, extended family in which virtually every relative has diabetes. She had witnessed parents, grandparents, aunts, and uncles who have blindness, heart problems, and multiple amputations as a result of the "family curse"; within the family, such dire consequences were considered inevitable, with no possibility of alternative outcomes. Having just found out that she too was now diagnosed with the same affliction, she was the first in her family to seek out a specialist and aim for a different outcome.

My goal here is to be in the best health possible . . . and if that means dying early by age 60, that's fine, just so I can have all my limbs. In my mind, I was being an optimist. . . . He said, "OK, I understand, but I don't think it has to be that way." The second time I saw Dr. Winner, I made up my mind that he is my doctor.

Gina was one of 16 patients we interviewed about living with a chronic illness in order to better understand two interrelated questions: What does it mean to be an "active/engaged" patient? and How does collaborative patient–provider communication occur in real time? Her story provides a good illustration of a model of active healthcare participation, resulting from our analysis of the interview data. The model consists of four themes, two attitudinal and two behavioral, that we depicted as dynamic continuums. Based on each participant's narrative elicited through the interview, we were able to map the individual within each continuum, resulting in a uniquely complex portrait of what active participation means for that person. While some had been constant within these continuums for years, for Gina and others, it was clear that their current positions had evolved over time, and were likely to continue changing. The four continuums include:

- **Centrality of illness,** how central the illness is in the individual's overall life story, ranging from peripheral to central.

- **Changeability of outcome,** how changeable the person believes the illness to be, ranging from fatalistic (resigned to whatever fate may await rather than seek alternatives) to changeable.

- **Engagement with illness,** the degree of illness-related activity a person engages in, ranging from passive to fully engaged.

- **Patient-Provider collaboration,** the role of partnership a person has with his or her healthcare provider in decision making and illness management, ranging from absolute patient control to absolute physician control with shared control as a midpoint.

As Gina continued with her illness narrative, she described her frustrations with family members who do nothing to improve the quality of their health, including responses to their doctors.

When the doctor tells my family something, they accept it for gold. You know, there's no questioning. I will question it.

(continued)

She also detailed her personal struggle with aspects of cultural upbringing that compromise her health:

> We're from Louisiana. In that area of the country, food and wine will probably be the top two vices for anybody.... I look at a list of things that they recommend that people should not eat in general and things that diabetics should not eat.... If you put those two lists together, everything on them is what we eat on a regular basis in our family.

The difference that Dr. Winner has made in Gina's story is helping her to envision a different outcome for herself.

> Usually, I would say that I am controlled by food and wine because I don't have the will power, but now the control is with Dr. Winner because he has information on his side and has been giving me better medications.

She described how he recognized her natural competitiveness, and encouraged her to make her walk to the parking lot a competitive event alongside other pedestrians, thus increasing her daily exercise efforts. In effect, Dr. Winner is collaborating with Gina to re-emplot her story and particularly to help her imagine a more empowered role for herself and a better ending. Returning to the four continuums, here is how we mapped her story:

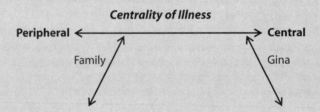

Diabetes affects everything I do; it's become a major part of my life.

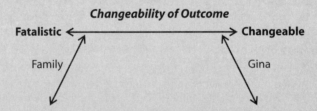

All I wanted to do was to try to correct it, and see if there was anything we could reverse... thought, "I don't want to be like everyone else."

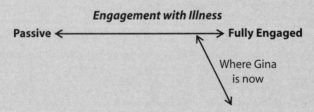

Because it's my disease, I have it. I should be the one because I have the capabilities ... to monitor my disease.

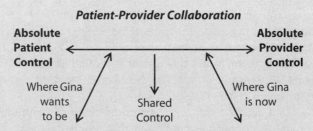

Patient-Provider Collaboration

> *We'll work back and forth. I still ask questions. He still gives me information he thinks is useful and will help me. But right now, he has to prod me, because I don't have control at the other end.*

In sum, Gina made considerable progress as an active patient by redefining her life goals in relation to diabetes, choosing to prioritize Dr. Winner's advice, asking questions and monitoring her health, and making lifestyle changes.

> *Because Dr. Winner and I work so closely together now, in the future I think I will have more control over the diabetes, which is very important to me. You probably can tell that I'm kind of a control freak. In the future, I will be able to be a major player in fighting the diabetes.*

QUESTIONS TO PONDER

1. Think back to your most recent significant visit with a healthcare provider, and consider your role in this interaction. Specifically,

   - Did you feel free to talk about your concerns?

   - Who spoke first?

   - Who spoke more often?

   - Did you plan in advance for this conversation or write down questions you wanted answered? Was the plan followed, questions answered?

   - Did the provider really listen to you?

   - At the end, were there still unvoiced issues?

2. How actively do you participate in the management of your own healthcare? Thinking of a personal chronic (continuing) health concern, map where you are along the four continuums and, if applicable, where you are now and where you may aspire to be. What does this exercise reveal about your own meanings and feelings concerning active participation?

3. What do you think are the benefits and outcomes of active healthcare participation? Might there be some drawbacks? Try to think of some specific examples.

Sources: Sharf, B. F., Haidet, P., & Kroll, T. L. (2005). "I want you to put me in the grave with all my limbs": The meaning of active health participation. In E. B. Ray (Ed.), *Health communication in practice* (pp. 39–51). Mahwah, NJ: Erlbaum. Haidet, P., Kroll, T. L., & Sharf, B. F. (2006). The complexity of patient participation: Lessons learned from patients' illness narratives. *Patient Education & Counseling, 62,* 323–329.

increasing shift of care of chronic illnesses to the home, bureaucratization of health-care systems, availability of health-related information through a variety of mass media, and questioning attitudes toward biomedical authority, patients as a group have concurrently assumed greater responsibility and voice concerning healthcare decisions affecting them. What this means is that an essential competency is to take some responsibility for our own active, health participation and not assume that our healthcare providers deliver it to us.

The idea that health communication competency is community-based is realized through the many nonprofits mentioned throughout our text. Each chapter offers insight into the ways that individuals rally together and create change.

National movements and nonprofits have sprung up across the nation in response to school shootings and other forms of youth violence. *Sandy Hook Promise*, in response to the two million acts of violence in schools, is devoted to building a national move-ment of parents, schools, and community organizations "engaged and empowered to deliver gun violence prevent programs and mobilize for the passage of sensible state and national policy" (http://www.sandyhookpromise.org/about#mission). Their website describes how this movement began:

> *Sandy Hook Promise* (SHP) was formed in the days immediately following the trag-edy at Sandy Hook Elementary School where 20 first graders and six adults were killed. From the moment it was formed, the goal was to create an organization for family members, if they chose, to have a platform to lead the change they wanted to see so that no other parent experiences the senseless, horrific loss of their child. (www.sandyhookpromise.org/how_was_sandy_hook_promise_formed)

In their view, it is not about guns; it is about mental illness. They emphasize that mental wellness involves competencies of coping skills, anger management, and other social-emotional skills; they suggest that most criminal gun violence is committed by individuals who lack mental wellness. Through Elizabeth's story in Chapter 1, we learned how often communicating about mental illness is stigmatized and that cul-tural conceptions of mental illness perpetuate secrecy and shame. As Yamasaki (Chapter 1) indicates, "More voices are calling for change in the way we think about, treat, and manage these disorders" (see p. 16); in this way, we can address the per-sonal, cultural, and political complexities surrounding mental illness that might help us to address the disorders before they lead to violence to self or others. As well, Chapter 6, which explores health and healing through art, stands in opposition to a deficit model of care, empowering participants by offering them opportunities to express through art what they find difficult or impossible to communicate.

One organization is taking steps to make visible in the community what is often invisible about social isolation, bullying, and in some cases violence. *Beyond Differences* is a student-led organization that trains high school students to go to middle schools to tell their stories of social isolation, which they see as an overlooked form of bullying. Ace Smith and Laura Talmus founded the organization after the passing of their daughter, who suffered from Apert Syndrome (premature fusing of certain skull bones), and from social isolation—she was often treated as if she were invisible. The organization focuses on building competencies of social inclusion through such programs as "No one eats alone," "Be kind online," and "Be the one" to speak up and include.

A second example of the way that communities can rally around a health cause is through nonprofit activism and advocacy. A charity saloon in Houston called OKRA (www.friedokra.org), which is run by "a collection of some of the city's best-known bars and restaurants" (Lozano, 2013), has become very popular as a way to give back. Each month, OKRA features four local charities that compete all month for votes (each drink buys a customer one vote). OKRA's bars and restaurant promote the stories of the four charities all month in various ways (social media, in-house presence) to rally for votes. The winning charity gets all proceeds the following month ($10,000–$40,000). OKRA bills itself as an advocacy group that enables its fellow community members an opportunity to be heard. The narrative ties activism and health citizenry together by emphasizing the storied voices of the members and volunteers of each organization. The benefits for one nonprofit are described in this way:

> For *A Simple Thread*, a small Houston nonprofit that distributes kits with everyday items such as socks, toothbrushes and books to homeless individuals, the $16,000 it got from the OKRA Charity Saloon allowed the group to do more. But it also empowered its volunteers, whose presence at the bar every day during the month it competed, helped convince many customers to vote for them. (Lozano, 2013)

The emphasis is on not only supporting nonprofit community organizations through fundraising, but also through its promotion, awareness, and empowerment. Each restaurant collaborates with the nonprofits to focus all attention on the charities each month. OKRA is a new concept for charitable organizing that is being developed in other states and countries, as well (Lozano, 2013).

A third example of the ways that communities can rally around a health cause is the Westside Health Authority (WHA) in Chicago. The West Side of Chicago contains neighborhoods with dilapidated buildings and overgrown vacant lots, drug dealers, gang warfare, a high crime rate, broken sidewalks, and rutted streets. Its discouraging health statistics include high infant mortality, low-birth-weight babies, teen mothers, and higher rates of sexually transmitted diseases, AIDS, and tuberculosis than the rest of the city. This is a deficit-, problem-focused description of this community.

In opposition to this typical emphasis on deficits, researchers emphasized assets and capacity-building (Kretzmann & McKnight, 1993; McKnight, 1995). Community resident and WHA founder, Jacqueline Reed, supported this perspective (see healthauthority.org/). Her plan mobilized the community by organizing block leadership; creating networks for employment opportunities, childcare, and transportation; and reaffirming community values and standards. WHA accomplishments over the past decade have included raising the funds necessary to purchase a neighborhood hospital that had closed; helping place nearly 300 young people in health career opportunities; helping local businesses gain access to potential hospital contracts; and reducing neighborhood violence by an impressive 20%.

In one of its newest initiatives called *Every Block a Village Online,* WHA has focused on Austin, one of its poorest, most troubled neighborhoods. The goals of this program include: (1) reducing maternal medical risk factors that complicate pregnancy, (2) reducing the proportion of low-birth-weight infants, (3) increasing first trimester initiation of prenatal care, (4) reducing emergency department visits through increased access to primary care, and (5) reducing annual crime (http://www.ebvonline.org/).

Supplying each block leader with a Web TV and a series of Web pages, "community members can provide information to others on their block, teach each other new skills, and become connected with other communities around the world" (ebvonline.org/faqs1.htm). Despite a litany of serious challenges facing this community, the program also recognizes a variety of assets including established, supportive block clubs and an array of educated, respected professionals in the area. In other words, while Austin has many social problems and a lack of material assets, it is rich in "human capital."

Using a capacities model of community development, and communication strategies that include local leadership development and recognition, personal networking, and computer interaction, the WHA is a successful role model of self-empowerment through community interaction: "This is not a question of holding hands out; it is the reality of holding hands together."

The fact that healthcare issues have emerged as some of the most prominent political themes and community activism over the past decade should come as no surprise to any of us. Topics that continue to be debated often focus on healthcare economics, include preserving choice of providers, access to primary and specialty care, economic availability of needed prescription medicines, continuity of care, provision of quality assurance standards, nondiscrimination in delivery of services, fair appeals mechanisms for healthcare denials, protection of patient confidentiality, and accountability of managed care organizations for patient outcomes (see www.senate.gov/). Often the issues and perspectives that take front and center stage often emanate from grassroots health communities, where ordinary citizens communicate with one another, create a movement to focus their advocacy on a particular health issue, and often end up influencing health policy.

One example of health advocacy is the updated International Symbol of Access (Chokshi, 2015; Young, 2015). The original image of a stick figure sitting in a wheelchair, designed in 1968 by a Danish art student, has been redesigned to depict the stick figure leaning forward in the wheelchair. The new image has generated controversy with some who think the image represents "Paralympic athletes, wheelchair races and speedy movements," while others suggest that the updated logo "is a metaphor for rethinking the enormously complex issue of how we treat people with disabilities" (Young, 2015).

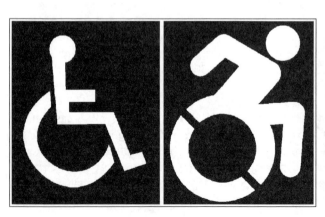

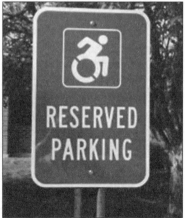

New York State has put into place the new symbol, and cities in Arizona, Texas, Massachusetts, and Connecticut are following the trend. Connecticut lawmakers want to replace the word "handicapped" with "reserved," and a disabilities nonprofit, the *Arch of Farmington Valley,* has put forward a new campaign to go with the rollout, which would state: "Change the sign. Change the attitude" (Young, 2015). The icon's graphic elements, including head position, arm angle, wheel cutouts, limb rendition, and leg position represent the metaphor "for taking action and rethinking disability" (Chokshi, 2014).

One of the most prominent examples of community activism has occurred among patients and providers with the campaign for death with dignity and the accompanying new state laws that have offered "physician assisted suicide," "compassionate choices," "Aid in Dying," and most recently the "End of Life Option Act"—all different names for the individual's choice to end his or her life when faced with a terminal or degenerative illness. While our book talks most about the choices individuals and communities make to communicate in ways to improve health, this competency focuses on individual, community, and organizational efforts to help people plan for and achieve a more dignified death. The nonprofit *Compassion and Choices* describes their mission as: "We work to change attitudes, practices and policies so that everyone can access the information and options they need to have more control and comfort at the end of life" (https://www.compassionandchoices.org/what-we-do/).

Twenty-nine-year-old Brittany Maynard became the emblem of this activism for a "good death." While Brittany's choice was a personal, individual example of empowerment as a key health competency, she wanted more. Before she died, she worked with the nonprofit *Compassion and Choices* to tell her story. Through Brittany's cooperation, The Brittany Maynard Fund was established as a website that offers an opportunity for people to learn about death with dignity, as well as opportunities to take action and donate money to the cause. The website offers a brief description of the steps Brittany and her family took to assist her in her choice to die with dignity:

> In the spring of 2014, 29-year-old Brittany Maynard learned that she had terminal brain cancer. After careful assessment of her prognosis and end-of-life options, she and her family reluctantly decided to move from their San Francisco Bay Area home to Oregon, one of five states (including Washington, Montana, Vermont, and New Mexico) that authorized death with dignity at the time. Aid in dying was legalized in California in October 2015.
>
> Brittany agreed to be interviewed on film regarding death with dignity because of her strong belief in the ethics of this basic healthcare and human right. Her first video, posted to TheBrittanyFund.org on October 6, 2014, was viewed more than 9 million times in its first month. Every member of the Compassion & Choices team was humbled by Brittany's courage and generosity, and continues striving to honor her gift to the end-of-life choice movement. Brittany Maynard's voice and her story did more than she could have known to advance end-of-life options and aid in dying across the country. It is a legacy to be proud of. (http://thebrittanyfund.org/about/)

Oregon's Death with Dignity Act was the first in the nation. The Oregon government website describes the act in this way: "On October 27, 1997, Oregon enacted the Death with Dignity Act which allows terminally-ill Oregonians to end their lives through the voluntary self-administration of lethal medications, expressly prescribed by a physi-

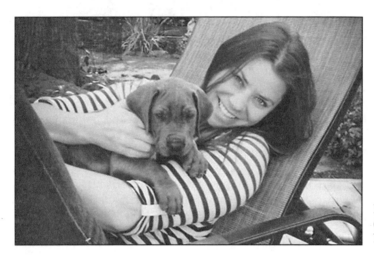

Brittany Maynard
(November 19, 1984–
November 1, 2014).

cian for that purpose" (https://public.health.oregon.gov/ProviderPartnerResources/EvaluationResearch/DeathwithDignityAct/Pages/index.aspx).

Individuals develop health communication competencies first and foremost through their stories. Your personal stories are a way for you to put into words your own suffering and the actions you feel you can or cannot take to relieve that suffering. As well, your stories may describe your joyful discoveries on your illness/wellness path. Often in that process of communicating your stories, you discover that you are not alone in your suffering and/or joy, and your individual competencies morph into citizenry and activism. Brittany Maynard's story is just one of many that represent personal empowerment constructed through resistance to cultural and political complexities. We hope that our text inspires you to tell your stories of health and illness and to discover the ways you are not alone—and even be compelled, like Brittany, to contribute to a community of activists for a personal cause.

Finally, we close this chapter with an invitation for you to consider your own *health citizenry* and the ways you may communicate to become an advocate or activist for health—your own, your family's and friends', or a community of strangers that you want to support. Now, after you've read the text, we hope you have envisioned some bright spots and lessons in terms of your own health, important public health issues, and the need for changes in health policy. We hope that today or in the near future you find the courage to name your own suffering or your desire to live life differently in some small or big way. As Siddhartha Mukherjee (2011), Pulitzer Prize winning author of *The Emperor of all Maladies: A Biography of Cancer*, suggests:

> To name an illness is to describe a certain condition of suffering—a literary act before it becomes a medical one. A patient, long before he [she] becomes the subject of medical scrutiny, is, at first, simply a storyteller, a narrator of suffering—a traveler who has visited the kingdom of the ill. To relieve an illness, one must begin, then by unburdening the story. (Mukherjee, 2011, 46)

We invite each of you to narrate your own suffering that in some ways restricts you from traveling with the passport for the Kingdom of the Well. And then in that

Kingdom of the Well, we hope that you enact the communication competencies that help you to construct a health citizenry for yourself and others.

■ Epilogue

As the murder case against Tony Hicks unfolded, and more information was gained about the 14-year-old, we begin to understand what the father of the victim, Azim Khamisa, meant when he stated, "There were victims at both ends of the gun." Children and adolescents like Tony, and even Tariq, are people without the life experience of adults. Like any other people, though, they move through life passages experiencing profound and formative biological, psychological, social, and spiritual changes. On a day-to-day basis they interact with "authorities" (e.g., parents, teachers, health professionals, grandparents, older siblings, or gang members), family, and friends in diverse contexts (e.g., home, preschool, school, clubs, athletic teams, homes of family and friends, providers' offices) who offer advice and support or, in some cases, communicate mandates concerning healthy and unhealthy behaviors. Throughout their lifetimes, children and adolescents may find themselves considering, resisting, and learning from the stories that others offer concerning "what is good for them," "what is the best medicine," what risks they might encounter if they do not heed the advice of these authorities, and what they can do to make good decisions for their own and others' well-being.

■ Conclusion

In this final chapter we have focused on the story of the formation of TKF, a foundation advocating for community and school efforts to teach nonviolence, forgiveness, and peace to eliminate youth violence (Khamisa, 1998, 2007, 2014; Khamisa & Quinn, 2009). Linking his story to personal, cultural, and political complexities that individuals and communities face in eliminating youth violence, Azim has become a health advocate, traveling throughout the world to spread the message of forgiveness. We have asked you to reflect on the health communication themes that have been offered throughout the book, and we have invited you to appreciate and practice the competencies that are important for communicating health. As health citizens, you can coordinate your own health information and advocate for yourselves and others as you navigate a wide range of health contexts. As members of communities, all of us can benefit by framing health issues within a capacities perspective, rather than a deficit perspective. At the macrolevel of health advocacy, individual citizens work together to formulate strategies of influence, develop interpersonal and organizational networks, build leadership, and affect policy decisions.

Discussion Questions

1. Have you experienced an incident in your life where you "went along with the crowd" doing something unhealthy, even though you knew it would detract from your health?

2. Have you experienced some type of tragedy in your life that led you to take action that contributed to your own or another's health?

3. Is there someone in your life who you have had difficulty forgiving for something he or she said or did? What changes do you think might occur if you were to forgive that person? (Consider what has happened to Azim when he forgave Tony.)

4. What health competencies do you feel you have practiced in your life? Did you learn them on your own or did someone teach them to you?

5. If you were to put into practice one change in the way you approach health or illness, what would it be? Who or what would be an obstacle to that change? Who or what might support you and help you put that change into practice?

REFERENCES

Bettencourt, M. F. (2015). *Triumph of the heart: Forgiveness in an unforgiving world.* New York, NY: Hudson Street Press.

Cantacuzino, M. (2015). *The forgiveness project: Stories for a vengeful age.* Philadelphia, PA: Jessica Kingsley Publishers.

Centers for Disease Control and Prevention. (CDC, 2012). Injury prevention & control: Data & statistics (WISQARS™). Retrieved from http://www.cdc.gov/injury/wisqars/fatal_injury_reports.html

Chokshi, N. (2014, July 29). The handicap symbol gets an update—at least in New York State. *The Washington Post.* Retrieved from https://www.washingtonpost.com/blogs/govbeat/wp/2014/07/29/the-handicap-symbol-gets-an-update-at-least-in-new-york-state/

Diamond, D. (2015a, August 26). More young Americans now die from guns than cars. *Forbes.* Retrieved from http://www.forbes.com/sites/dandiamond/2015/08/26/americas-gun-violence-problem-in-three-charts/#5cf9e8ab58b7

Diamond, D. (2015b, October 1). How to reduce gun violence: Treat it as a public health problem. *Forbes.* Retrieved from http://www.forbes.com/sites/dandiamond/2015/10/01/gun-violence-is-a-public-health-problem-heres-why/#1f9b54d24c86

Frank, A. (1995). *The wounded storyteller: Body, illness, and ethics.* Chicago, IL: University of Chicago Press.

Freemantle, F. (2001). *Luminous emptiness: Understanding the* Tibetan Book of the Dead. Boston, MA: Shambhala.

Gebreyes, R. (2015, September 15). Surgeon General Vivek Murthy highlights 5 crucial health issues facing Americans. *HuffingtonPost Healthy Living.* Retrieved from http://www.huffingtonpost.com/entry/surgeon-general-vivek-murthy_us_55f67ab7e4b042295e36b2d1

Goss, R. E., & Klass, D. (1997). Tibetan Buddhism and the resolution of grief: The *Bardo-thodol* for the dying and the grieving. *Death Studies, 21,* 377–395.

Hanne, M. (1994). *The power of the story: Fiction and political change.* Providence, RI: Berghahn Books.

Harrington, A. (2008). *The cure within: A history of mind-body medicine.* New York, NY: Norton.

Honkasalo, M. (2001). Vicissitudes of pain and suffering: Chronic pain and liminality. *Medical Anthropology, 19,* 319–353.

Jackson, J. E. (2005). Stigma, liminality, and chronic pain: Mind-body borderlands. *American Ethnologist, 32,* 332–353.

Khamisa, A. (1998). *Azim's bardo: From murder to forgiveness.* La Jolla, CA: ANK Publishing.

Khamisa, A. (2007). *From forgiveness to fulfillment.* Bend, OR: Rising Star Press.

Khamisa, A. (2014). *From fulfillment to peace.* Online: CreateSpace/Amazon.

Khamisa, A., & Quinn, J. (2009). *The secrets of the bulletproof spirit: How to bounce back from life's hardest hits.* New York, NY: Ballantine Books.

Kretzmann, J. P., & McKnight, J. L. (1993). *Building communities from the inside out: A path toward finding and mobilizing a community's assets.* Evanston, IL: ABCD Institute.

Lozano, J. A. (2103, December 23). OKRA charity saloon, Houston bar, donates 100% of profits to charity. *HUFFPOST IMPACT.* Retrieved from http://www.huffingtonpost.com/2013/12/23/okra-charity-saloon_n_4492734.html

McKnight, J. L. (1995). *The careless society: Community and its counterfeits.* New York, NY: Basic Books.

Miller, M. Z., Geist-Martin, P., & Beatty, K. C. (2005). Wholeness in a breaking world: Narratives as sustenance for peace. In L. M. Harter, P. M. Japp, & C. S. Beck (Eds.), *Narratives, health, and healing: Communication theory, research, and practice* (pp. 295–316). Mahwah, NJ: Erlbaum.

Mukherjee, S. (2011). *The emperor of all maladies: A biography of cancer.* New York, NY: Simon and Schuster.

Nathanson, C. A. (1999). Social movements as catalysts for policy change: The case of smoking and guns. *Journal of Health Politics, Policy and Law, 24,* 421–488.

Parrott, R. (2004). Emphasizing "communication" in health communication. *Journal of Communication, 54,* 751–787.

Rey, L., & Extremera, N. (2015). Forgiveness and health-related quality of life in older people: Adaptive cognitive emotion regulations strategies as mediators. *Journal of Health Psychology, 93,* 1–11.

Rinpoche, S. (1993). *The Tibetan book of living and dying.* San Francisco, CA: Harper.

Row, K. A. (2008). Forgiveness, physiological reactivity and health: The role of anger. *International Journal of Psychophysiology, 68,* 51–58.

Sanchez, R. (2015, October 3). Death and guns in the USA: The story in six graphs. *CNN.* Retrieved from http://www.cnn.com/2015/10/03/us/gun-deaths-united-states/

Sandoval, E., & Pearson, E. (2015, December 13). For Newtown, 2012 Sandy Hook Elementary School shooting is still painful. *New York Daily News.* Retrieved from http://www.nydailynews.com/news/national/newtown-forget-sandy-hook-shooting-tragedy-article-1.2464074

Sontag, S. (1978). *Illness as metaphor.* New York, NY: Farrar, Straus, & Giroux.

Svalina, S. (2012). Forgiveness and health among people in outpatient physical therapy. *Disability and Rehabilitation, 34,* 383–392.

TKF celebrates years of preventing youth violence. (2015, September 25). Retrieved from tkf.org/tkf-celebrates-years-of-preventing-youth-violence

Toussaint, L., Owen, A. D., & Cheadle, A. (2011). Forgive to live: Forgiveness, health, and longevity. *Journal of Behavioral Medicine, 35,* 375–386.

Webb, J. R. (2013). Forgiveness and health: Assessing the mediating effect of health behavior, social support, and interpersonal functioning. *The Journal of Psychology, 147,* 391–414.

Webb, J. R., Toussaint, L., & Conway-Williams, E. (2012). Forgiveness and health: Psycho-spiritual integration and the promotion of better healthcare. *Journal of Health Care Chaplaincy, 18,* 57–73.

Worthington, E. L., Jr. (2007). Forgiveness, health, and well-being: A review of evidence for emotional versus decisional forgiveness, dispositional forgivingness, and reduced unforgiveness. *Journal of Behavioral Medicine, 30,* 291–302.

Worthington, E. L., Jr., Van Oyen Witvliet, C., Pietrini, P., & Miller, A. J. (2007). Forgiveness, health, and well-being: A review of evidence for emotional versus decisional forgiveness, dispositional forgivingness, and reduced unforgiveness. *Journal of Behavioral Medicine, 30,* 291–302.

Young, S. (2015, October 22). Advocates for the disabled differ on new symbol. 2007 *Health Care Communication News.* Retrieved from http://www.healthcarecommunication.com/Main/Articles/13682.aspx

Zoller, H. M. (2005). Health activism: Communication theory and action for social change. *Communication Theory, 15,* 341–364.

Name and Subject Index

D'Agostino, T. A., 65
Dahl, R., 315
Dana, W., 12
Dancing Wheels, 213
D'Andrea, W., 209
Daredevil masculinity, 214
Das, J. K., 277
Davidson, R., 67
Davies, D., 42
Davin, S., 288
Davis, C. S., 191, 197, 199–200, 213, 215
Davis, L. E., 159
Dawson, N. V., 66
de Fossard, E., 294, 296
De Haes, H. C., 66
de Souza, R., 244
Dean, M., 53, 59–60, 62, 66, 68, 288
Dean, M., 58
Death with dignity, 375–376
Deci, E. L., 67
Defenbaugh, N., 105
Deficit-based model of healthcare, 136, 141
DeKlerk, N. H., 191
Del Piccolo, L., 68
Delynko, K. M., 213
Demeris, G., 94, 179, 227
Denison, J., 282
Dennett, T., 150
DeSantis, A. D., 282
Desire Map, The (LaPorte), 183
Despres, C., 90
Developmental disabilities, 136–137
Deviance
    dehumanization of, 199–200
    and normality, medicalization of, 314
    social emphasis on productivity linked to, 204
Devil terms/god terms, 325
Dewey, J., 137, 139–141, 147, 153
Diamond, D., 358
Diem, S. J., 288
Digital divide, 129
Digital storytelling workshop about sexuality, 350–351
Digitized healthcare
    complexities of, 128–130
    computerized prognosis and treatment plans, 110–112
    digital doctors, 113–116
    digital patients, 117–127
    "smart" diagnoses, 107
    technological advancements in, 107–110
Dignan, M. B., 274
Dillman, L., 226

Dillon, B. L., 176
Dillon, P. J., 338–339
Disability(ies)
    communicating through wheelchair rugby, 213–215
    hidden, 205–206
    and separation from broader community life, 292
Discrimination and stigma, 201–202
Disease mongering, 314
Disease vs. illness, 62
Disease, scientific perspective vs. subjective experiences of, 2
Disempowerment, 365
Disenfranchised domestic workers, storytelling by, 333–354
Disenfranchised grief, 244–245
Diversity among team members, 83–84
Dlouhy, S., 135–136, 142
DNR (do not resuscitate) order, 238
Doctor–patient communication, 113–115
Dominguez-Cherit, G., 96
Domoff, S. E., 204
Donaghue, N., 198
Doolan, D., 111
Doshi, M. J., 235, 237
Doty, L., 204, 207
Dougal, S. D., 208
Dougherty, D. S., 175
Dougherty, S. B., 163
Dozier, D., 152
Drachman, R. H., 277
Dual diagnosis, 9, 12, 16
Dualisms, 139–140
Dubois, M., 239
Dubriwny, T. N., 316–317
Duggan, A. P., 64, 69, 72
Duggan, P. S., 64
Duncan, J., 143
Dunn, D. S., 163
Dunn, S. M., 68
du Pré, A., 59–61, 111, 118
Durable power of attorney for healthcare, 238
Dutcher, G. A., 125
Dutta, M. J., 333–336, 339–340, 342–343, 345–346, 353
Dwamenta, F. C., 61
Dziegielewski, S. F., 179

Easterbrook, G., 42
Ebola Virus Disease (EVD), 319
Eckstein, D., 239
Ecological model of communication in medical encounters, 57, 59–61

Economic development, importance to public health, 317
Ecowellness, 160, 177–178, 181–183
Edington, D. W., 170
Edley, P., 178
Edu-tainment. *See* Entertainment-education
Eggleston, R., 197, 204
Egilman, D., 322
Ehlke, D., 321, 324, 327
Einarsen, S., 175
Elaboration Likelihood Model (ELM), 293
Electronic health records (EHRs), 108, 111–112, 114
Electronic medical records (EMRs), 111
Elite theories of policy making, 315
Ellen, P. S., 278
Ellingson, L. L., 34, 79, 82, 85–86, 91, 95–96, 98–99, 159, 193
Ellis, K. J., 239
Emanuel, E. J., 40
Embedded teamwork/joint work, 95
Emend, 125
Emerson Literacy Education and Empowerment Project (eLEEP), 121–122
Empathic response, 229, 245
Empathy, 229–230
Emperor of All Maladies, The: A Biography of Cancer (Mukherjee), 376
Employee Assistance Programs (EAPs), 177
Empowerment, 366
Encarnacion, B., 212
Endevelt, R., 294
End-of life communication, 241, 243
End-of-life planning, Five Wishes model for, 239
Engel, G. L., 61–62
Engeln-Maddox, R., 192
English, M., 171
Engström, I., 96
Engström, K., 96
Entertainment, 285–288
Entertainment-education
    campaigns, 285–296
    designing, 295–296
    in developing countries, 289–290
    history of, 288–289
    impact on society, 286–288
    obstacles to, 294–295
    theories of, 293–294
Environmental theories of illness, 307, 308, 310
Epstein, L., 193
Epstein, R. M., 66–68, 72

conveying prosocial health messages through, 273–274, 279, 286
and cultural narrative of weight, fat, and obesity, 308–310
impact on patient–provider interaction, 59
media agency for at-risk urban youth, 120–122
narratives about health in, 310, 316–317, 319
portrayals of prophylactic mastectomy narratives, 316–317
social. *See* Social media
television, mediated view of reality created by, 293–294
theories outlining media effects, 279
Medicaid, 327–328
Medical care reform, 320–328
Medical interviewing, patient-centered vs. clinician-centered, 62–63
Medical professionalism, 85
Medical proxy co-owners, 48
Medical records, electronic, 111–112
Medicalization
definition of, 314
of fat/obesity, 195–198, 204, 212
model for end-of-life care, 238
politics of, 313–314
of work, 163–164
Medicine
biomedical model of, 61, 147, 197, 361
humanizing through illness narrative, 33
integrative, 92–93
Medved, C. E., 178
Meghji, R. K., 181
Menachemi, M., 111
Mental illness, 9–11, 17, 150
Merkakis, K., 229
Meyers, R. A., 95
Microaggressions, transgender, 202–203
Millar, F. E., 224, 231
Miller, A., 89
Miller, A. J., 367
Miller, A. N., 244
Miller, B., 286
Miller, K., 233–234
Miller, K. I., 177
Miller, K. L., 98
Miller, L. E., 127–128
Miller, L. J., 202–203
Miller, M., 191
Miller, M. Z., 360

Miller, W., 228–229, 231
Miller-Day, M., 18, 20, 231
Milligan, R. A., 99
Mills, C. W., 315
Mills, M. E., 67
Mindfulness, 227
Mingé, J. M., 105
Minuchin, S., 231
Mirivel, J., 165
Mischler, E., 212
Mishel, M. H., 68
Mitchell, G. J., 98
Mitchell, P., 135–136, 142, 146–148, 153
Modern Family, 273, 279, 285, 293, 295
Montgomery, K. C., 295
Moody, C., 328
Moore, J., 138
Moorhead, S., 125
Morahan-Martin, J. M., 118
Moran, M. B., 283
Morgan, D. G., 98
Morgan, J. M., 84
Morgan, S. E., 282
Morone, J. A., 321, 324, 327
Morra, D., 111
Morris, D. B., 2, 6, 40
Morris, J., 136
Morrone, A., 163
Morton, J. M., 212
Moser, R. P., 89
Moss-Racussin, C. A., 208
Mouffe, C., 148
Moy, B., 239
Moyer-Gusé, E., 293–294
Mukherjee, S., 376
Mullener, B., 239
Multidisciplinary teams, 90
Murderball, 214–215
Murphy, L. T., 279
Murphy, S., 283
Murray-Johnson, L., 278, 281
Murrock, C. J., 143
Murthy, V., 358
"My Voice" awareness campaign about HPV, 312
Myers, J. E., 160, 181
MyHealthVet (MHV), 129

Nabi, R. L., 294
Nacinovich, M. R., 239
Namie, G., 172
Naming and word choice, 325–326
Narayanan, V., 225
Narcan/naloxone, 2, 12
"Narrative turn" in the social sciences, 32

Narratives of health and illness
analysis of, 34–36
community, and the culture-centered approach to health disparities, 335–336
cultural, about aging, 37–43
essential nature of, 32–34
functions of, 33
influence on healthcare policy agenda, 324
inverting narrative structures and expectations, 343
preservation of personal identity through, 33, 37
restitution narratives, 34
scholarship on, 34
story elements in, 32–33
types of, 33–34
See also Stories; Storytelling
Nash, J. M., 90–91
Nathanson, C. A., 359
Nattinger, A. B., 288
Naus, M. J., 72
Nazi, K. M., 129
Negotiation and sensemaking, 337
Neill, A., 149
Nelson, N., 339, 343
Neoliberalism
cultural narrative of, 336
and globalization, as cause of health disparities, 334
negative impacts on developing countries, 320
Nestle, M., 318
New Recovery Advocacy Movement, 15
Next US, The, 179
Nguyen, N. T., 192
Nicklas, J. C., 279
Nielsen, M. B., 175
Nielsen-Bohlman, L., 118
Nobel, J., 145
Noguchi, Y., 164
Nonlinearity, 228
Nonverbal communication, in patient–physician encounters, 114
Norander, S., 136
Nørgaard, B., 99
Normal People Scare Me, 142
Normality and deviance, medicalization of, 314
Novak, D. K., 136
Novak, D. R., 178
Nowak, G., 295
Nowson, C. A., 209
Nurse–team interactions, managing role tensions in, 87–89
Nussbaum, J. F., 160–162